REM DIES

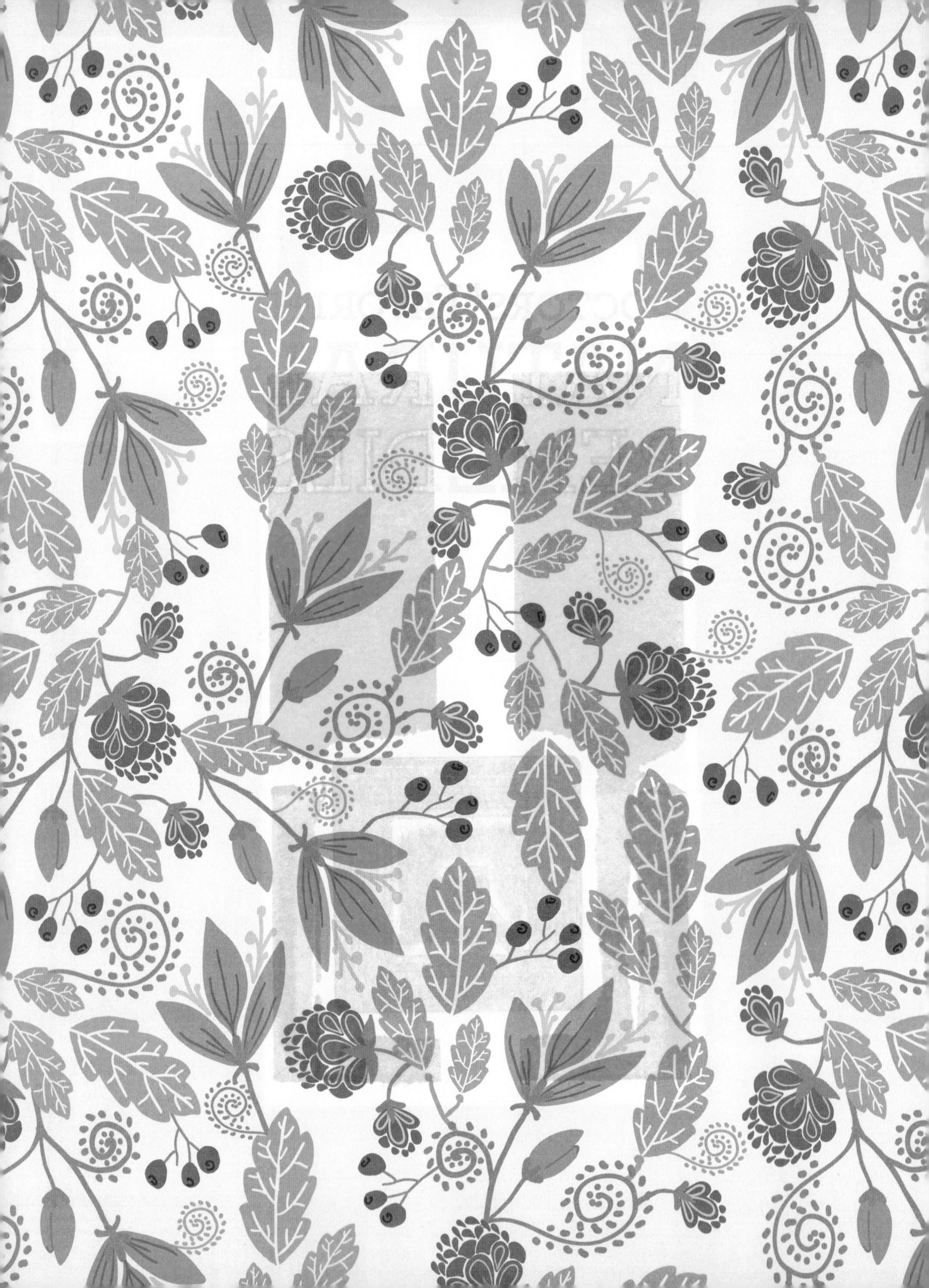

Doctors' Favorite NATURAL REMEDIES

The Safest and Most Effective Natural Ways to Treat More Than 85 Everyday Ailments

Reader's digest

Montreal/New York

Contents

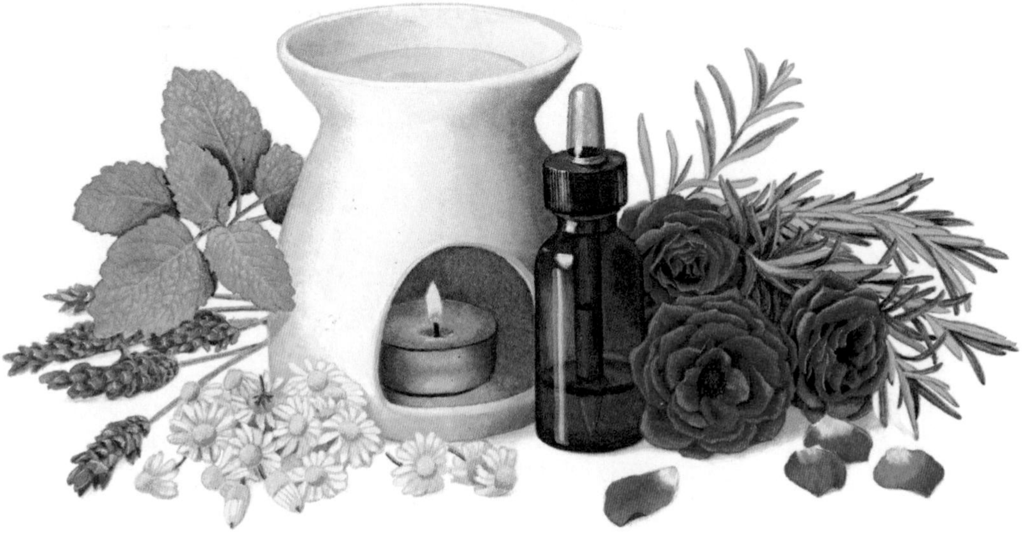

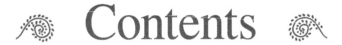

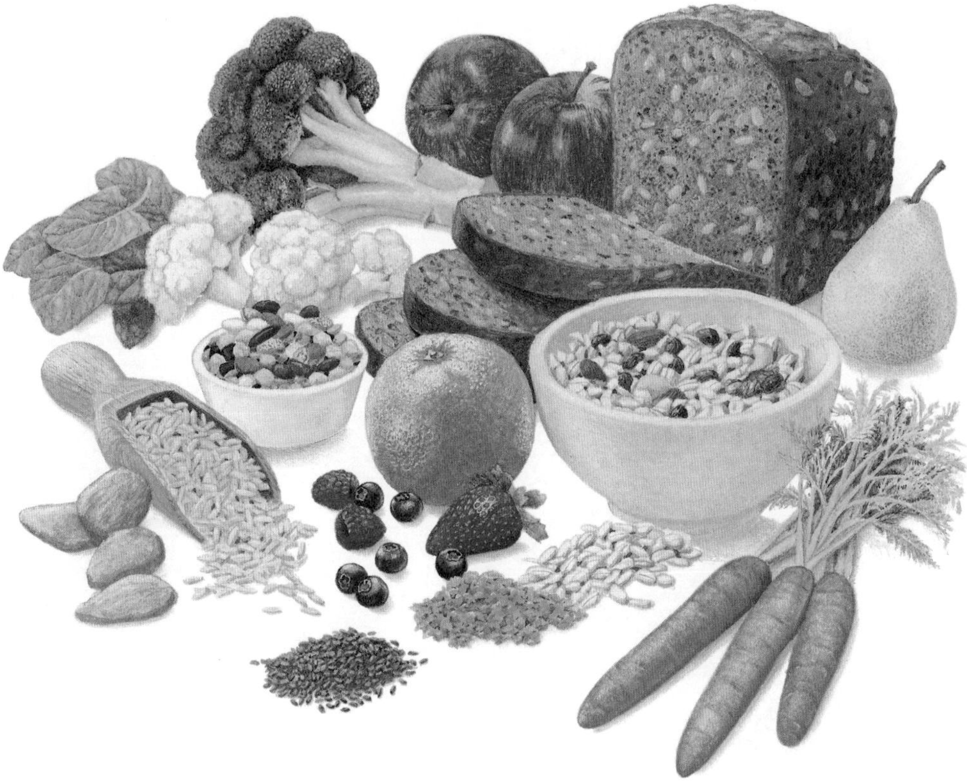

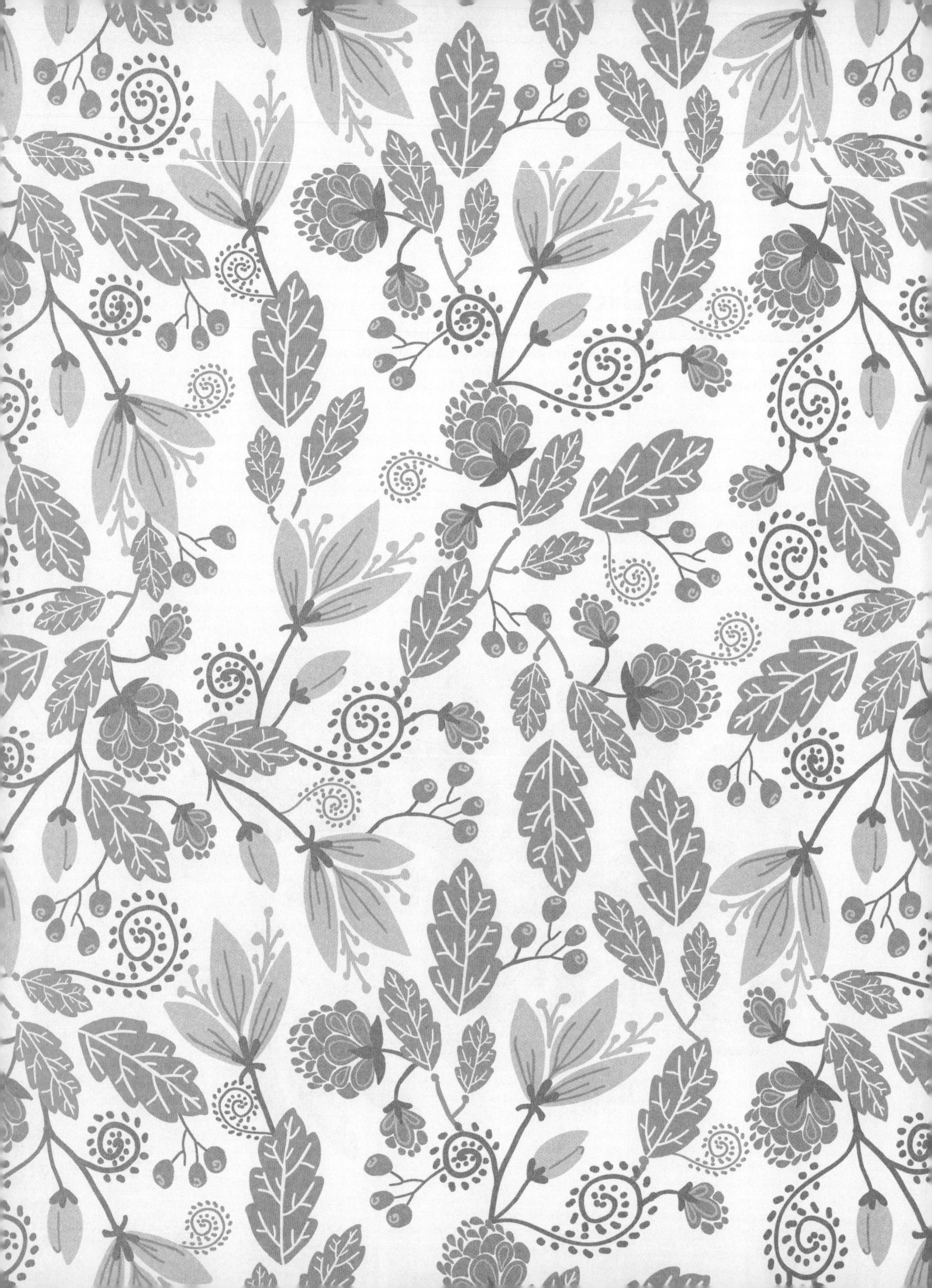

Foreword

WELCOME TO *Doctors' Favorite Natural Remedies,* a comprehensive guide to the natural remedies and therapies that really work to improve your health and well-being. With an emphasis on holistic health, we compiled a list of common everyday ailments and set about finding the most effective natural remedies, based on medical science and traditional usage. There were many to choose from and we hope that you will find the final selection helpful, enlightening and interesting. You'll find well-known favorites, such as garlic and ginger, acupuncture and Pilates, along with less obvious yet powerful remedies such as laughter and dancing.

As our consultant, Professor Marc Cohen, explains in the introduction, wellness is made up of several elements, including emotional, physical and mental health. By looking at the bigger picture of what is going on in your life, you may find that simple changes to your lifestyle—such as tackling stress or quitting smoking—can produce big results. Your diet, too, plays a significant role in keeping your body fueled and healthy. This is why for each ailment, we begin with some general advice on diet and lifestyle.

Next we have provided a list of suggested remedies. We chose them from the hundreds available based on the most proven and medically approved for the particular ailment. They are the sorts of remedies a doctor would prescribe. Most have a long history of traditional use that is gradually being backed up by science; some are more modern and have emerged from recent research. As we compiled the book, there were remedies that came up time and time again for numerous ailments. For example, two of the most commonly referenced remedies are sleep and exercise. It seems that most people don't get enough of either. Simply improving your sleeping habits and taking up regular exercise will do wonders for your general health.

When deciding to go down the route of natural therapies, the choice can be overwhelming. Every day, an article on the Internet or in a newspaper reports on the latest new remedy or "wonder" herb—but how can you be sure that what you are reading is trustworthy? Well, we've done the research for you. We have selected the remedies based on how effective they are. Many have scientific studies to support them, while the traditional remedies have a significant history of safe usage behind them.

Holistic health requires you to take charge of your health and well-being. This book provides a sensible and balanced approach to the world of natural remedies. We hope that it will provide you with many paths to wellness and a happier and healthier life.

THE EDITORS

About this book

DOCTORS' FAVORITE NATURAL REMEDIES is a guide to the best natural remedies for common health problems. Some have a long and respected traditional use, while many are backed up by modern science. They include the most effective healing therapies, nutritional supplements and home remedies available—all presented in an easy-to-read format.

A to Z of Ailments

The first section of the book lists common ailments with a wide range of entries from acne to memory problems and warts. Each ailment is briefly described followed by a list of suggested natural remedies. You will also find general advice on dietary measures and lifestyle factors that can play a big part in preventing or remediating an ailment. The "Quick fix" feature offers a remedy that may bring instant relief, while the "Did you know?" feature provides snippets of additional useful or intriguing information connected to the ailment. Occasionally, a "Watch out!" box warns of a potential hazard to avoid.

A to Z of Remedies

In the second section of the book, we have listed the natural remedies and treatments in alphabetical order by common name. Readers will find a diversity of treatments, therapies, herbs and nutritional

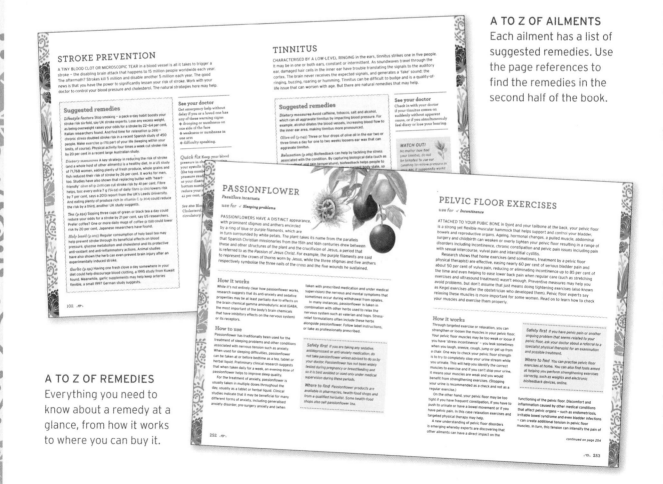

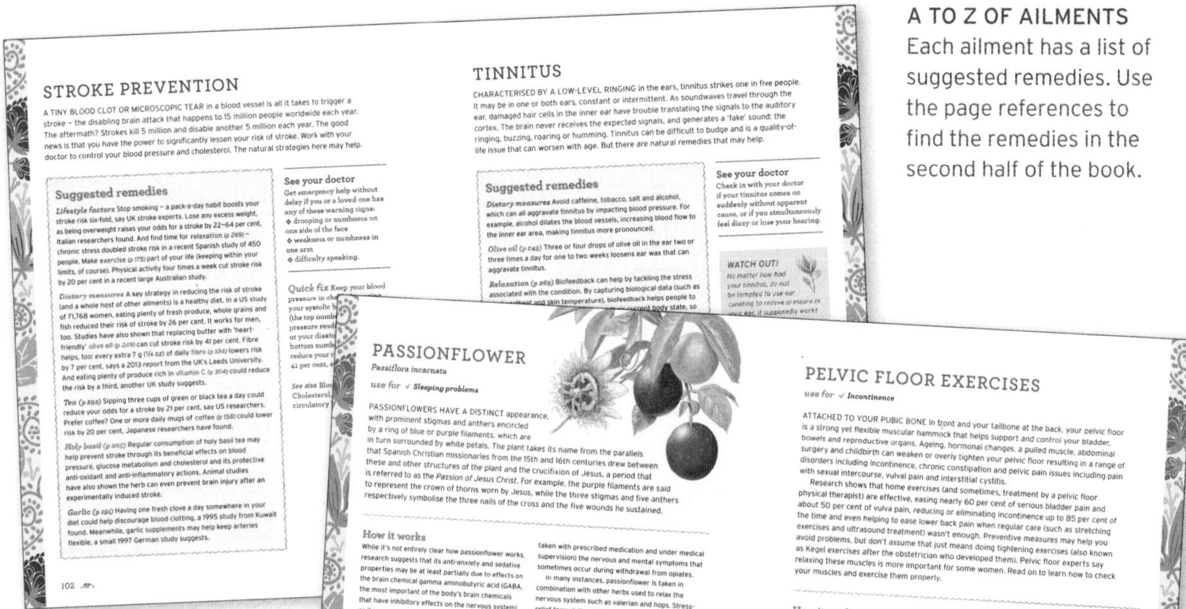

STROKE PREVENTION

A TINY BLOOD CLOT OR MICROSCOPIC TEAR in a blood vessel is all it takes to trigger a stroke – the disabling brain attack that happens to 15 million people worldwide each year. The aftermath? Strokes kill 5 million and disable another 5 million each year. The good news is that you have the power to significantly lessen your risk of stroke. Work with your doctor to control your blood pressure and cholesterol. The natural strategies here may help.

TINNITUS

CHARACTERISED BY A LOW-LEVEL RINGING in the ears, tinnitus strikes one in five people. It may be in one or both ears, constant or intermittent. As soundwaves travel through the ear, damaged hair cells in the inner ear have trouble translating the signals to the auditory cortex. The brain never receives the expected signals, and generates a 'fake' sound: the ringing, buzzing, roaring or humming. Tinnitus can be difficult to budge and is a quality-of-life issue that can worsen with age. But there are natural remedies that may help.

PASSIONFLOWER

Passiflora incarnata

PASSIONFLOWERS HAVE A DISTINCT appearance, with prominent stigmas and anthers encircled by a ring of blue or purple filaments, which are in turn surrounded by white petals. The plant takes its name from the parallels that Spanish Christian missionaries from the 15th and 16th centuries drew between these and other structures of the plant and the crucifixion of Jesus, a period that is referred to as the *Passion of Jesus Christ*. For example, the purple filaments are said to represent the crown of thorns worn by Jesus, while the three stigmas and five anthers respectively symbolise the three nails of the cross and the five wounds he sustained.

PELVIC FLOOR EXERCISES

ATTACHED TO YOUR PUBIC BONE in front and your tailbone at the back, your pelvic floor is a strong yet flexible muscular hammock that helps support and control your bladder, bowels and reproductive organs.

A TO Z OF AILMENTS
Each ailment has a list of suggested remedies. Use the page references to find the remedies in the second half of the book.

A TO Z OF REMEDIES
Everything you need to know about a remedy at a glance, from how it works to where you can buy it.

CAUTION!

This book is not intended to be a substitute for medical advice. Some natural remedies are not suitable for people under certain circumstances, or may interact with prescription medications. If you suffer from a diagnosed illness, are taking prescribed medicines, or are pregnant or breast-feeding, talk to your doctor before using any natural remedy. While the creators of this book have made every effort to be as accurate as possible, medical and pharmacological knowledge is constantly changing. Readers are advised to consult a qualified medical professional for individual advice. The writers, researchers, editors and publishers of this book cannot be held liable for any errors, omissions or actions that may be taken as a consequence of information contained in this book.

supplements. For each remedy there is information on its origins and how it works, followed by information on how it should be used. The "Safety first" feature reminds readers of important safety issues associated with the remedy and "Where to find" tells readers the best place to access the remedy.

Using the remedies

Herbal remedies and nutritional supplements should be viewed as medicines and as such there are some common sense guidelines to keep in mind:

- Unless otherwise stated, the remedies are intended for adult use. Extra caution should be taken when treating babies and children and you should seek specific advice from your doctor or other trained health practitioner.
- Always keep supplements and herbal remedies out of reach of children.
- Never take essential oils internally.
- Before taking a new remedy, ask your doctor or pharmacist about possible interactions with other medications you are taking.
- If you experience any uncomfortable symptoms after taking a remedy, discontinue use and seek medical assistance as appropriate.
- Shop carefully, choosing reputable brands.

Where we have used illustrations to depict an exercise sequence, please note that the pictures are for guidance only. It is best to seek instruction from a qualified practitioner.

Abbreviations used in this book

cm = centimeter

g = gram

IU = International Unit (40 IU = 1 mcg)

kg = kilogram

L = liter

lb = pound

mcg = microgram (there are a million micrograms in a gram)

mg = milligram (there are a thousand milligrams in a gram)

ml = milliliters (there are a thousand milliliters in a liter)

ng = nanogram (there are a billion nanograms in a gram)

nmol = nanomole (there are a billion nanomoles in a mole)

oz = ounce

YOUR HEALTH IS YOUR RESPONSIBILITY

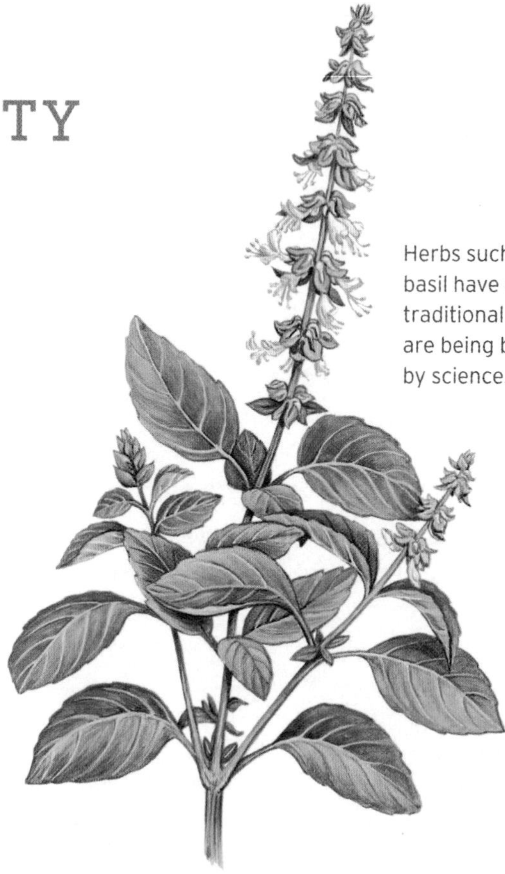

Herbs such as holy basil have many traditional uses that are being backed up by science.

EVERY CULTURE THROUGHOUT history has developed its own approach to health and healing and we are living in a time when the wisdom of many different cultures and philosophies is becoming readily available. Over time, two general approaches to health have emerged. The orthodox or conventional approach is to define specific diseases by their symptoms or underlying disease processes, and attempt to develop drugs or surgical procedures to treat or prevent the disease. The natural or complementary approach, in contrast, attempts to initiate and support natural healing mechanisms within the body by addressing any current symptoms, along with the emotional, social, cultural and spiritual aspects of a person's well-being.

While the two approaches may have more relevance for certain conditions or be of more use during particular phases of life, they are not mutually exclusive. As the name suggests, complementary therapies are meant to complement conventional treatment and when used in this way can achieve good results. Furthermore, while it is clear that conventional doctors and complementary practitioners train for years to develop their expertise, the person with the greatest ability to positively impact your health is *you*.

Understanding your health and taking responsibility for looking after yourself will ensure that you have the best chance of enjoying good health now and well into the future.

Understanding your health and taking responsibility for looking after yourself will ensure that you have the best chance of enjoying good health now and well into the future. This involves adopting a strategy of actively seeking wellness in its fullest sense, rather than just fire-fighting the ailments as they arise.

A lot of people pass the responsibility for their health to their doctor or health practitioner. They adopt unhealthy lifestyles and then expect to be cured from any illness by simply taking pills or undergoing surgery. Mainstream medicine generally supports this approach by developing drugs and therapies for curing or managing disease rather than promoting well-being. For example, within Western medical practice it is considered normal for doctors to treat coronary heart disease by stripping a vein from the leg, opening the chest, placing the vein across a blocked artery and then repeating the procedure every 10 years. It is considered less usual, however, to prescribe relaxation, exercise, eating good food and sharing feelings, despite the fact that research has proven the success of this latter approach.

A focus on illness rather than wellness has led to a crisis in health care with an epidemic of lifestyle-related diseases such as obesity, diabetes, heart disease and cancer. A 2005 World Health Organization report suggests that the most common causes of death are chronic lifestyle-related diseases that are the result of over-indulgence in sugar, fat, salt, alcohol and tobacco, as well as exposure to pollution and toxic chemicals. It is becoming increasingly obvious that conventional medicine is not going to deliver wellness—we need to create it for ourselves.

What is wellness?

Wellness is much more than just being free of disease; wellness means enhanced health, and includes looking, feeling and being well. This implies having healthy skin, hair and nails, mental clarity, physical strength and stamina, along with maximum resistance to stress, disease and the ravages of aging. Wellness, therefore, naturally leads to longevity and achieving the most enjoyment and fulfillment from life.

At a basic level, wellness can be equated with health, which, according to the World Health Organization, is "a state of complete physical, mental and social well-being and not merely the absence of disease or infirmity." The notion of wellness may be extended further to include not only physical, mental and social factors but also emotional, spiritual, sexual, occupational, financial and environmental aspects. If any one of these dimensions is lacking, then complete wellness cannot be achieved.

Yet while our health and well-being are arguably the most valuable things we possess, they are very difficult to measure accurately. Perhaps the best way is to think of health as a spectrum, with wellness and illness at opposite ends. Health can then be classified into three broad areas: ill health, average health and enhanced health (see below).

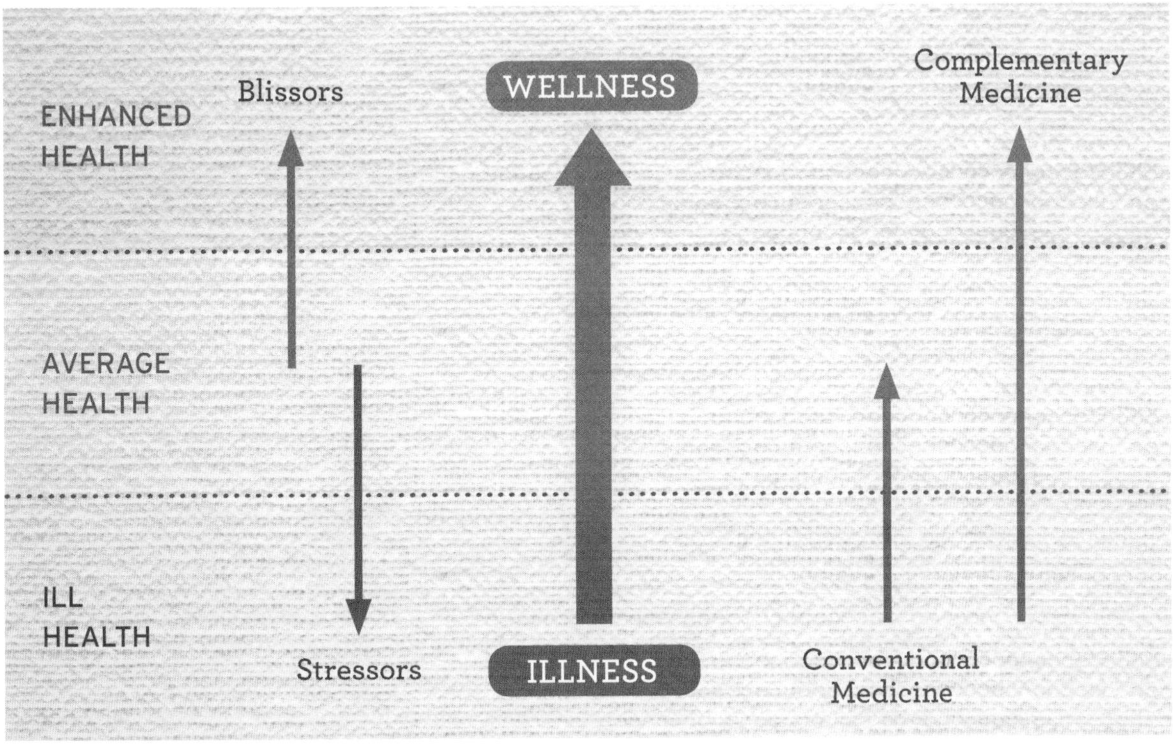

A SPECTRUM OF WELLNESS Conventional medicine moves a person from ill health to average health by tackling stressors. Complementary therapies take a person to enhanced health via a holistic approach that embraces blissors.

FIND OUT WHAT WORKS FOR YOU

It is important to personalize any treatment to your specific needs. In some cases it is possible to determine the most appropriate therapy by conducting scientific experiments on yourself through the so-called "n of 1 study." These studies, which have a single patient in them (you), involve keeping a careful record of your symptoms over a period of time (see Journaling, *p. 215*) and then noting whether your symptoms get better or worse while you try different treatments. An example of this approach is an elimination diet *(p. 171)* to determine which foods aggravate your symptoms and are best avoided. But the method can be applied to other situations. For example, you may keep track of your pain symptoms and note how they change when you try different remedies. This self study may help you to document any side effects that you experience and therefore determine which therapy is the safest and most effective for you.

The divide between ill health and average health is defined by different diseases. In medical terms these are referred to as raised blood pressure, poor control of blood glucose or other specific symptom patterns. Conventional medicine uses a bottom-up approach that concentrates on moving people across this division by developing drugs and surgery to treat or prevent specific symptoms of disease and control "stressors" that reduce well-being.

From average health to wellness

The divide between average health and enhanced health is less distinct as it incorporates the many factors that determine physical, psychological, emotional, social, economic, environmental and spiritual health. In many Eastern philosophies, the idea of enhanced health can be extended to the concept of perfect health or "enlightenment," whereby a person is in a state of "nirvana" or bliss. Such traditions adopt a top-down approach by attempting to elicit bliss through meditation and other practices that enhance well-being.

Moving up the spectrum from illness to wellness gives you greater resilience so that you are better able to cope with the stressors of life. The best form of prevention is, therefore, to be as high on the wellness spectrum as possible. While stressors such as depression, disease, disability, divorce, dementia, disappointments, debt and other unsettling influences tend to drag us down toward illness, blissors such as joy, play, engagement, intimacy, community, connectedness, mindfulness and security all enhance our life and elevate us toward greater well-being. While we can't always avoid the stressors in life—if we actively pursue the blissors then the balance will be shifted upward toward wellness.

Many complementary therapies and natural remedies aim to improve resistance to disease as well as improve overall health. Such therapies vary widely with respect to their level of scientific validation, safety and cost, yet they generally share common principles. These include taking advantage of the wisdom within traditional medical systems, the use of food as medicine, regular consumption of adaptogenic herbs that support the body's natural healing forces and a daily routine of mindfulness and movement practices.

Integrative medicine: the best of both worlds

While there are certainly some diseases and emergencies that will always need conventional medical treatment, natural remedies can complement the treatment of many ailments and can sometimes offer help where conventional medicine can't. The practice of integrative medicine aims to make sense of natural therapies and apply them alongside conventional treatments. When choosing between different therapies, practitioners of integrative medicine adopt certain principles such as the Hippocratic ethic of "first do no harm," and respect for a patient's preferences. They also consider each treatment's practicality, cost, availability and the scientific evidence supporting its safety and efficacy. When these principles are applied in the full context of a person's life, including their mind, body and spirit, medicine may be said to be truly holistic.

The therapeutic relationship

More and more doctors are now adopting a holistic, integrative approach and there is a rapidly expanding body of scientific research that attests to the benefits of such an approach. This research also highlights important safety concerns that can arise when conventional and complementary approaches interact. For this reason it is very important to develop a good therapeutic relationship with your health practitioners; if you have more than one practitioner, you must keep them well-informed about all the medications and natural remedies that you are taking. It is also a good idea to encourage your practitioners to work together for your benefit and to communicate with each other about your current treatments and future health strategies. You also need to ensure that your practitioners include you as an active (and the most important) participant in your own care and that you are well-informed about decisions concerning your health.

The therapeutic relationship or "helping alliance" has been shown to have a beneficial impact on treatment outcomes.

Developing a good therapeutic relationship with your practitioners not only provides the best foundation for informed decisions about your health, it may actually be therapeutic in itself. The therapeutic relationship or "helping alliance" has been shown to have a beneficial impact on treatment outcomes. Furthermore, while scientific research and traditional wisdom can suggest treatments that may be appropriate for a given situation, a good relationship with your practitioner will best enable you to adapt any treatment to your specific needs.

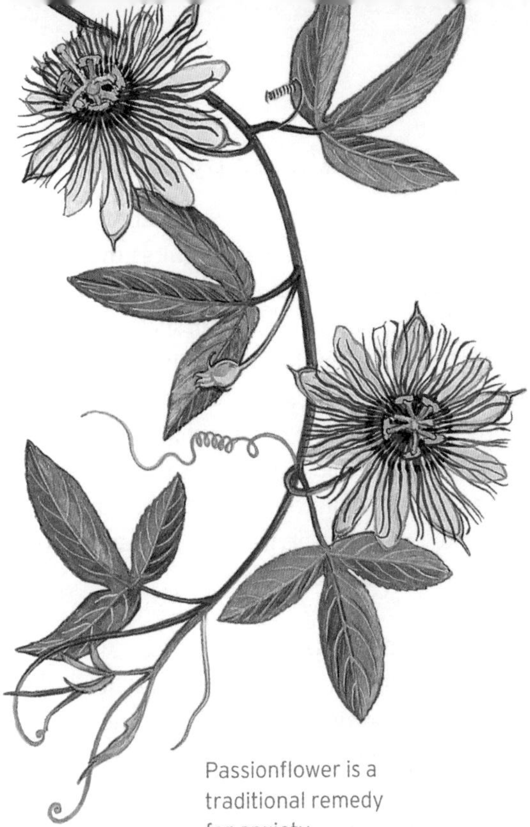

Passionflower is a traditional remedy for anxiety.

Toward individualized care

Each one of us is an individual with a unique genetic makeup, life history and social circumstance. Our symptoms and risk factors are also unique. Accounting for individual differences is a cornerstone of many ancient systems of medicine. Traditional Chinese medicine, Ayurvedic medicine and Western herbal medicine all have sophisticated systems of categorizing people in order to guide treatment selection. In comparison, conventional medicine has been slow to accept and use this individualistic approach. But this may be changing; the relatively recent fields of pharmacogenomics and nutrigenomics, which emerged out of the Human Genome Project, are providing a scientific basis for individualized treatments. They emphasize the importance of individual responses to medicines and nutrients, and the roles of dietary and genetic interactions in patient health.

Building a wellness pyramid

Wellness has an impact on every aspect of our lives and experiencing wellness requires the integration of multiple factors that determine physical, psychological, emotional, social, economic, environmental and spiritual health. If we want enhanced health, we must address the key life activities that determine our health. Using the model of a "wellness pyramid" can help us to achieve this. Layer by layer, the different aspects build and work together to create a healthier, balanced and more enjoyable life (see below).

Share your feelings

Sharing your feelings and building social networks to support yourself is the foundation of the wellness pyramid. Love and relationships are by far the most important factor in building a happy and fulfilling life. This is the conclusion of the Harvard Grant Study that followed a group of Harvard undergraduates for 75 years and looked at growth and change over the participants' lives. Devoting ourselves to quality time with others and fostering love and intimacy in all our personal relationships does wonders for our well-being. This can be expanded to include developing an ethic of service to others and a sense of social and civic responsibility through volunteer and community work.

Certainly, the most joyous and important times in our lives come from our connection with people rather than from possessions, places, pills, etc. It seems that when pain is shared it decreases, while joy shared increases. It is extremely beneficial to have people in your life with whom you are able to discuss your deep and intimate thoughts and feelings and who rely on you to have empathy with their own. Simply telling your story to a sympathetic listener can help you understand the causes and implications of your disease, as well as provide much needed psychosocial support. While sharing your feelings with sympathetic friends and family can greatly reduce your mental burden, you may also benefit from sharing your feelings with a trusted practitioner

THE WELLNESS PYRAMID To reach a state of wellness we need to tend to many aspects of our lives. The wellness pyramid is a reminder of how the different aspects work together to create overall health and well-being. With the pyramid in place, ailments are less likely to arise, and when they do we have the physical and mental resources to cope with them.

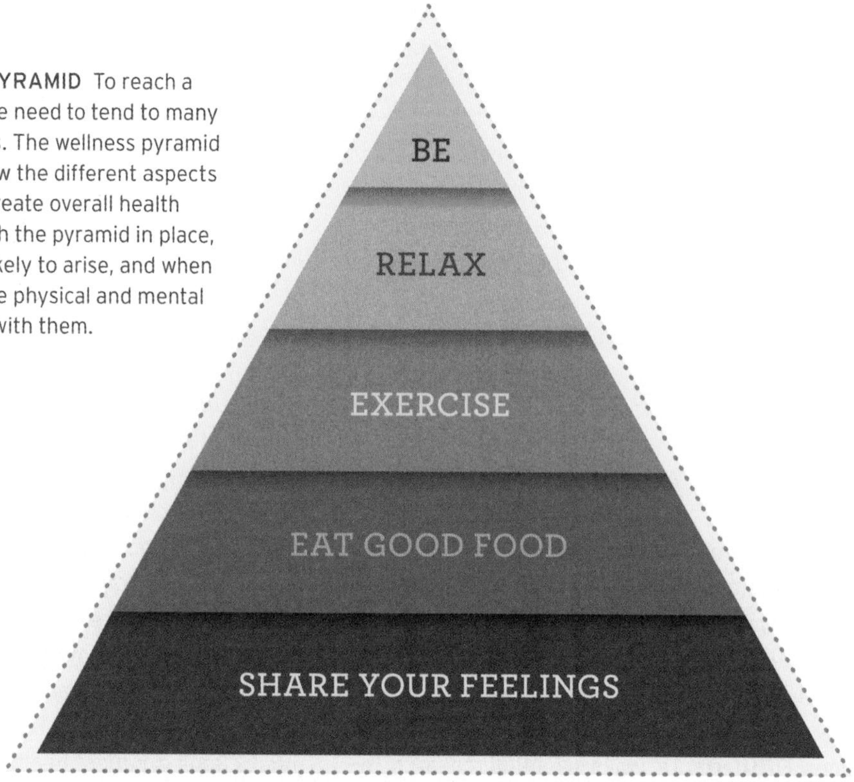
BE
RELAX
EXERCISE
EAT GOOD FOOD
SHARE YOUR FEELINGS

with whom you can create a therapeutic relationship. It is also possible to benefit from sharing feelings with yourself through **journaling** *(p. 215)*.

Sharing feelings does not have to involve words as it is also possible to share feelings through the power of touch. Since Harlow's famous experiments with monkeys in the 1950s that found that baby monkeys preferred motherly touch to food, it has been clear that physical touch is vital for health and well-being. "Skin hunger" or the craving for human contact is common in modern low-touch societies with the elderly and disabled being especially at risk. The need to touch may be satisfied through simply reaching out to others for a back rub or hug, stroking a beloved pet **(see pet therapy,** *p. 257*) or regularly seeking or giving a **massage** *(p. 230)*.

Eat good food

Food is the body's fuel and so it makes sense that if you want a healthy body, you need to eat healthy food. However, while eating good food is critical for health, the vast amount of conflicting information on different diets makes determining what is good for your individual circumstances extremely challenging. While it makes sense to try to avoid excessive sugar, fat, salt, alcohol and tobacco, and to minimize exposure to pesticides and other environmental toxins by choosing organic produce where possible, it is less clear how to construct a healthy balanced diet.

For many years nutritional advice has been based on various regimes that divide food into various food groups, with an emphasis on their nutritional merits and a recommendation to keep the fat content low. But this approach is being challenged. In 2013, the Swedish Council on Health Technology Assessment published an Expert Committee Review of 16,000 studies that suggests the low-fat diet dogma needs to be reconsidered in favor of low-carbohydrate, high-fat nutritional advice.

Brazil has taken this further and in 2014 produced the first national dietary guidelines that emphasize *meals* rather than nutrients. These evidence-based guidelines have been widely acknowledged as providing a common sense approach to eating that can be summarized in 10 basic steps.

SLOW FOOD

When deciding on which foods to include in your diet, think SLOW: Seasonal, Local, Organic and Whole. This approach to eating assures that the food you eat is more likely to be fresh and have the highest nutritional content by minimizing storage times, distance traveled and processing. The best way to embrace seasonal and local produce is to grow at least some of your food yourself. The next best way is to obtain food from local producers and "shake the hand that feeds you." Seeking out local food sources is not only important for ensuring the nutritional quality of food, it also has social and environmental benefits through contributing to your local food economy.

1. Prepare meals using fresh and staple foods.
2. Use oils, fats, sugar and salt in moderation.
3. Limit consumption of ready-to-eat food and drink products.
4. Eat at regular mealtimes and pay attention to your food instead of multitasking. Find a comfortable place to eat. Avoid all-you-can-eat buffets and noisy, stressful environments.
5. Eat with others whenever possible.
6. Buy food in stores and markets that offer a variety of fresh foods. Avoid those that sell mainly ready-to-eat products.
7. Develop, practice, share and enjoy your skills in food preparation and cooking.
8. Decide as a family to share cooking responsibilities and dedicate enough time for healthy meals.
9. When you eat out, choose restaurants that serve freshly made dishes. Avoid fast-food chains.
10. Be critical of food industry advertising.

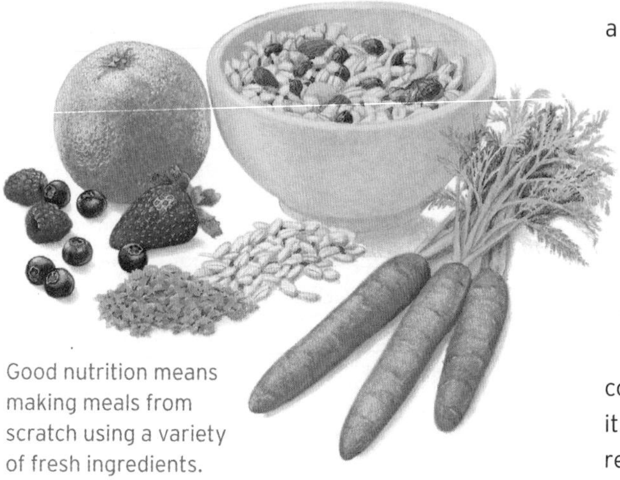

Good nutrition means making meals from scratch using a variety of fresh ingredients.

Basing dietary guidelines on meals rather than nutrients is a straightforward approach that can be extended to include following a particular cuisine rather than a "diet." This is based on the fact that cuisines, which have developed over hundreds of generations in areas such as the Mediterranean and regions of Asia, include meals that naturally balance a blend of different foods in healthy proportions. Such cuisines also often involve regular consumption of adaptogenic and health-enhancing herbs and spices such as holy basil, turmeric, garlic, green tea, ginger and olive oil.

Recent research shows that eating mostly organic food for as little as a week can reduce your exposure to organophosphate pesticides by as much as 90 percent.

Adopting a cuisine is much more likely to lead to a complete approach to nutrition than the modern counting of calories, macronutrients (fat, carbohydrate and protein) or micronutrients (vitamins, trace minerals and phytochemicals). There may be, however, specific deficiencies or ailments that can benefit from nutrients at higher doses than those that can be obtained through the diet. In these cases supplements can be beneficial, with the best supplements containing natural forms of various vitamins and trace minerals. Michael Pollan, a celebrated food author and Professor of Journalism at the University of California, Berkeley, has analyzed many diets and come up with some simple rules for healthy eating. These include the much-quoted seven-word adage: "Eat food. Not too much. Mostly plants." This adage distinguishes "food" from "edible food-like substances," which are the highly processed results of industrial food-processing technologies.

While it is important to consider your food's content, it is also important to consider what is *not* in it. Organic food has fewer pesticides and antibiotic-resistant bacteria and while the nutritional benefits of organic food are debated, recent research shows that eating mostly organic food for as little as a week can reduce your exposure to organophosphate pesticides by as much as 90 percent. Foods that are more susceptible to pests are more highly sprayed, while foods with greater natural protection from pests due to thicker skins, for example, require much less pesticide use. The Environmental Working Group in the US identified the Dirty Dozen (the foods that have high pesticide loads), including berries, apples, salad greens and potatoes. The Clean Fifteen, on the other hand, are foods that have less need for pesticides. These generally include onions, pineapples, avocados and corn. However, agricultural practices, and hence use of pesticides, can vary considerably in different countries and you should check with your local environmental agency.

Exercise

As the third tier of the wellness pyramid, exercise is at the center of a healthy lifestyle. Our modern lifestyles have become extremely sedentary so it is important to build physical activity into our regular routines. Engaging in regular physical activity ensures that both the musculoskeletal system and the cardiovascular system get a regular workout. The best exercise for you is the one that you enjoy and are able to include as a regular part of your routine **(see Exercise, *p. 175*)**.

Not only is exercise important to burn calories and maintain a healthy weight, it has also been shown to be extremely effective in boosting mood and combating depression. The adage "use it or lose it" further suggests that if we don't continually use our bodies, they will begin to deteriorate.

For many people **walking** *(p. 309)* is the easiest and most accessible exercise; however, it is a good idea to include exercise that engages your full range of physical movement as this will maintain your flexibility. You should also aim to engage your cardiovascular system from time to time through aerobic exercise that raises a sweat.

Relax

If you want to counter stress, you need to bring more relaxation into your life. This includes getting sufficient sleep **(see Sleeping strategies,** *p. 281***)**, as well as taking the time to release pent-up mental stress and muscle tension. Relaxation evokes the parasympathetic nervous system and the "rest and digest" response. This is an important counter to the "fight or flight" response that is brought on by the frantic pace of modern living.

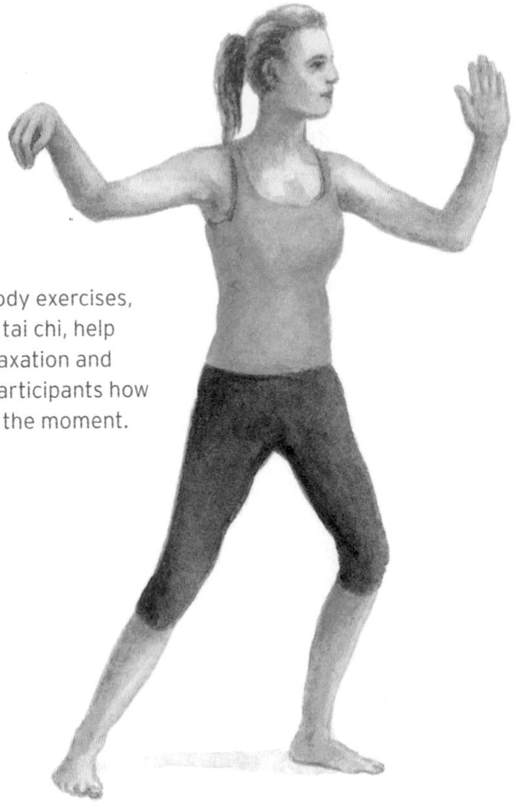

Mind-body exercises, such as tai chi, help with relaxation and teach participants how to be in the moment.

There are many activities that promote **relaxation** *(p. 269)*, including meditation, breathing techniques, progressive muscle relaxation and massage. But relaxation can also be gained from activities done simply for enjoyment such as hobbies, taking a nap, walking in nature or anything else that infuses life with creativity, humor and fun. One of the most effective ways to combat stress is to find an activity that completely absorbs you when you are doing it so that you lose track of time. Such "single-minded" activities include creative pursuits, gardening, sports, playing music, dancing and reading. When fully absorbed in the present it is impossible to mull over the past or worry about the future and so during these activities it is possible to relax fully and experience moments that are truly free of stress.

Be

At the top of the pyramid is the simple activity of "being." This includes "being balanced," "being positive" and "being at peace" with yourself and your surroundings. Being requires you to be fully engaged in the present moment. This may sound simple, yet it is the ultimate goal of many ancient techniques—such as **meditation** *(p. 234)*, **qi gong** *(p. 266)*, **tai chi** *(p. 290)* and **yoga** *(p. 316)*—that are designed to integrate mind and body. Perhaps the easiest way to experience just being is through spending time in nature. Nature is inherently healing and a recent review of research suggests, "access to nature plays a vital role in human health, well-being and development that has not been fully recognized."

A state of being can also be cultivated through various mindfulness practices that can include mindfulness meditation, mindful eating, mindful walking, and so on. While regular practice of these activities may involve some degree of discipline, they are often activities that people enjoy. It seems that loving an activity enhances the ability to lose oneself completely and simply "be."

PROFESSOR MARC COHEN
MBBS(Hons), PhD,
BMedSc(Hons), FAMAC, FICAE

AILMENTS

ACNE

THE CURSE OF TEENAGERS AND MANY young adults, acne—in the form of pimples, blackheads or small cysts—is caused by overgrowth of normal skin bacteria that may be triggered by hormonal changes, heat, greasy cosmetics or certain prescription medications. It usually occurs on the face or shoulders when pores become blocked with excess sebum (an oil your skin glands produce) and dead skin cells. Acne may be a mild inconvenience or become serious and lead to secondary infection and permanent scarring. Many cases, however, are treatable with natural remedies.

Suggested remedies

Lifestyle factors Wash your skin once or twice a day and immediately after exercise when sweat can build up, using a gentle, non-drying soap. Don't scrub as that can encourage sebum production. If you use makeup, find a brand that is water-based and remove it at night. Don't scratch or squeeze spots and try not to touch an acne-prone area.

***Tea tree** (p. 293)* Applied topically, tea tree essential oil can limit an outbreak of acne and reduce its severity. In one Australian study of 124 patients, a 5 percent tea tree oil gel was as effective as a 5 percent benzoyl peroxide lotion—with fewer side effects.

***Niacin** (p. 245)* In gel form, nicotinamide, a topical vitamin B_3 preparation, is a good alternative to conventional antimicrobial creams to which patients may develop a resistance. A 2013 Iranian study suggests it works best with oily skins.

***Ayurveda** (p. 127)* A herbal combination with aloe, turmeric and ashwagandha used orally and topically significantly improved acne symptoms in an Indian study. Oral treatment with the Ayurvedic herb guggul may also be effective, particularly for oily skin.

Retinoids For severe acne, doctors may prescribe a cream or pills containing retinoids, a synthetic form of vitamin A, to reduce the amount of sebum produced. **(See Vitamin A, *p. 301.*)**

See also Eczema and dermatitis, Psoriasis, Skin rashes

See your doctor

Consult a doctor if the acne persists for months, gets worse or leaves scars.

Quick fix Health and beauty experts recommend ice (see Cold therapy, *p. 161*) to calm an angry spot and reduce redness and swelling. Cleanse the area, then wrap two or three ice cubes in a clean washcloth and apply for up to 10 minutes.

DID YOU KNOW?

Contrary to popular belief, chocolate and greasy foods probably don't cause acne, but a healthy diet, in particular the low-glycemic index diet, may reduce its severity, according to recent Korean and Australian studies. However, it is genes that largely determine who gets spots. If acne runs in your immediate family, there's an almost 80 percent chance that you'll be susceptible, too.

ALLERGIES

ACROSS THE WORLD ALLERGIES ARE ON the rise. Increasing numbers of us are becoming susceptible to triggers such as pollen, certain foods, chemicals, dust or pet dander. Once the body perceives these substances as harmful, the immune system goes into overdrive, releasing chemicals that cause reactions such as rashes, itching and sneezing. Occasionally allergies can cause life-threatening anaphylactic reactions.

It may take time to identify an allergen; even then, you can't always avoid it. However, there are several natural remedies that can help to alleviate symptoms, while the first (see below) may provide a lasting cure.

Suggested remedies

***Sublingual immunotherapy** (p. 289)* This therapy can combat a range of allergies from dust mites to olives. You will need to be referred to a practitioner by your doctor. After testing to identify the allergen, a vial of the substance is prepared. The patient takes this as drops under the tongue and builds up resistance as the dose is gradually increased. It may take time to develop immunity and several years' treatment may be required.

***Butterbur** (p. 139)* The herb worked as well as the antihistamine fexofenadine in a 2005 Swiss study involving 330 patients with allergic rhinitis (sneezing, watery eyes and runny nose).

***Vitamin C** (p. 304)* Taking extra vitamin C reduced allergic rhinitis symptoms in a 2013 study of 4,554 Korean children.

Quercetin Laboratory studies show that quercetin stops certain immune cells from releasing histamine, a chemical that triggers allergic reactions. (See Flavonoids, *p. 187.*)

***Elimination diet** (p. 171)* While a food intolerance may cause discomfort and digestive problems, the symptoms of a food allergy–perhaps to nuts or shellfish–are usually much more immediate and severe. Even so, it can be tricky to identify the cause as potential triggers include not only foods but a range of common food preservatives, including sulfites and benzoates. An elimination diet can help you pinpoint the culprit.

***Perilla** (p. 256)* In Japan, the leaves of *Perilla frutescens* are used to treat fish and crabmeat allergies; a 2003 animal study suggests perilla constituents have a powerful antiallergy action.

See also Asthma, Eczema and dermatitis, Food intolerances, Hay fever, Insect bites and stings

See your doctor

Anaphylaxis—a reaction where swelling or breathing problems rapidly worsen—requires immediate medical attention. People with an extreme sensitivity—perhaps to a type of food or bee stings—are often prescribed a device such as an EpiPen that provides an injectable adrenaline dose in emergency situations.

Quick fix The stuffy nose that comes with many allergies can be cleared with nasal irrigation *(p. 242)*. With a bulb syringe, squeeze bottle or neti pot, you introduce a saline solution into one nostril and let it flow through the nasal passage and out.

DID YOU KNOW?
Worldwide, up to 50 percent of school-aged children suffer from one or more allergies. More than 4 million Australians (19.6 percent of the population) and 20 percent of Americans have at least one allergy. It is thought that as many as half of all Europeans could be affected by at least one allergy.

ANEMIA

IF YOU'RE PALE, CONSTANTLY FEEL tired and suffer from headaches, you may have anemia, which affects at least 2 billion people across the world. It is caused by having too few red blood cells or too little hemoglobin, the iron-based protein within them, to carry the oxygen the body needs. Iron-deficiency anemia is the most common type; others include B_{12}-deficiency anemia and foliate-deficiency anemia. Once diagnosed, anemia can usually be treated successfully with a healthy diet and supplements, though some forms, such as aplastic anemia or sickle cell anemia, require specialist care.

Suggested remedies

Dietary measures To prevent and treat anemia, you need to ensure your diet includes foods that are rich in iron *(p. 214)*. Tea and coffee can block iron absorption, so avoid caffeinated beverages at meal times. Also make sure you are getting plenty of foods containing vitamin B_{12} *(p. 303)* and folic acid *(p. 189)*. Try to eat vitamin C-rich foods *(p. 304)* along with iron-rich foods as this vitamin helps your body to absorb more iron. The blue-green algae supplement spirulina can be especially helpful for older people. In one US study, spirulina boosted hemoglobin levels and immune function in 30 people aged 50 or more with a history of anemia.

Taking the following vitamin and mineral supplements may be helpful. Check with your doctor first.

Iron (p. 214) Taking extra iron, especially as ferrous fumerate, glycerate or sulfate, which are easily absorbed, will replenish your body's supplies.

Vitamin B_{12} (p. 303) If you are very deficient, your doctor may recommend B_{12} injections, followed by supplements, which you may need to take for life.

Folic acid (p. 189) To correct foliate-deficiency anemia, you may need supplements for up to four months.

Quick fix If you suspect that you may have anemia, a simple blood test can verify this and determine the cause. Armed with this knowledge, your doctor can advise on appropriate treatment.

See also Celiac disease, Fatigue, Headaches

See your doctor

Seek immediate medical advice if you develop a very rapid or irregular heartbeat, which can signal a severe deficiency that could limit your heart's ability to function properly.

DID YOU KNOW?

Teenage girls and menstruating women often have low iron levels due to the monthly loss of menstrual blood. Pregnant women may become anemic because they need more iron to support their growing child. Vegetarians and vegans are also at risk as iron from animal sources is better absorbed than iron from plants. Those suffering from celiac disease may not absorb enough iron or folate from food. Older people may suffer from pernicious anemia, an autoimmune disorder that interferes with the absorption of vitamin B_{12}.

ANXIETY

BETWEEN 14 AND 18 PERCENT OF THE population (and more women than men) struggle with anxiety. You may experience a racing heart, muscle tension, trembling, hyperventilation, trouble breathing or concentrating or a headache; or you may have trouble falling or staying asleep. There are several remedies that may ease anxiety.

Suggested remedies

Lifestyle factors Take steps to lessen the stress in your life and make sure you are getting enough sleep. Loss of sleep can lead to irritability and raises risks of developing anxiety disorders. Sleeping strategies *(p. 281)* may help.

Rebreathing Breathing into a bag will help raise carbon dioxide levels in the blood and reduce symptoms of a panic attack such as hyperventilation and tingling.

Pet therapy (p. 257) Pet owners have long known the benefits of a canine or feline companion and now research is backing them up. A pilot study by Kean University in the US suggests that five minutes with a therapy dog reduces the levels of cortisol—a stress marker chemical—in the blood and saliva.

Aromatherapy (p. 122) Place a few drops of chamomile *(p. 147)*, lemon balm *(p. 221)*, bergamot *(p. 129)* and jasmine essential oils on a cotton ball and inhale, or add them to a warm bath. Alternatively, book yourself an aromatherapy massage *(p. 230)*.

Relaxing teas Teas or tinctures containing soothing herbs, such as ashwagandha *(p. 124)*, chamomile *(p. 147)*, hops *(p. 206)*, lavender *(p 219)*, lemon balm *(p. 221)* and holy basil *(p. 205)*, can assist in calming nerves and inducing relaxation.

Relaxation (p. 269) There are several breathing methods that help to calm the mind. Yoga *(p. 316)* and meditation *(p. 234)* are also well-trodden paths to tranquility. But if none of these appeal to you, try listening to your favorite music *(p. 241)* once in a while. Scientists are discovering it is a powerful antidote to anxiety.

Social contact (p. 283) Go see your friends. Caring for others and forming social alliances have been shown to increase oxytocin and endorphin levels—the "feel-good" brain chemicals.

Cognitive behavioral therapy (p. 159) You can learn strategies to change your reactions in anxiety-causing situations by learning to use this powerful technique.

See your doctor

When anxiety is ongoing and interferes with work or relationships, leads to depression or a substance abuse problem, or is linked to a physical problem, see your doctor. If you have thoughts of harming yourself, talk to someone or call a help line such as The Samaritans or Lifeline.

Quick fix Breathe in for two counts, then exhale for four. Longer exhalation triggers your vagus nerve, activating the parasympathetic nervous system, which puts the brakes on fight-or-flight symptoms such as a rapid heartbeat.

See also Concentration, improved, Depression, Phobias

WATCH OUT!

Kava, long suggested as a first-line remedy for anxiety, may have only modest short-term effects, and long-term use has been linked with liver damage. Check with your doctor before using kava, and never use it for longer than 24 weeks.

ASTHMA

MORE THAN 300 MILLION PEOPLE AROUND the world suffer from asthma, according to the World Health Organization. Asthma is a respiratory disorder triggered by allergens, stress, smoke, cold air or exercise. As the bronchial tubes become inflamed and clogged with mucus, and the small muscles around them contract, it can be frighteningly difficult to breathe. Conventional medicines include bronchodilators, which relax the muscles, and anti-inflammatory medicines to reduce the swelling. Natural remedies can help but should not replace prescribed medications.

Suggested remedies

Lifestyle factors Remove dust and other triggers through regular vacuuming with a High Efficiency Particulate Air (HEPA) filter vacuum cleaner, washing linen with **eucalyptus oil** *(p. 173)* to kill dust mites, using allergen-proof pillow covers and minimizing the use of carpets and soft furnishings in your home.

Boswellia (p. 136) German research has shown that the Indian herb *Boswellia serrata*—known for its anti-inflammatory effects—can improve breathing and regular use may reduce the frequency of asthma attacks.

Maritime pine (p. 229) An extract from the bark of the French maritime pine may help by improving lung function and limiting the number of inflammation-causing compounds released by the immune system during an asthma attack.

Eucalyptus (p. 173) Taking eucalyptus oil in capsule form could help asthma sufferers to reduce their steroid medication levels by more than a third, according to German research.

Fish oils High in **omega-3 fatty acids** *(p. 250)*, fish oils may be especially effective for treating exercise-related asthma. Pregnant women who take fish oils may also protect their children against future asthma, according to a large Danish study.

Green-lipped mussels (p. 201) Extracts of New Zealand green-lipped mussels can help treat allergic asthma by blocking the production of substances that irritate the lungs.

Relaxation (p. 269) Calming breathing exercises can help to relieve asthma symptoms. A number of studies have also shown the benefits of **yoga** *(p. 316)*.

See also Allergies

See your doctor

Seek emergency help if you have difficulty breathing that is not relieved by medication or your symptoms become severe.

Quick fix If you are without your inhaler, drinking a couple of cups of strong **coffee** *(p. 158)* could help you breathe more freely during an attack and for up to four hours. Caffeine has a similar structure to theophylline, an early asthma medication.

WATCH OUT!

Ephedra, the Chinese herb "ma huang," is effective for mild asthma, but its active ingredient ephedrine can cause rapid heartbeat, high blood pressure and stroke. Supplements containing ephedrine alkaloids are banned in the US, Australia and some European countries, though they are available on the Internet.

BACK AND NECK PAIN

VARIOUS MUSCULAR, JOINT AND DEGENERATIVE problems can cause back and neck pain that plagues many people. But often tension, poor posture, bad lifting or bending are equally to blame. Natural remedies can provide a gentler alternative to standard anti-inflammatory drugs, while lifestyle adjustments can help prevent the pain from recurring.

Suggested remedies

Lifestyle factors In the past, bed rest was prescribed for back pain, yet it is now known that being inactive can make matters worse. Moving your spine as much as possible, while avoiding movements that cause severe pain, is likely to speed up your recovery. To avoid recurrent problems, check your posture. Keep your back supported against an office chair and don't slouch when standing. Sleep on your side or back, using a pillow that doesn't raise your neck out of line. Gentle stretching *(p. 286)* may help.

Heat therapy/Cold therapy (p. 204/p. 161) A hot-water bottle or wheat pack applied to the affected area or a hot bath can provide some temporary relief as can a cold pack applied to an inflamed area or alternating between hot and cold treatments.

Massage (p. 230) A gentle massage can relax tight muscles, improve circulation and enhance mobility.

White willow bark (p. 312) A daily dose of willow bark extract (with an active ingredient similar to aspirin) relieves chronic back pain, according to Israeli researchers; it may treat neck pain, too.

Comfrey (p. 162) In one Czech study involving 215 patients, concentrated comfrey cream greatly reduced myalgia pain in the lower and upper back.

Chiropractic (p. 152) The hands-on therapy favored by many back pain sufferers was declared both safe and effective in a recent systematic review of research.

Acupuncture and acupressure (p. 112) In one Chinese study of 129 patients with back pain, a month of acupressure worked better than physical therapy and kept people pain-free for six months.

Bodywork Therapies such as the Alexander Technique, Bowen Technique, Feldenkrais Method and pilates *(p. 115, p. 138, p. 180 and p. 258)* can address tension problems and improve your posture.

Devil's claw (p. 168) The herb's anti-inflammatory properties make it a useful agent in easing back and neck pain.

See your doctor

See a doctor if the pain persists or if it is sudden or severe, especially if you have a fever, numbness, swelling or unexplained weight loss.

Quick fix For fast pain relief, try capsaicin cream (see Cayenne, *p. 145*). In a 2010 German study, capsaicin cream provided significantly more relief than a placebo. A special capsaicin plaster can be highly effective for nonspecific low back pain.

See also Chronic pain, Frozen shoulder

BAD BREATH AND BODY ODOR

THEY'RE UNPLEASANT IN OTHER PEOPLE and embarrassing if they're your own. But as bad breath and body odor become better understood, they become easier to treat and avoid. For instance, scientists now know that the sulfur compounds that make breath smell bad are waste products produced by certain strains of bacteria munching on food leftovers in our mouths. Body odor can be genetic but is also affected by diet, hygiene and what you wear.

Suggested remedies

Lifestyle factors Regular tooth brushing, flossing and tongue scraping will remove the food particles that bacteria feed on and help prevent gum disease, which adds to breath problems. Similarly, washing sweat-prone areas, such as armpits and feet, regularly with an antibacterial soap will minimize unpleasant body odor. Wearing natural fibers, such as cotton or extra fine merino wool, allows your skin to breathe so sweat evaporates faster.

Dietary measures Avoid, garlic, onions and spicy foods as they can affect your breath and the odor of your perspiration, as do smoking and excessive alcohol intake. Eating red meat also makes body odor more intense. Chewing on a few fennel seeds (see Carminative herbs, *p. 143*) provides an aromatic scent and acts as a digestive aid that also helps reduce bad breath. Other herbs such as parsley, spearmint, rosemary and cardamom can also help freshen breath, while crunchy foods such as carrots and celery will help reduce odor-causing plaque.

Holy basil (p. 205) Drinking and/or rinsing the mouth with holy basil tea after a meal can reduce oral bacteria and prevent plaque, gum disease and mouth ulcers. A number of studies have shown the herb to be as effective yet more pleasant than antibacterial mouthwashes containing chlorhexidine or other chemical agents.

Green tea For freshening the breath, green tea is more effective than chewing gum, mint or parsley-seed oil, according to recent Canadian research. (See Tea, *p. 292*.)

Essential oils Korean research suggests that mouthwashes prepared from diluted tea tree *(p. 293)*, peppermint *(p. 255)* or lemon *(p. 220)* essential oils may be effective for reducing mouth odor. Try adding a few drops of each to 1 cup (250 ml) of water. Consider mouthwashes containing eucalyptus *(p. 173)*, or its active ingredient cineole, as this not only keeps breath fresh but may also prevent dental plaque and gum disease.

See your doctor

Consult a dentist if you have bleeding gums or dental pain. For severe body odor, a doctor might suggest treatment to control your sweat glands.

Quick fix If you have nothing else on hand, banish bad breath with a solution of salt water *(p. 275)* or bicarbonate of soda *(p. 130)*. Rinse for 15–30 seconds, then spit it out.

DID YOU KNOW?
New Zealand researchers have been developing oral probiotics *(p. 261)* containing *Streptococcus salivarius* K_{12}, a strain of "good" mouth bacteria that counteract the effects of malodorous ones.

See also Tooth and gum disorders

WATCH OUT!
Commercial alcohol-based antiseptic mouthwashes may temporarily mask unpleasant odors but can also wipe out all bacteria, good or bad, dry out your mouth and even affect your sense of taste.

BLOOD PRESSURE, HIGH

YOUR BLOOD PRESSURE READING IS AN indication of how much pressure your blood exerts on your arteries as it is pumped around your body by your heart. It consists of two numbers; the first is your systolic blood pressure (the pressure in your arteries when your heart contracts) and the second is your diastolic blood pressure (the pressure as your heart relaxes). Blood pressure of less than 120/80 is considered normal, and between 120/80 and 140/90 is classified as high-normal. High blood pressure (also known as hypertension) is diagnosed when blood pressure is consistently greater than 140/90, and is considered severe when it exceeds 180/110.

High blood pressure doesn't always cause symptoms, and may be present even if you feel well. Nevertheless, it increases your risk of developing some serious health problems (including heart attack, stroke and kidney disease) and requires ongoing treatment by your doctor. The following remedies may help you manage your blood pressure.

Suggested remedies

Lifestyle factors If you have high blood pressure, your doctor may recommend that you quit smoking, eat more fruit and vegetables, cut back on salt and alcohol and/or reduce your body weight. You should also follow a healthy diet.

Meditation (p. 234) Regular meditation–transcendental meditation in particular–has been shown in numerous studies to reduce blood pressure, most likely by reducing stress and balancing the autonomic nervous system.

Relaxation (p. 269) Methods that encourage slow, deep, rhythmic breathing may be as effective as some medications in treating high blood pressure. Numerous studies have shown the benefits of **yoga** *(p. 316)*, **qigong** *(p. 266)* and other forms of exercise that involve slow, deep breathing for lowering high blood pressure. Simply listening to **music** *(p. 241)* can help, too.

Isometric exercises Hand-grip and other isometric exercises have been shown to reduce blood pressure over time, but may also cause transient increases in blood pressure, so caution is required in people with extremely high blood pressure.

Coenzyme Q_{10} (p. 157) In a review of the scientific evidence for a range of natural therapies for hypertension published in 2008, CoQ_{10} supplements were shown to lower blood pressure more significantly than any other therapy studied.

Garlic (p. 191) Extensive research suggests that garlic may be of some help in lowering blood pressure in people with hypertension.

See your doctor

If you suspect you have high blood pressure, talk to your doctor, who can recommend appropriate treatment for you. Seek immediate medical assistance if you notice you have extremely high blood pressure (180/110 or higher), or if you experience:

- chest pain
- blurred vision
- nausea or vomiting
- severe headache.

Quick fix If you feel your blood pressure rising in a stressful situation, simply taking some slow, deep breaths may help.

See also Heart and circulatory health

BRONCHITIS

INFLAMMATION OF THE BRONCHI (the airways of the lungs) and the hacking cough, sore throat, wheezing and breathlessness that often go with it are usually caused by a viral infection, though bronchitis can be bacterial, too. Pollution, smoking and exposure to tobacco smoke make you more susceptible. Plenty of rest and lots of fluids will speed recovery and a number of herbs and supplements can ease your symptoms.

Suggested remedies

Lifestyle factors Quit smoking–as many as 40 percent of smokers develop chronic bronchitis. If you have bronchitis, it is best to stay home and let your body rest and recuperate rather than trying to "soldier on" at work and risk spreading your infection throughout your workplace. Making sure your body has adequate hydration *(p. 209)* and using a humidifier or steam inhalation (see Quick fix) helps to loosen and expel phlegm.

Cough tea Boil a wedge of lemon *(p. 220)* with some grated garlic *(p. 191)* and ginger *(p. 192)*. Then add herbs such as echinacea *(p 169)*, thyme and holy basil *(p. 205)*. When cooled, add some manuka honey *(p. 228)* to taste. This antimicrobial tea will help to soothe a sore throat that comes from coughing and help your immune system to fight off infection.

Mullein (p. 239) Try a soothing mullein tea made with dried leaves and flowers or inhale the steam. The herb contains saponins, which help to loosen mucus and ease congestion.

Peppermint (p. 255) The menthol in peppermint helps to clear congestion, thins mucus and loosens phlegm. Make tea from the leaves or use an inhalation of peppermint oil.

South African geranium (p. 284) The extract is widely used in Germany to relieve respiratory symptoms. In one double-blind study of 468 adults with bronchitis, those who took it returned to work two days earlier than the control group.

N-acetyl cysteine The dietary supplement helps to thin mucus and also has antioxidant properties that may help to protect against further bronchitis attacks. (See Amino acids, *p. 118.*)

Aromatherapy (p. 122) To help you sleep, use a home humidifier alone or with a prescribed combination of aromatic essential oils, such as jasmine, lavender *(p. 219)*, tea tree *(p. 293)* or marjoram, which help thin mucus.

See your doctor

Consult a doctor if:

- your cough does not clear up after a week or so
- the cough becomes severe
- you have a high temperature for more than three days
- you cough up any blood.

You should also consult your doctor if you get bronchitis and suffer from other conditions such as asthma, chronic obstructive pulmonary disease (COPD) or heart disease.

Quick fix An inhalation of eucalyptus oil *(p. 173)* can fight infection and clear congestion, enabling you to breathe more easily. Add a few drops of oil to a bowl of boiling water, put a towel over your head, close your eyes and gently inhale for several minutes.

See also Asthma, Colds and flu, Frequent illness, Sinusitis

BRUISES

A BUMP, FALL OR COLLISION WITH a hard object—we all get bruises from time to time. The fairer your skin, the more perceptible they are as tiny blood vessels are broken and leak into soft tissue, causing discoloration, swelling and pain. Older people and people taking steroid medications often have thinner skin and more fragile tissue and therefore bruise more easily. Natural remedies can speed healing and relieve pain.

Suggested remedies

Elevation Raising (above the level of the heart) and resting the bruised area to reduce the blood flow to it will make it less painful and reduce discoloration.

Arnica *(p. 121)* The plant has been widely used to treat bruises and soothe aches and pains for more than 500 years. Until recently few human studies supported its efficacy. But US research has now shown that a 20 percent arnica ointment and also homeopathic arnica can reduce bruising.

Bromelain Taking bromelain, an enzyme found in pineapples, can help to reduce swelling and tenderness. It is often used with other enzymes to help injured athletes and postoperative patients to recover faster. (See Enzymes, *p. 172*.)

Flavonoids *(p. 187)* Flavonoid supplements, including hesperidin, can help control inflammation and strengthen capillaries. When combined with enzymes, such as bromelain, they may be even more effective. In one study of 44 people with sports injuries, the combination treatment reduced time away from training by half.

Comfrey *(p. 162)* Try a soothing comfrey gel. Applied several times a day, comfrey can reduce swelling and speed healing.

Horse chestnut *(p. 207)* A gel containing 2 percent aescin, the active ingredient in horse chestnut, can help to relieve tenderness. It should be applied as soon as possible.

See your doctor

You should consult a doctor as soon as possible if:

❖ the impact was forceful and you have pain and swelling but no skin discoloration—you may have deeper, internal bruising
❖ the area is very painful and you suspect you may have broken a bone
❖ you receive a powerful blow to the head or face
❖ the bruise is severe or painful and you're on blood-thinning medication
❖ you notice bruising but don't know the cause
❖ the bruise persists for more than two weeks.

Quick fix Stem bleeding under the skin and reduce swelling with Cold therapy *(p. 161)*. Apply ice cubes, an ice pack or even a packet of frozen vegetables, wrapped in a towel (do not place ice in direct contact with the skin), to the site of bruising for 20 minutes at a time. Repeat as necessary over the next day or so.

BURNS

WHETHER CAUSED BY FIRE, BOILING WATER, chemicals or sunlight, burns require immediate first aid. Superficial (first-degree) burns affecting only the top skin layer are largely treatable at home with natural remedies, but partial thickness (second-degree) burns, which penetrate deeper and cause blistering, may need expert attention. Full-thickness (third-degree burns), where tissue and sometimes muscle, bones and organs beneath the skin are also damaged, are medical emergencies.

Suggested remedies

Lifestyle factors Where there is no broken skin, mild burns and sunburns can be left uncovered after the initial water treatment (see Quick fix). Don't prick blisters but do put a nonadhesive dressing over any that burst.

Aloe vera *(p. 117)* Herbalists recommend fresh gel from aloe leaves or in a cream. In one recent Iranian study aloe helped second-degree burns heal faster than the antibacterial cream silver sulfadiazine.

Tea tree (p. 293) Gels containing tea tree oil can be effective first aid for minor burns. Tea tree oil has antibacterial, antifungal and anti-inflammatory properties that can assist the healing of burns.

Gotu kola (p. 199) A herb used in the ancient Indian healing system called Ayurveda *(p. 127)*, gotu kola applied as a cream may be helpful. Laboratory and animal studies have shown that gotu kola plant chemicals, called triterpenoids, can strengthen skin and boost the blood supply to an injured area.

Manuka honey (p. 228) Indian and New Zealand research shows that honey dressings help burns heal faster and can reduce scarring. Honey is also very effective in preventing and fighting a wide range of infections. Manuka honey is best because it has a more powerful antibacterial action than other types of honey.

Quick fix As soon as possible, remove jewelry or clothing near the burn and run cool water over the wound for up to 30 minutes. This is essential to limit skin damage. Then cover the burn with a cloth or plastic wrap to keep it clean.

See your doctor

Get urgent help if:

- ❖ the burn is larger than an inch (3 cm) across or located on the hands, face or groin area
- ❖ the burn is not painful (this indicates a full-thickness burn that has damaged nerve endings—superficial burns are usually more painful)
- ❖ there is significant peeling or blistering of the skin, or the wound is weeping
- ❖ the burn is fullthickness
- ❖ the flesh is black or charred with white or yellow tissue
- ❖ it is a chemical or electrical burn.

WATCH OUT!

Whatever your grandmother said, don't use butter on burns. "Butter may contain bacteria that could cause an infection," says Dr. Leila Cuttle, a scientist at the Royal Children's Hospital in Brisbane, Australia. Cool running water is the only effective immediate treatment, she says.

BURSITIS AND TENDONITIS

PAINTING, GARDENING AND PLAYING tennis are among the many activities that can trigger bursitis and tendonitis; both are caused by repetitive movements and can affect an arm, leg or shoulder. In bursitis, the small sac of fluid (bursa), which cushions a joint, becomes inflamed. In tendonitis, the tendon, which attaches muscle to the joint, becomes swollen and painful. A variety of natural remedies may help reduce the swelling and pain.

Suggested remedies

Lifestyle factors Rest and avoid whatever action caused the problem until the pain and swelling ease. A joint support, sling or splint can immobilize the affected area, while using knee pads or a stool can allow activities such as gardening or cleaning to be performed without putting pressure on painful areas.

White willow bark *(p. 312)* White willow's active ingredient salicin has pain-relieving effects similar to those of aspirin, but doesn't irritate the stomach in the same way.

Boswellia *(p. 136)* To reduce pain and swelling, try *Boswellia serrata*. The gummy resin of this herb has an anti-inflammatory action, making it suitable for treating both bursitis and tendonitis.

Acupuncture *(p. 112)* Studies show that acupuncture can reduce pain and increase mobility in patients suffering from both tennis elbow and tendonitis of the shoulder. In one recent Swedish study, acupuncture plus exercise was as effective for healing shoulder tendonitis as corticosteroids combined with exercise.

Yoga *(p. 316)* Classes can help prevent bursitis recurring by stretching tendons and muscles around the bursa.

Bodywork Therapies such as the Alexander Technique *(p. 115)*, Bowen Technique *(p. 138)*, Feldenkrais Method *(p. 180)* or pilates *(p. 258)* aim to correct poor posture and awkward movement, so could help you change or avoid the repetitive action that has led to bursitis or tendonitis.

See also Back and neck pain

See your doctor

If either condition persists and becomes very painful, or you develop a fever, see a doctor.

Quick fix First apply an ice pack, wrapped in a towel, for 20–30 minutes every few hours (see Cold therapy, *p. 161*). After about 48 hours, a heat pad or moist heated towel may bring better relief (see Heat therapy, *p. 204*).

DID YOU KNOW?

Leech therapy is an effective, if unconventional, bursitis treatment. Leech saliva contains enzymes that help reduce pain and inflammation and dissolve blood clots that form when tissue is damaged. In a recent German study, a single treatment with two to four leeches worked better for healing tennis elbow than a 30-day course of a topical cream (diclofenac).

CANCER SUPPORT

ONE IN THREE OF US WILL DEVELOP some form of cancer in our lifetime. This large group of related diseases—where malignant cells proliferate, invade and damage normal tissue—remains a challenge for doctors, but with screening programs and increased education, more cancers are being spotted at an early stage with better outcomes.

While no single natural remedy will prevent or cure cancer, some can be protective and others appear to enhance the effects of conventional treatments, alleviate side effects or boost the immune system and speed recovery.

Key defense strategies

Living well offers powerful protection against many cancers. A healthy diet, regular exercise *(p. 175)*, avoiding tobacco and moderating alcohol and salt intake can help prevent more than 30 percent of all cancers, says the World Health Organization, while some US researchers estimate that up to 95 percent of cancers are related to environment or lifestyle.

Eating plenty of fruit and vegetables can reduce your risk of mouth, esophagus and lung cancer plus some types of stomach cancer, according to the European Prospective Investigation into Cancer and Nutrition (EPIC). Nutritionists recommend seven servings a day. The natural fiber *(p. 184)* present in fresh produce and whole grains *(p. 313)* could help to reduce your risk of bowel cancer, too, by as much as 40 percent.

A major 2013 review of cancer studies found that one or two portions of oily fish a week could be protective, reducing the risk of breast cancer in later life by 14 percent. The omega-3 fatty acids *(p. 250)* in the fish may also help to prevent colorectal cancer.

By contrast, eating too much red meat and especially red or white processed meats, such as sausages and burgers, can raise your risk of bowel cancer. Stomach cancer, the fourth most common type, has been linked to excessive salt intake.

Avoiding exposure to toxic environmental chemicals can also help to lower your cancer risk. Chemicals in many plastics, pesticides and exhaust fumes have been identified as carcinogens. You can avoid them through simple lifestyle choices.

Quick fix When taken before chemotherapy, ginger *(p. 192)* may help to reduce nausea; peppermint *(p. 255)* and spearmint oils work well, too. Techniques that encourage relaxation *(p. 269)*, such as guided imagery, may help to reduce anxiety and help you to cope with pain.

WATCH OUT!

There is no "magic bullet" to cure cancer but plenty of contenders. They include laetrile—a synthetic form of amygdalin, a plant compound found in the kernels of bitter almonds and apricots—which has been promoted as a cancer cure. A Cochran Review of 2011 concluded that there was no scientific evidence supporting the claims. Laetrile can be metabolized in the body to cyanide so there are toxicity concerns, too. Doctors also warn against taking Essiac. As formulations vary, it may interact with conventional cancer treatments and there are no clinical studies to support its efficacy.

Suggested remedies

Turmeric (p. 298) Small trials show that turmeric, or supplements of its key ingredient curcumin, may help prevent colon and pancreatic cancers and boost the general health of patients with colorectal cancer.

Garlic (p. 191) When taken regularly, fresh or in supplement form, garlic may protect against colon and stomach cancers.

Green tea The powerful antioxidants in green tea appear to suppress the proliferation of cancer cells and may offer some protection against gastrointestinal tract, ovarian, prostate and breast cancer. (See Tea, *p. 292*.)

Tomato paste (p. 297) Tomato products, such as pastes and sauces, are concentrated sources of lycopene, an antioxidant carotenoid that one US review of studies suggests could reduce prostate cancer risk by up to 30 percent.

Holy basil (p. 205) This herb may help in preventing cancer through its antioxidant properties and ability to help the liver detoxify many cancer-causing chemicals. It may also help cancer patients cope with cancer treatments through its stress-relieving, immune-boosting and radio- and chemoprotective actions.

Boswellia (p. 136) The supplement *Boswellia serrata* appears to help shrink the swelling around brain tumors in patients receiving radiation.

Medicinal mushrooms (p. 233) Taken in extract form maitake mushrooms may boost the immune system. Lentinan, a substance found in shiitake mushrooms, has been shown to boost survival in stomach cancer patients receiving chemotherapy. Turkey tail has been shown to boost the immune systems of breast cancer patients.

Melatonin (p. 237) Taking this supplement may improve tumor response to chemotherapy, radiotherapy and hormonal therapy and extend patient survival times. Discuss with your doctor.

The following mental therapies and practitioner-based therapies can support patients going through the shock of a cancer diagnosis and the trauma of cancer treatments.

Meditation (p. 234) Through calming the mind, this may help patients tolerate aggressive cancer treatments. Hypnotherapy *(p. 211)* can help by changing a patient's expectation of pain and so can reduce the experience of postoperative pain.

Acupuncture (p. 112) This therapy has long been used to relieve pain, nausea and anxiety. In one small 2011 UK study, 82 percent of cancer patients receiving acupuncture reported relief from peripheral nerve pain.

Massage (p. 230) A 2009 review of classical Swedish massage suggests it may improve well-being, relieve pain, ease anxiety and lift depression in cancer patients.

Yoga (p. 316) For people with acute and chronic health conditions, including cancer, there are physical and mental benefits to be gained from yoga. This was the finding of a 2013 review of 13 studies—eight in the US and one each in Slovenia, Italy, the UK, Canada and Turkey.

Qigong (p. 266) This gentle mind-body exercise has been shown to help cancer survivors and those undergoing treatment cope with the anxiety that often accompanies the disease.

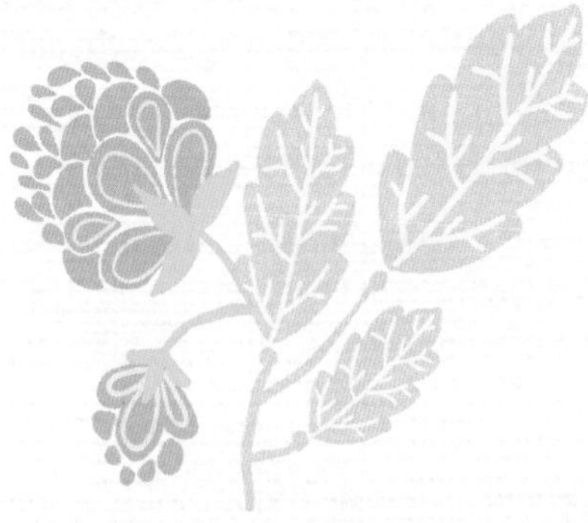

CHOLESTEROL, HIGH

OUR BODIES NEED A CERTAIN AMOUNT of cholesterol, but high levels are a risk factor for heart attack and stroke. Cholesterol is carried in the blood by two types of protein: low-density lipoprotein (LDL, the "bad" cholesterol) and high-density lipoprotein (HDL, the "good" cholesterol). If a blood test shows your total cholesterol is too high, you will need to reduce your levels of LDL and blood fats called triglycerides. By contrast, you should boost your levels of HDL, which carries cholesterol back to the liver for disposal in waste products.

You may need medication, but lifestyle adjustments and natural remedies can be highly effective at reducing and controlling cholesterol levels. Metabolic syndrome is the term given when high cholesterol exists along with high blood pressure, high blood glucose and obesity. This condition may affect more than 25 percent of adults in developed countries.

Suggested remedies

Lifestyle factors Lose weight if necessary and take regular exercise *(p. 175)*.

Dietary measures Cut down on cholesterol-containing foods such as fatty meats, cakes, cheese and chips. Instead follow a healthy diet such as the Mediterranean diet with its emphasis on olive oil *(p. 249)* and fresh vegetables. Try also to include more soy *(p. 285)* foods in your diet.

Niacin (p. 245) US studies show that taking niacin (vitamin B_3) can reduce LDL cholesterol by 10 percent, triglycerides by 25 percent and raise HDL cholesterol by 20–30 percent.

Fish oil Taking fish oil appears to bring down triglyceride levels, reducing total cholesterol. (See Omega-3 fatty acids, *p. 250*.)

Garlic (p. 191) This culinary herb has long been known to thin the blood and lower cholesterol levels.

Holy basil (p. 205) Studies suggest that the herb has a beneficial effect on cholesterol levels, blood glucose levels and blood pressure, making it particularly suited for people with metabolic syndrome.

Psyllium (p. 264) The soluble fiber in psyllium helps to lower cholesterol by reducing its absorption into the bloodstream.

Red yeast rice (p. 268) The traditional Chinese herbal medicine contains cholesterol-lowering chemicals similar to statins that may be equally effective, according to a 2011 review of research.

See also Blood pressure, high, Diabetes and insulin resistance, Heart and circulatory health

See your doctor

Have a cholesterol test if you:

- have suffered any kind of stroke, have a heart problem or family history of early cardiovascular disease
- are overweight, have high blood pressure or diabetes
- have a family history of hypercholesterolemia, a genetic condition affecting about one in 500 people.

Quick fix If you smoke, quit. A substance in cigarette smoke called acrolein stops "good" HDL from transporting excess cholesterol back to the liver, encouraging a buildup of "bad" LDL cholesterol and consequent artery narrowing.

DID YOU KNOW?

Oats are full of cholesterol-lowering soluble fiber *(p. 184)*. A serving of cooked oats makes a good start to the day, supplying more than half the daily recommended amount; top it with a chopped banana to add even more soluble fiber.

CHRONIC PAIN

PAIN IS THE BODY'S WARNING SIGN THAT something is wrong and it should never be ignored. Treating the underlying ailment usually resolves pain, but ongoing pain can sometimes be an inevitable component of conditions such as osteoarthritis or cancer. In some cases, nerve pain may also persist long after an injury has healed. There are a number of natural solutions that can help reduce pain and lessen your intake of conventional painkillers and the unwanted side effects they can bring.

Suggested remedies

Acupuncture (p. 112) This works by stimulating nerves, muscles and connective tissue, boosting blood flow and activating natural pain-relieving endorphins. In one 2013 Japanese study, almost 90 percent of patients with neck pain found it effective.

TENS and electroacupuncture (p. 294) These hand-held devices can be used at home. They work by delivering small pulses of electrical current through pads applied to affected areas.

Massage (p. 230) Hands-on therapy may be particularly helpful for muscle, arthritic and back pain, though the effect is temporary. It brings respite and pleasure, helping sufferers to relax, according to a 2005 Swedish study.

Anti-inflammatories Herbs such as boswellia *(p. 136)*, butterbur *(p. 139)*, devil's claw *(p. 168)* or white willow bark *(p. 312)* may help.

Vitamin D (p. 305) Studies have shown that many people who suffer with chronic pain are deficient in vitamin D and that long-term supplementation with vitamin D can significantly improve chronic pain in some people.

Cognitive behavioral therapy (p. 159) Learning to control thought patterns helps people to manage many types of pain.

Music (p. 241) Guided listening to favorite music can relieve pain and anxiety, a recent US review of studies confirmed.

Hypnotherapy (p. 211) Hypnosis can help mask the perception of pain. In one example, an Italian woman allergic to anesthetics had a skin tumor removed under hypnosis and felt no pain at all.

Stretching (p. 286) A tailored program of stretches can help ease many types of chronic pain, including joint pain.

See your doctor

Your particular disorder will dictate which remedies to try. Discuss them with your doctor. If you find chronic pain hard to tolerate, ask for a referral to a pain specialist, or pain clinic; many offer both physical and mental therapies. Seek immediate help if pain suddenly worsens or if your pain makes you feel morbidly depressed.

Quick fix Watch a funny film. Laughter *(p. 218)* helps you relax, enhancing your brain's responsiveness to the body's natural pain relievers—endorphins. In one US study, children who saw a funny video tolerated pain much better; other research suggests this works for adults, too.

See also Back and neck pain, Cancer support, Menstrual problems, Migraines, Neuralgia, Osteoarthritis, Rheumatoid arthritis, Shingles

CELIAC DISEASE

AFFECTING AROUND ONE IN A HUNDRED people, celiac disease does not always cause symptoms. This inherited autoimmune disorder is triggered by an intolerance to gluten, a protein in wheat, rye and barley. It can cause painful inflammation in the lining of the small intestine, preventing nutrients from being digested and absorbed, eventually leading to weight loss and symptoms resulting from nutritional deficiencies. Other symptoms include bloating, constipation and diarrhea. Though it cannot be cured, following a gluten-free diet should control it and bring considerable relief within weeks.

Suggested remedies

Supplements Once diagnosed, medical tests may reveal nutrient deficiencies. You may initially require supplements, which you should take as prescribed (see **calcium**, *p. 140;* **iron**, *p. 214;* **folic acid**, *p. 189;* **vitamin B_{12}**, *p. 303;* **vitamin D**, *p. 305;* **vitamin K**, *p. 308;* and **zinc**, *p. 319).*

Dietary measures You will need to follow a **gluten-free diet** *(p. 198).* Don't be dismayed by all the foods you must avoid such as bread, pasta, cereals, cakes, pies and sauces. The gluten-free food market is rapidly expanding with an increasing number of substitute products. Naturally gluten-free foods include fruit and vegetables, meat and fish, rice and most dairy products.

Probiotics (p. 261) If you enjoy probiotic dairy foods, look out for those that contain bifidobacterium strains. Early research suggests that the "friendly bacteria" may help to heal gut damage caused by celiac disease.

Aloe vera (p. 261) If you have developed dermatitis herpetiformis, a rash that can be caused by gluten intolerance, creams or gels containing aloe vera may help to relieve the itching.

Quick fix The first essential step is to remove gluten from your diet. This means no wheat, rye and barley. You may also want to avoid oats, which contain no gluten but may be contaminated by contact with other cereals. The Celiac Disease Foundation website (www.celiac.org) has a wealth of information and resources including a downloadable gluten-free marketplace smart phone app.

See also Food intolerances, Inflammatory bowel disease, Irritable bowel syndrome

See your doctor

To avoid severe vitamin and mineral deficiencies, an early diagnosis is crucial. So if you suspect that you may have celiac disease arrange to see your doctor without delay. Your doctor is likely to order a blood test and may arrange for a small bowel biopsy to confirm the disease. You may be referred to a dietitian to help you plan a healthy gluten-free diet.

WATCH OUT!

Celiac disease is a serious disorder, which requires a professional medical diagnosis. Talk with your doctor before you consider trying any unorthodox testing, such as Vega testing, iridology or hair analysis, which may produce misleading results and lead to ineffective treatment.

COLDS AND FLU

A SORE THROAT, RUNNY NOSE AND general sense of feeling unwell all signal the start of a cold, the world's most common infection. A flu virus, which attacks the respiratory system, can be more dangerous, particularly for the very young and very old. Flu is usually accompanied by fever and can produce chills, sweats and muscular aches. In both cases, natural treatments can be as helpful as medication for reducing symptoms. Some of the remedies may have a preventive action, too.

Suggested remedies

Dietary measures Drink plenty of liquids to replace sweat and also moisture lost through your nose (see Hydration, *p. 209*). Several studies show Chicken soup *(p. 150)* can help reduce cold symptoms. You might also look for probiotics *(p. 261)* that contain both lactobacillus and bifidobacterium strains; research suggests they help prevent colds and reduce their duration.

Cough tea Boil a wedge of lemon *(p. 220)* with some grated garlic *(p. 191)* and ginger *(p. 192)*. Then add herbs such as echinacea *(p. 169)*, thyme and holy basil *(p. 205)*. When cooled, add a spoonful or so of manuka honey *(p. 228)* to taste. This antimicrobial tea will help to soothe a sore throat that comes from coughing and aid your immune system in fighting off infection.

Zinc (p. 319) Zinc lozenges ease sore throats and coughs, while supplements reduce the duration of colds, and help prevent colds and flu in elderly people who are often zinc deficient.

Ginseng (p. 194) American ginseng helps prevent colds and may protect against flu in elderly people.

Vitamin C (p. 304) Taking high doses of vitamin C throughout the winter can help reduce the duration and severity of colds and may be particularly effective for athletes in training.

Eucalyptus (p. 173) In cough lozenges and vapor rubs, this herb eases cold symptoms and its essential oil makes an effective steam inhalation. Other helpful essential oils for inhalations include tea tree *(p. 293)*, peppermint *(p. 255)*, rosemary *(p. 272)* and marjoram.

Elder (p. 170) Elderflower tea and elderberries have been shown to be helpful against respiratory illnesses.

See your doctor

Consult a doctor if you:

- ❖ have breathing problems
- ❖ suffer chest pains
- ❖ cough up blood
- ❖ experience severe swelling of glands in your neck or armpit.

Quick fix Rest is the best cure for a cold or a fever, so don't try to soldier on. Try andrographis *(p. 119)*, which reputedly curtailed the 1919 flu epidemic in India. The powerful herb prevents and treats the common cold. Another proven remedy is astragalus *(p. 125)*, which has been a stalwart of traditional Chinese medicine for over 2,000 years.

See also Asthma, Bronchitis, Fever, Sinusitis

CONCENTRATION, IMPROVED

ATTENTION DEFICIT HYPERACTIVITY DISORDER (ADHD), dementia, low blood glucose, menopause or depression can cause poor concentration. Muddled thinking can also be the result of head trauma or intoxication, or may just be a sign of old age. In our modern, fast-paced world, multitasking is concentration's biggest foe. Slow down and follow some of these strategies to bring your thoughts into clearer focus.

Suggested remedies

Lifestyle factors Keep track of hours spent on the computer. A Swedish study found unrestrained time on the web–pathological Internet use (PIU)–is associated with increased symptoms of ADHD, especially in men.

Dietary measures Never skip breakfast. Studies show that breakfast eaters score higher on visual searches, accuracy and reaction time. A diet that keeps your blood glucose levels steady throughout the day is best for cognitive performance.

Ginkgo (p. 193) Placebo-controlled UK research found a 120 mg dose of standardized *Ginkgo biloba* extract quickened performance on tasks requiring attention.

Ginseng (p. 194) A small placebo-controlled Korean study found 4,500 mg of red ginseng a day for two weeks improved participants' reaction times and brain power.

Vitamin B_6 (p. 302) Make sure you're getting enough B_6. A Tufts University study linked low vitamin B_6 concentrations in the blood to decreased attention and ability to plan.

Sleep One night of sleep deprivation can reduce concentration on a visual tracking exercise by more than 40 percent. If sleep is eluding you, try some sleeping strategies *(p. 281)*.

Coffee (p. 158) Compounds in coffee (not just caffeine) stimulate the brain's innate antioxidant system, improving cognitive function and reducing age-related cognitive decline.

Dark chocolate (p. 167) Eating dark chocolate has been shown to improve cognitive function and increase driving accuracy and reduce collisions in clinical studies.

Meditation (p. 234) A month of meditation training has been shown to decrease reaction time and increase the ability to concentrate without exerting any extra effort.

See your doctor

Seek immediate medical attention if you have recently bumped your head. Visit your doctor if poor concentration is having a significant impact on your life.

Quick fix Sharpen your wits with a sniff of peppermint *(p 255)*. A randomized *International Journal of Neuroscience* study of 144 adults found the scent of peppermint enhanced memory, increased alertness and improved reaction times.

See also Dementia, Diabetes and insulin resistance, Memory problems, Menopausal symptoms

CONSTIPATION

NORMAL BOWEL MOVEMENTS VARY greatly between once a day or more for some people, to a few times a week for others. If yours become more infrequent than usual, the stools are hard, you're straining and also feel bloated, you are probably suffering from constipation. In most cases some simple lifestyle and dietary adjustments can solve the problem and keep you regular. There are some natural remedies that can help, too.

Suggested remedies

Lifestyle factors Get moving with some kind of exercise *(p. 175)*. Cycling, walking *(p. 309)* or simply climbing stairs all help. Exerting your heart and lungs speeds up your metabolism and stimulates the muscles that propel food through your intestine.

Dietary measures Modern food processing often removes fiber *(p. 184)*, the roughage that helps transport waste products out of the body. Try to include more fiber-rich foods in your diet such as fruit, flaxseed *(p. 188)*, whole grains *(p. 314)* and vegetables. The soluble fiber of oats, fruit and pulses may be especially helpful. Check the fiber content of breakfast cereals—bran cereals can have up to 20 times the fiber of highly processed cereals. When introducing extra fiber into your diet, do so gradually as too much too soon can cause bloating, gas, or make your bowels loose and uncomfortable. Make sure you get plenty of fluids, too: Drinking around 2 pints (1.2 L) of water a day helps roughage on its way (see Hydration, *p. 209*).

Psyllium (p. 264) Taken with water, the soluble fiber in psyllium husks swells to form a mucilaginous gel that helps transport waste matter through the intestine.

Glucomannan This fiber supplement, found in health food stores, expands in a similar way to psyllium, increasing stool bulk and the number of helpful gut bacteria. Follow label instructions.

Probiotics (p. 261) Taken alone or combined with prebiotics, these friendly bacteria are worth a try. In one UK study of several hundred women, eating yogurt containing *Bifidobacterium animalis* and the prebiotic fructo-oligosaccharide twice a day for two weeks increased the frequency of bowel movements and relieved straining and pain. Researchers have found probiotics equally effective for children and elderly people.

See your doctor

If a fiber-rich diet plus exercise does not help, see your doctor, who may advise tests to check for other disorders. Consult your doctor immediately if you notice blood in your stools. This could indicate bowel cancer, which is highly treatable if diagnosed early.

Quick fix Natural stimulant laxatives such as senna *(p. 279)* and cascara work quickly by making the bowel contract more often. But they should only be used in the short term as long-term use can cause serious health problems.

See also Hemorrhoids, Irritable bowel syndrome

CRAMPS, MUSCLE

THE SUDDEN SEARING PAIN OF A CRAMP in your calf or thigh, though intense, is usually quite disproportionate to its seriousness. The spasm tends to pass within seconds or minutes, though the area can remain tender for a few hours. You may have strained a muscle or the cause may be unknown; cramps often occur during pregnancy. They can be triggered by mineral deficiencies, dehydration (sometimes caused by diuretics), or by other medicines such as statins, which regulate high cholesterol. In most cases, natural strategies quickly bring relief.

Suggested remedies

***Stretching** (p. 286)* After a cramp in the leg, gently massage the area. Then, sit with your affected leg extended and pull the top of the foot toward you, or stand, keeping the leg straight, then bending the knee while breathing slowly and deeply. Regular stretching keeps muscles flexible; always stretch after exercise and drink plenty of water.

***Heat therapy/Cold therapy** (p. 204/p. 161)* Applying a hot pad or ice pack, or taking a warm bath may help to ease tight muscles.

Dietary measures To avoid mineral deficiencies that might be causing cramps, eat plenty of foods rich in potassium *(p. 260)*, calcium *(p. 140)* and magnesium *(p. 227)*.

Taking vitamin and mineral supplements may be helpful; discuss it with your doctor.

***Multivitamins** (p. 240)* Taking vitamin B complex can reduce the frequency of nocturnal cramps and may be safer than prescribed quinine for elderly people.

***Magnesium** (p. 227)* Magnesium lactate or citrate can help relieve cramps in pregnancy, according to a 2002 UK study.

Quick fix Cramps in the foot or calf can sometimes be relieved by pressing firmly on an acupressure *(p. 112)* point known as "bigger rushing," located on the top of the foot in the notch between the bones of the big toe and second toe. Pressing on this point can relieve headaches, too.

See your doctor

Get immediate advice if a cramp:

- ❖ lasts longer than 10 minutes and stretching does nothing to relieve it
- ❖ occurs after contact with a toxic substance, or when a cut has become infected
- ❖ disrupts sleep
- ❖ is associated with numbness or tingling.

See also Back and neck pain

CUTS AND SCRAPES

A COMMON FACT OF LIFE, CUTS AND SCRAPES can happen at any moment—from a sudden slip of a bread knife to a stumble on the curb. Most of these injuries won't require a trip to the doctor and can easily be handled at home with natural remedies that lessen discomfort and speed up the healing process.

Suggested remedies

Dietary measures Following a healthy diet rich in nutrients such as zinc *(p. 319)* and vitamin C *(p. 304)* will help your body to repair itself and fight infection.

Aloe vera *(p. 117)* The active compounds in aloe soothe inflammation, relieve pain and help to repair and regrow skin.

Calendula (p. 141) Creams containing calendula may stimulate tissue regrowth, prevent or relieve minor infections and encourage healing by triggering greater blood flow to wounds.

Echinacea (p. 169) A tincture with 15 percent pressed *Echinacea angustifolia* herb juice (not root) applied daily can help to hasten the healing of abrasions, ulcerations, boils, sores and cuts.

Lavender (p. 219) Add a few drops of lavender oil to almond or olive oil and use to swab wounds, making use of the herb's antimicrobial action.

Manuka honey (p. 228) Honey has been used for millennia in wound care due to its broad spectrum antimicrobial and anti-inflammatory activities. Medical-grade honey preparations are widely available for treating wounds.

Salt water (p. 275) A warm salt-water solution, with 1 teaspoon (5 ml) of table salt per 2 cups (500 ml) of water, can help irrigate the wound and keep it clean.

Tea tree (p. 293) Long hailed for its antibacterial healing properties, tea tree oil will keep cuts clean. Neat tea tree oil can cause irritation so dilute it first in a carrier oil.

Holy basil (p. 205) A unique combination of analgesic, anti-oxidant, anti-inflammatory and antimicrobial activity makes this herb particularly effective in dealing with minor wounds and assisting in healing. It can be taken as a tea and applied to the wound as a paste, made by crushing fresh leaves.

See your doctor

Visit a doctor or emergency room if the wound:

- is on your face
- is deep or bleeds heavily
- is numb
- has a jagged edge
- has debris embedded in it
- was sustained from an animal or human bite.

Quick fix If you need to stop minor bleeding, swabbing with witch hazel *(p. 315)* can help. The tannins in witch hazel help relieve minor skin irritation, reduce inflammation, repair the wound and repel bacteria.

DEMENTIA

AS WE AGE, SOME COGNITIVE DECLINE is normal, but a person has full-blown dementia when problems with thinking, learning and memory start to impact his or her daily functioning. Most cases of dementia can be attributed to Alzheimer's disease, but dementia is also linked to many other conditions such as Parkinson's, diabetes and heart disease. Luckily, there are several natural remedies that may help us stave off cognitive decline, if not prevent the worst of it.

Suggested remedies

Lifestyle factors Try to remain active with regular exercise *(p. 175)* that is within your limits. US research shows that brain-derived neurotrophic factor (BDNF), released during exercise, "fertilizes" your brain. BDNF adds new brain cells, speeds your reaction time and makes you feel happier. Just 30 minutes of exercise can increase your recall of faces and names.

Dietary measures Older people can sometimes neglect their diet. A healthy diet is important at any stage in life and the Mediterranean diet, in particular, may prevent cognitive decline or at least help slow the progression into Alzheimer's.

Cognitive challenge (p. 160) Engaging the brain in leisure activities such as reading, playing board games and playing musical instruments has been associated with a reduced risk of dementia. Social contact *(p. 283)* is important, too, so make time to see friends. In one dementia-prevention study, freestyle social dancing *(p. 165)* was found to reduce the risk of cognitive decline more than any other physical or mental activity.

Aromatherapy (p. 122) Soothe memory-stealing stress with lavender *(p. 219)* essential oil while lemon balm *(p. 221)* regulates the nervous system and treats anxiety. Together they ease depression that can lead to cognitive decline.

Vitamins Since vitamin B_{12} *(p. 303)* and folic acid *(p. 189)* are typically deficient in Alzheimer's patients, it might be worth taking supplements. Discuss it with your doctor.

Omega-3 fatty acids (p. 250) These essential fatty acids can reduce anxiety and improve cognitive function immediately.

Green tea Substances in tea boost mental acuity and a flavonoid in green tea is thought to fend off the development of amyloid plaques associated with Alzheimer's disease. (See Tea, *p. 292*.)

See your doctor

Check in with a doctor if:

- you have trouble with everyday tasks such as paying bills or driving
- your personality becomes flat and you lose interest in things you once loved
- you often use the wrong words without realizing it
- you become angry, striking out (sometimes due to hallucinations)
- you forget key details of your life history and find reading and writing very difficult.

Quick fix Having a purpose was found in a study from Rush Medical Center to guard against Alzheimer's. People with scores of 4.2 out of 5 on the purpose-of-life scale were about two and a half times more likely to remain free of Alzheimer's than people who scored a 3.

See also Anxiety, Concentration, improved, Depression, Memory problems

DEPRESSION

ACCORDING TO THE WORLD HEALTH ORGANIZATION (WHO), depression is the leading cause of disability worldwide. It can be mild and transient or severe and long lasting. Depressed people lose interest in normal activities and have problems with sleeping. They may become irritable, angry, tearful or withdrawn and may have trouble concentrating or making decisions. While depression requires medical attention, there are self-help remedies that can provide some relief.

Suggested remedies

Lifestyle factors Try to maintain good social contact *(p. 283)* with friends and family. WHO cites relationships as protective factors against the onset or recurrence of depression. Find a form of exercise *(p. 175)* you enjoy and do it regularly. Aerobic exercise releases brain chemicals that improve mood and relieve depression. Qigong *(p. 266)*, which acts on the body and mind, may also offer relief, while dancing *(p. 165)* is another activity that research is revealing to be a serious antidote to depression.

Dietary measures Following a healthy diet that keeps blood glucose levels steady is a good long-term strategy against depression. It might be worth taking supplements of omega-3 fatty acids *(p. 250)* and vitamin B_{12} *(p. 303)*. Taking omega-3s twice a day for 60 days has been linked with a 45 percent reduction in depression. Low blood levels of vitamin B_{12} are linked with higher depression scores. Try to reduce the use of alcohol, which can exacerbate depression. Dark chocolate *(p. 167)* may help lift mood.

Sleep Depression is associated with insomnia, while sleep improves mood. If sleep is eluding you, try some sleeping strategies *(p. 281)*.

SAMe (p. 276) This supplement may be as effective at treating depression as tricyclic antidepressants, according to research.

St. John's wort (p. 274) Numerous studies suggest St. John's wort may assist in mild to moderate depression.

Pet therapy (p. 257) US researchers found pets increase the "cuddle hormones" oxytocin and prolactin, and elevate mood.

Yoga (p. 316) Through diaphragmatic breathing (pranayama) and relaxation, this gentle form of exercise may help ease tension.

Cognitive behavioral therapy (p. 159) As effective yet longer lasting than medication, this talking therapy examines emotions, thoughts and behaviors that aggravate depression.

See your doctor

Depression always requires medical attention, especially intense sadness accompanied by feelings of helplessness or hopelessness, or trouble sleeping or eating. If you ever consider hurting yourself, call a help line, such as The Samaritans or Lifeline, or seek medical attention without delay.

Quick fix If you are feeling blue, try some brisk walking *(p. 309)* or other physical activity. One short burst of activity can relieve a depressed mood for several hours, just like taking an aspirin relieves a headache.

See also Menopausal symptoms, Seasonal affective disorder, Sleeping problems

DIABETES AND INSULIN RESISTANCE

AROUND 90 PERCENT OF PEOPLE WITH DIABETES have type 2, a chronic disease in which the body can no longer effectively use insulin, a hormone that regulates blood glucose. In prediabetes, or "insulin resistance," the body is showing signs of not being able to regulate blood glucose levels and glucose builds up in the blood instead of being absorbed by the cells. Insulin resistance is also a key symptom of "metabolic syndrome" a combination of disorders that may include raised blood pressure, obesity and high cholesterol.

Many people are unaware that they have high blood glucose, a condition that is silently damaging their organs and body systems, before progressing into full-fledged diabetes. If it is not managed well, diabetes can lead to heart disease, stroke, kidney failure, impotence, limb amputations and blindness.

Key defense strategies

The good news is that most cases of insulin resistance and type 2 diabetes can be prevented or improved with simple lifestyle changes. A Harvard study found that quitting smoking, losing 5 percent of your body weight every two years (if overweight/obese), participating in some form of **exercise** *(p. 175)* for at least 30 minutes a day, eating a healthy diet, with fewer than three servings a week of red meat and at least two servings a day of **whole grains** *(p. 313)*, drinking two or more cups of **coffee** *(p. 158)* a day, drinking a small amount of alcohol a day, and drinking less than one fizzy drink a week, more than halved the risk of diabetes for middle-aged women.

An Italian study published in *Diabetologia* found that people who combined low-glycemic index principles (restricting refined sugars and grains, eating more vegetables, fruit, nuts and legumes) as part of a Mediterranean-style diet were 20 percent less likely to develop diabetes than people who did not follow either of those eating strategies.

A study in the *New England Journal of Medicine* showed those with diabetes who ate about 2 ounces (50 g) of **fiber** *(p. 184)* a day—especially from fruit and vegetables—were able to control their blood glucose better than those who ate less. Taking **psyllium** *(p. 264)* can help you to increase your daily consumption of soluble fiber. Some studies have also shown that intermittent fasting may offer some protection against developing diabetes. Fasting for two non-consecutive days per week may slow progression to diabetes, while lowering blood pressure and cholesterol.

See your doctor

If either insulin or blood glucose is not controlled well, diabetes can be life-threatening and you must seek help.

When insulin is too high, blood glucose plummets, and can cause insulin shock, characterized by:

- a fast pulse
- headache
- numbness in extremities
- pasty, sweaty, pale skin
- trembling and weakness.

When insulin is too low, high blood glucose can trigger a diabetic coma. There may be:

- confusion
- drowsiness
- faint, rapid pulse
- nausea
- warm, dry, flushed skin
- wobbly walk
- eventual fainting.

Suggested remedies

Chromium (p. 154) A mineral found in whole grains, lean meats, cheese, black pepper and thyme, chromium may help lower blood glucose in people with diabetes.

Cinnamon (p. 155) A placebo-controlled study of people with diabetes found about 1 teaspoon (6 g) of cinnamon a day for 40 days reduced fasting blood glucose by 29 percent, triglycerides by 30 percent, LDL ("bad") cholesterol by 27 percent and total cholesterol by 26 percent. Even taking as little as 1/4 teaspoon (1 g) per day made a difference.

Fenugreek (p. 182) Studies have shown that fenugreek seed extract can decrease blood glucose and cholesterol levels in people with diabetes.

Bitter melon (p. 132) This fruit is a traditional remedy that can suppress the appetite and may help to reduce blood glucose levels.

Gymnema sylvestre *(p. 202)* Known as the "sugar destroyer" in Hindi, the leaves of this traditional Ayurvedic remedy plant, when chewed, block the taste of sweetness and stimulate the body to produce more of its own insulin.

Holy basil (p. 205) Research has shown that regular consumption of holy basil not only helps glucose control but also improves other aspects of metabolic syndrome including cholesterol and blood pressure. It can be taken as a tea or used to flavor food.

Magnesium (p. 227) Magnesium plays an important role in metabolizing glucose. Increasing your intake of magnesium by 100 mg/day could decrease your risk of diabetes by 15 percent.

Omega-3 fatty acids (p. 250) Omega-3s can lower high triglycerides and raise "good" HDL cholesterol, reversing common afflictions in diabetes.

Coffee (p. 158) Regular coffee intake has an inverse association with the risk of type 2 diabetes. Coffee's phytochemicals may keep blood vessel linings healthy, improve circulation and glucose metabolism, and block oxidative stress and inflammation.

Vitamin D (p. 305) People with higher levels of vitamin D may be less likely to develop (or die from) diabetes-related heart disease or kidney disease.

Apple cider vinegar (p. 120) Like other vinegars, apple cider vinegar may help lower blood glucose and so may be of benefit to people with type 2 diabetes.

Quick fix What is the fastest way to balance blood glucose? Exercise *(p. 175)* after meals. Exercise allows your muscles to take up more glucose, leaving less in the blood. A US study found a 15-minute walk 30 minutes after each meal lowered blood glucose more effectively than a single 45-minute walk midday.

DID YOU KNOW?
Early diagnosis and careful blood glucose monitoring may reduce the risk of eye or kidney disease, nerve problems, heart disease or stroke. Be sure your annual health checkup includes a blood test for fasting blood glucose. If you are even borderline high, redouble your lifestyle strategies, then request an HbA1c test at your following checkup, to see a more accurate picture of your blood glucose levels over time.

See also Cholesterol, high, Heart and circulatory health, Overweight and obesity, Stroke prevention

DIARRHEA

THE MOST COMMON CAUSES of diarrhea are bacterial, viral or parasitic infections. It may also be a symptom of irritable bowel syndrome, food intolerances, other digestive or intestinal problems, or a side effect of taking antibiotics. Where there is no underlying disorder, diarrhea usually clears up in a few days. Natural strategies can help prevent it recurring, relieve symptoms and get your system back to normal.

Scrupulous hygiene stops diarrhea infections from spreading. Wash hands before handling food and after visiting the toilet; disinfect the toilet after use. If there's infection in the home, don't share towels or utensils. When traveling in a country where hygiene is poor, drink bottled water and avoid raw foods such as salad that could be contaminated.

Suggested remedies

Hydration *(p. 209)* Diarrhea can leave you dangerously dehydrated with reduced levels of electrolytes (sodium, potassium and chloride). Sip constantly on homemade or proprietary rehydration drinks and water to ensure the regular passing of clear or pale straw-colored urine.

Calming teas Sipping mild herbal teas such as chamomile with honey added to taste helps to maintain hydration and may help to ease cramping.

Probiotics *(p. 261)* By encouraging high levels of helpful gut bacteria, active culture yogurts can help you recover faster and protect against future infections. If diarrhea is the result of taking antibiotics, which can wipe out good microbes along with the bad, probiotics can replace them.

Bovine colostrum *(p. 137)* Colostrum from cows may protect against various forms of diarrhea, in particular infectious traveler's diarrhea.

See also Celiac disease, Food intolerances, Gastroenteritis, Irritable bowel syndrome

See your doctor

Infants, elderly people and those with weakened immunity should see a doctor if:

- there is severe pain
- they appear dehydrated (sunken eyes, dry mouth, listless, passing little or concentrated urine)
- they are unable to drink or keep down fluids
- there is blood in the feces
- there is both diarrhea and vomiting
- the condition does not improve after a day.

Otherwise healthy adults should see a doctor if symptoms are very severe, last more than a few days or there is:

- blood or pus in the feces
- persistent vomiting
- high fever.

Quick fix More usually prescribed for constipation, psyllium *(p. 264)* can be a useful remedy for diarrhea by absorbing fluid in the digestive tract, slowing the passage of stools and making them firmer.

ECZEMA AND DERMATITIS

THE TWO MOST COMMON TYPES OF eczema are atopic and contact dermatitis, both characterized by itchy, inflamed patches of skin and sometimes scaling and cracking. While atopic eczema usually starts in infancy, often in people with a family history of allergies and asthma, contact dermatitis is a reaction to an irritating substance. Recognizing and avoiding an eczema trigger is key—whether it is a food, detergent or other substance. Natural remedies can help reduce rashes and swelling, and tackle allergies and irritants.

Suggested remedies

Dietary measures Following an elimination diet *(p. 171)* may help you to identify if there are foods that trigger your eczema. Probiotics *(p. 261)* may reduce the severity of symptoms in children, according to recent Korean research.

Emollients To keep your skin moist and protected against infection, you will need emollient soap substitutes, creams and lotions. Look for products that contain calendula *(p. 141)*, chamomile *(p. 147)* or chickweed *(p. 151)*.

Compress (p. 163) A strong tea of chamomile and calendula with a few drops of lavender oil applied as a cool compress can give symptomatic relief.

St. John's wort (p. 274) For mild to moderate atopic dermatitis, a St. John's wort preparation may help. In one German study, 21 patients used the cream and a placebo for a month to compare results. The St. John's wort cream was greatly superior, reducing inflammation and bacterial infection.

Vitamin B_{12} (p. 303) B_{12} creams work by reducing levels of nitric oxide, which plays a role in the immune response and inflammation. A 2004 study suggests they can reduce the extent and severity of dermatitis in both adults and children.

Evening primrose (p. 174) Research suggests that topical preparations containing gamma-linolenic acid (GLA), the oil in evening primrose and borage *(p. 135)*, may be effective. In one study of 32 Japanese children with dermatitis, those who wore undershirts coated in borage oil for two weeks had significantly less redness and itching.

Light therapy (p. 223) Harnessing the therapeutic effects of ultraviolet (UV) rays, specialists sometimes treat dermatitis with light therapy, which can also prevent the bacterial infections that often accompany the problem.

See your doctor

A doctor can diagnose the problem and prescribe a treatment if eczema becomes infected. Seek specialist help if you can't identify the cause, or if natural treatments don't help.

Quick fix Take a vacation. Sunshine, especially seaside sunshine, can be surprisingly effective for mild to moderate atopic dermatitis and may make it temporarily disappear.

DID YOU KNOW?

Some suspect that substances in infant formula trigger atopic dermatitis. In a study of more than 17,000 women in Belarus, the incidence of eczema in children who were breastfed was half that of those who had been given infant formula.

See also Allergies, Psoriasis, Skin rashes

EYE DISORDERS

FROM THE ITCHY DISCOMFORT OF DRY eyes to vision-robbing conditions such as diabetic retinopathy, glaucoma, cataracts and age-related macular degeneration (AMD), many eye disorders become more of a concern with age. To protect your eyesight, it's important to see an eye doctor for regular vision and eye-health exams. That said, research shows that adding well-chosen natural remedies helps lower the risk for some eye conditions and may help ease symptoms of others such as dry eyes.

Suggested remedies

Lifestyle factors You may need to shed excess weight. Extra weight can double the pace of AMD progression and increase cataract risk by 36 percent. Make sure you incorporate exercise *(p. 175)* into your day. A regular briskly paced routine can cut the risk for advanced AMD by 25 percent, University of Wisconsin scientists say. It can also reduce eye pressure in glaucoma.

Dietary measures Increase your intake of foods containing lutein and zeaxanthin *(p. 225)*. These antioxidants concentrate in the yellow spot of the retina (the macula) where most light is focused. Damage to this area causes the loss of central vision that occurs with AMD. Regular consumption of oily fish and the omega-3 fatty acids they contain *(p. 250)* has been shown to significantly lower the risk for dry eyes and AMD.

Nuts (p. 247) Eating more nuts and keeping your blood glucose levels steady may help to stem the progression of existing AMD.

Relaxation (p. 269) A good add-on for glaucoma, relaxation techniques may help lower vision-threatening eye pressure, according to German research.

Multivitamins (p. 240) If you already have AMD, a specially formulated AMD supplement could cut the risk of further vision loss by 33 percent. It contains vitamin E *(p. 307)* and vitamin C, also shown to protect against cataracts. Supplements containing lutein, zeaxanthin and omega-3 fatty acids may also be helpful.

Sunglasses and a sun hat Protecting your eyes from the sun's damaging ultraviolet rays can slow the development of cataracts according to the US National Eye Institute. Wraparounds also block out wind and dry air, keeping dry eyes more comfortable.

See your doctor

Get emergency help for sudden blindness, double vision, low or distorted vision (especially if your eyes are red or painful). Call your doctor for an eye exam if you experience:

- difficulty with night vision
- trouble seeing colors
- blurriness
- itchy eyes
- discharge.

Quick fix To soothe dry eyes, apply a warm compress *(p. 163)* made from tea bags containing chamomile or regular tea. This will loosen blockages in glands on your eyelids that add moisturizing oils to the tears that bathe your eyes. A cup of coffee *(p. 158)* or tea *(p. 292)* may help as both beverages increase tear production in the eyes within hours.

EYE INFECTIONS

COMMON EYE INFECTIONS INCLUDE STYES (inflamed oil glands at the edge of your eyelid), conjunctivitis (or "pink eye" caused by bacteria, viruses, allergies or chemical exposure) and blepharitis (irritated, itchy eyelids). Natural remedies may help soothe affected eyes and help prevent a recurrence. If the infection or irritation is mild, home treatment may be enough. For more serious infections, your doctor may prescribe medication, such as antibiotic creams, drops or pills, and may suggest an eyelid scrub for blepharitis.

While you have an eye infection, skip contact lenses and eye makeup and protect your eyes from dust and bright light with sunglasses and/or an eye patch. Conjunctivitis can be highly contagious. Wash your hands after touching your eyes, don't share towels with others and follow your doctor's advice about staying home from work or school.

Suggested remedies

Lifestyle factors Take steps to boost your immune system through a healthy diet, exercise *(p. 175)* and other lifestyle changes. A weak immune system can make eye infections more severe and difficult to treat, say US vision experts.

Eyelid massage Recommended by the US National Institutes of Health for people with "posterior blepharitis" that affects the inner surface of the eyelid, a careful massaging of the eyelids helps to clean out clogged oil glands.

Preservative-free saline eye drops Available in most pharmacies, these simple eye drops soothe irritation caused by pink eye in children according to US natural health expert and pediatrician William Sears, MD. They work for adults, too.

Acupuncture (p. 112) Practitioners of this form of traditional Chinese medicine report that acupuncture may reduce the recurrence of styes and other eye infections.

Quick fix Recommended by the American Optometric Association, a warm compress *(p. 163)* helps soothe the pain and discomfort of blepharitis, styes and bacterial conjunctivitis. Use a cold compress for viral or allergic conjunctivitis. Tea bags containing cooled chamomile or regular black tea can be used for this purpose.

See also Frequent illness

See your doctor

Call your doctor if:

- symptoms last more than a day
- you have eye pain
- your vision changes
- there is a yellow or greenish discharge from the eye
- you become extremely sensitive to light.

WATCH OUT!

Don't try to remove an object that's large or embedded in your eye–seek medical help. For smaller things–such as an eyelash or a speck of dirt–first clean around the eye with a clean, wet cloth to remove other particles. Then gently wash the surface of the eye with sterile saline solution. Make sure your hands are clean when touching your eye to avoid introducing infection.

FALL PREVENTION

EVERY YEAR, ONE IN THREE PEOPLE over the age of 65 has a fall. These stumbles send millions to the hospital and are a leading cause of broken bones including hip fractures—a serious injury that can steal independence and even shorten a person's life span.

The good news? At-home strategies—from clearing clutter to simple balance and strength exercises—offer significant protection from trips and falls.

Suggested remedies

Lifestyle factors After making your home safe (see Quick fix) try to remain active and take up a form of exercise *(p. 175)* you enjoy. A routine that builds balance and strength is best. In a 2007 German study, a regular exercise program reduced fall risk by 23 percent. Walking *(p. 309)* is a good low-impact option.

Minerals Thinning bones boost the risk for falls and fractures. A daily supplement containing 1,000 mg of calcium *(p. 140)* and 400 IU of vitamin D *(p. 305)* reduced falls by 12 percent in a 2005 study by Denmark's Aarhus University Hospital. Foods rich in magnesium *(p. 227)* and vitamin K *(p. 308)* keep bones strong. Getting at least 110 mcg of vitamin K daily lowered fracture risk by 30 percent in one large Harvard School of Public Health study.

Tai chi (p. 290) The gentle, graceful movements of this ancient Chinese exercise routine cut stumble risk by 55 percent in a 2005 study of 256 people from the Oregon Research Institute. The related exercise form called qigong *(p. 266)* may also be beneficial.

Feldenkrais Method (p. 180) Bodywork therapies such as Feldenkrais teach you how to move correctly, improving your balance and so lessening the risk of a fall.

Quick fix Most falls happen at home; simple measures can cut the risk by 61 percent says a 2005 study of 391 people from New Zealand's Otago Medical School. Keep floors and stairs free of clutter; remove throw rugs; use nonslip mats in the bath, shower and on the bathroom floor; add grab bars in the bathroom and handrails on stairs; improve lighting and ensure outside paths are kept clear and well lit. Repair or clearly mark any uneven or cracked paths or other potential trip hazards.

See also Osteoporosis

See your doctor

Get help right away if you've fallen and injured yourself (a good reason to keep your mobile phone in your pocket and invest in an emergency alert service). If you feel unsteady on your feet, talk with your doctor. Some medications (including some antidepressants and anti-anxiety drugs) can cause dizziness and drowsiness. Get regular vision checks, too.

DID YOU KNOW?

Well-fitting shoes may lessen the likelihood of a stumble. In contrast, high heels and shoes with thick rubber soles may boost the risk, says the World Health Organization. Add a "traction aid" for extra grip on snow or ice; these devices attach to the soles of your shoes and may lower the risk of a fall outdoors by as much as 60 percent, according to one study.

FATIGUE

FEELING WEARY? MOST TIREDNESS IS CAUSED by factors within your control such as sleep or your diet. Natural remedies can reverse this garden-variety fatigue. However, persistent tiredness could be a medication side effect or a symptom of a more serious health condition (such as chronic fatigue syndrome, diabetes, anemia or depression) and should be investigated by your doctor.

Suggested remedies

Lifestyle factors Try to do at least some exercise *(p. 175)* every day. Regular, mild activity reduced fatigue by 65 percent in a small US study of people who frequently felt tired. Try to get eight hours of sleep a night, too. Sleeping strategies *(p. 281)* may help.

Dietary measures Eat regular meals (starting with breakfast). Drink plenty of water (see Hydration, *p. 209*), as even slight dehydration can cause mental fatigue, says a 2013 US study. You are drinking enough if you pass clear or pale straw-colored urine several times each day.

Holy basil (p. 205) Considered by many naturopaths to be the ultimate adaptogen herb, holy basil has been shown to increase physical stamina, boost mental clarity and reduce feelings of exhaustion and stress.

Coffee (p. 158) Caffeine blocks the sleep-inducing brain chemical adenosine. Sip a cup slowly through the morning and early afternoon for maximum alertness, says a 2008 study from Boston's Brigham and Women's Hospital. Don't overdo it, though, as you may find it hard to sleep later on.

Green tea In a Dutch study, L-theanine in green tea boosted alpha brain waves (associated with relaxed alertness). (See Tea, *p. 292.*)

Magnesium (p. 227) This mineral supports energy production in cells. It may ease the tiredness of chronic fatigue syndrome, 2001 UK research review says.

Dark chocolate (p. 167) Consumption of dark chocolate has been shown to enhance exercise capacity, delay fatigue and improve brain function and arousal.

Iron (p. 214) A daily, 80 mg supplement reduced fatigue by 48 percent for women with low iron levels in a French study.

Ginseng (p. 194) American ginseng *(Panax quinquefolius)* lifted fatigue in cancer patients in a recent Mayo Clinic study.

See your doctor

Seek immediate help if you also:

- feel confused or dizzy
- have blurred vision
- cannot urinate
- have abnormal bleeding
- have severe pain.

Otherwise, see your doctor in two weeks if natural remedies don't help.

Quick fix A short snooze boosted alertness and reduced sleepiness in a ground-breaking 1995 NASA study of long-haul airline pilots. After a nap, splash your face with cold water or stand in bright sunlight for a minute for even more energy, Japanese researchers suggest.

WATCH OUT!

Skip the energy drinks. Often laced with herbal stimulants and up to five times more caffeine than a can of cola, these drinks were associated with kidney failure, seizures, high blood pressure, heart attacks and even death in a 2011 University of Miami study.

See also Anemia, Chronic pain, Depression, Menopausal symptoms

FEVER

A FEVER IS PART OF THE HUMAN BODY'S natural defenses against infection, helping to fight off invading bacteria and viruses. Most of the time children and adults with a mild to moderate fever will stay safe and comfortable with home remedies (including plenty of fluids).

Suggested remedies

Dietary measures Keep a check on hydration *(p. 209)* during a fever. Children who refuse fluids can be tempted with watermelon, grapes or ice blocks made with frozen juice, which will all help to replace fluids. If you often catch colds and flu, you may need to look closely at your diet and lifestyle with the aim of boosting your immunity (see Frequent illness, *p. 55*).

Andrographis *(p. 119)* In a 2010 study from India's King George Medical University, when *Andrographis paniculata* was given to people with upper respiratory tract infections, it reduced fever and other symptoms longer than a placebo.

Holy basil *(p. 205)* As an adaptogen herb, holy basil boosts the immune system and has broad-spectrum antimicrobial activity against viruses, bacteria and fungi. It can be taken as a tea, hot or cold, to replenish fluids and assist the body to fight off infection.

Echinacea *(p. 169)* Some natural healers recommend this popular herb to cool mild fevers below 100°F (37.8°C).

Elder *(p. 170)* Black elderberry *(Sambucus nigra)* extracts have eased flu symptoms, including fever, in several studies.

Onion or garlic foot poultice Onion poultices were adopted by early American settlers from Native Americans including the Cherokee. Similarly, crushed garlic applied to the feet can be effective and tasted in the mouth shortly after application. Garlic can be an irritant to tender feet if left on for too long and care should be taken not to apply garlic directly to the soft feet of infants (see Compresses and poultices, *p. 163*).

See also Colds and flu, Frequent illness

See your doctor

Call emergency services if a fever is associated with confusion, difficulty breathing or signs of bacterial meningitis, which may include a bad headache, stiff neck or bruise-like rash.

Call a doctor if the fever:

- is over 102.2°F(39°C)
- lasts more than 48 hours
- is associated with dehydration such as low urine output, listlessness or difficulty drinking or retaining fluids.

Quick fix For every 1.8°F (1°C) rise in body temperature, sip at least an extra ½ cup (125 ml) of water per day. A high fever, especially with vomiting or diarrhea, could deplete electrolytes—minerals that regulate body chemistry. Juice, broth or rehydration drinks given directly or frozen and sucked as ice blocks can help.

FLATULENCE

THE AVERAGE ADULT PASSES GAS 13 TO 21 times per day. Tough-to-digest foods, air swallowing and food intolerances can increase the number of embarrassing and inconvenient "personal emissions" you experience. Natural remedies and dietary changes can reduce or eliminate many causes of excess gas. Start by eating more slowly so that you swallow less air with each bite.

Suggested remedies

***Low-FODMAP diet** (p. 224)* This eating strategy has been proven to ease flatulence and other symptoms of irritable bowel syndrome, according to researchers at Australia's Monash University. It works by restricting FODMAPs—foods that contain these poorly absorbed carbohydrates: fermentable oligosaccharides, disaccharides, monosaccharides and polyols.

***Fiber** (p. 184)* Increasing dietary fiber may help, yet it should be increased slowly over a few weeks to prevent increased gas production and bloating. If excess gas remains a problem, changing the type of fiber you are taking may provide a solution.

***Carminative herbs** (p. 142)* Fennel *(Foeniculum vulgare)*, dill *(Anethum graveolens)*, anise *(Pimpinella anisum)* and caraway *(Carum carvi)* seeds hold a special place in botanical medicine as digestion-promoting herbs that ease flatulence. Crunch a handful after a meal or take them in teas.

***Globe artichoke** (p. 195)* People with digestive complaints who took an extract of globe artichoke leaves for six weeks enjoyed a 68 percent reduction in flatulence.

***Probiotics** (p. 261)* In supplements and in foods like live yogurt and kefir, "friendly bacteria" may reduce flatulence by replacing gas-producing bacteria in the digestive system. In a 2005 Mayo Clinic study of 48 people, those who took a probiotic supplement for four weeks reduced flatulence by half.

See also Celiac disease, Irritable bowel syndrome

See your doctor

Contact your doctor if you also experience:

- stomach or rectal pain
- heartburn
- nausea or vomiting
- diarrhea or constipation
- weight loss
- oily, foul-smelling or bloody stools.

Quick fix Do you love foods like beans, cabbage and onions, but loathe the explosive aftermath? Start your meal with a few drops of alpha-galactosidase. This enzyme breaks down complex carbohydrates before gas-producing bacteria can digest them. In a small Italian study, the supplement significantly reduced flatulence in people who consumed a large serving of beans. (See Enzymes, *p. 172.*)

WATCH OUT!

Artificial sweeteners such as sorbitol, xylitol, mannitol and maltitol are partially digested by gas-producing bacteria in the gut. Overindulging can cause bloating and increase embarrassing emissions.

FOOD INTOLERANCES

FOOD SENSITIVITIES ARE GAINING new recognition. About one in eight adults cannot digest lactose, the natural sugar in dairy products, and up to eight in 100 may have a sensitivity to gluten, a compound in many grains. Still others are sensitive to food additives or to naturally occurring salicylates and amines in foods.

Food intolerances are not the same as food allergies. An intolerance usually develops gradually, may cause symptoms only if you eat a lot of the offending food and isn't life-threatening. (In contrast, a food allergy triggers a fast reaction every time you eat even a tiny amount of a food and can be life threatening.) Symptoms of food intolerance can include diarrhea, nausea, vomiting, cramps and bloating, heartburn, headaches and irritability. Natural approaches can help you pinpoint, avoid and minimize food culprits.

Suggested remedies

Journaling *(p. 215)* Wondering what's causing your symptoms? Find clues by keeping a food diary; list what you eat and when, along with details of any discomfort you experience afterward.

Elimination diet *(p. 171)* Once you've narrowed down suspected culprits, try removing them from your diet for two weeks. Then add them back, one at a time. If you react, the food is likely a trigger for you. Common triggers include wheat, dairy, citrus and food additives such as colorings, preservatives and monosodium glutamate (MSG).

Dietary measures Once you have identified your trigger foods, steer clear of them while continuing to eat a healthy diet that includes plenty of foods that are rich in antioxidants, such as green vegetables and berries, and minimal processed foods or foods high in sugar, fat and salt. If you are lactose intolerant, probiotics *(p. 261)* may help. In one Italian study, people with lactose intolerance who took a probiotic supplement of *Lactobacillus reuteri* showed signs of better lactose digestion.

Bromelain This pineapple-derived enzyme may aid digestion. Some alternative medicine practitioners recommend it to help ease reactions if you have a food sensitivity. (See Enzymes, *p. 172*.)

Gluten-free diet *(p. 198)* If bread or other foods containing grains exacerbate your symptoms, you may need to exclude gluten from your diet. This isn't as difficult as it may seem.

See your doctor

Get immediate help if you're having trouble breathing, have swelling of your throat or tongue or have signs of shock after eating a food. You may be having a severe allergic reaction known as anaphylaxis. See your doctor if food reactions interfere with your quality of life.

Quick fix If you have trouble digesting dairy products, reach for lactose. This enzyme—taken before a meal or added to milk—breaks down the lactose in the milk for you, reducing or even eliminating digestive discomfort. (See Enzymes, *p. 172*.)

See also Allergies, Celiac's disease

FREQUENT ILLNESS

THE AVERAGE ADULT GETS TWO TO FOUR colds per year; millions contend with stomach flu annually. But if you're battling more than your fair share of coughs and sneezes or simply feel constantly run-down, your immune system may need a tune-up. Healthy lifestyle changes and natural remedies can often bolster natural defenses worn down by stress, lack of sleep and nutritional gaps.

Suggested remedies

Lifestyle factors Take steps to reduce stress. In a Spanish study of 1,149 people, those who felt the most stressed were twice as likely to catch colds. Try to take time for relaxation *(p. 269)*. Exercise *(p. 175)* helps, too. Physical activity activates virus-killing antibodies, according to US research.

Dietary measures Follow a healthy diet that includes plenty of fresh produce. A produce-packed diet boosted immune response to the pneumonia vaccine in a 2012 study from the UK. You may also need to consider including foods or supplements containing zinc *(p. 319)* and vitamin D *(p. 305)*. Try probiotics *(p. 261)*, too. Beneficial bacteria revved up respiratory-system immune cells, shortening colds by two days in a 2005 German study.

Holy basil (p. 205) As the ultimate adaptogen herb, holy basil tea can be taken two or three times daily to help the body cope with stress and provide a natural boost to the immune system.

Tai chi (p. 290) The ancient Chinese martial art doubled immune response to the shingles vaccine in a 2007 study of older adults.

Ashwagandha (p. 124) This traditional immune booster stimulated white blood cell activity in a recent US study.

Astragalus (p. 125) Saponins and polysaccharides in astragalus stimulate the body's immune cells, several studies show.

Medicinal mushrooms (p. 233) Compounds in reishi boost the activity of immune system cells, research shows.

Acupuncture (p. 112) This traditional modality enhances T-cells and white blood cell counts, says the US National Cancer Institute.

Laughter (p. 218) Watching a comedy video energized the body's infection-fighting cells in a 2001 study.

Echinacea (p. 169) This herb supports the immune system and, taken during winter, may boost resistance against colds and flu.

See your doctor

Visit your doctor if you have:

- a persistent fever
- painful congestion
- coughing
- trouble swallowing
- can't keep fluids down.

Check in if you continue to have frequent illnesses despite making healthy dietary and lifestyle changes.

Quick fix Getting fewer than seven hours of sleep per night can triple the risk for catching a cold, says a 2009 study from Carnegie Mellon University. If sleep eludes you, sleeping strategies *(p. 281)* may help.

See also Bronchitis, Colds and flu, Diarrhea, Fever, Nausea and vomiting, Sinusitis

FROZEN SHOULDER

PAIN AND STIFFNESS ARE THE MOST common symptoms of frozen shoulder, which affects up to 5 percent of the population, often women and usually people in their fifties and sixties. It occurs when tissue around the joint becomes thickened and inflamed, sometimes as a result of injury, a stroke or long periods of immobility. People with diabetes, heart, thyroid or lung disease are also more susceptible. Frozen shoulder starts with aching and pain when you reach upward and the joint becomes increasingly stiff. There are natural remedies that can help speed recovery.

Suggested remedies

Lifestyle factors Avoid slouching over a computer, which can place pressure on the shoulder, and try sleeping with a pillow between your sore arm and your body to keep your shoulder joint gently stretched.

Acupuncture and acupressure *(p. 112)* A number of Chinese studies claim that various forms of acupuncture bring relief, even in the earliest painful stage. A 2008 review of studies suggests that acupuncture treatment can offer some short-term benefits and that acupuncture plus exercise *(p. 175)* is helpful for up to five months. In one large recent Chinese study, acupoint massage was superior to both electroacupuncture and TENS (transcutaneous electrical nerve stimulation) for relieving frozen shoulder.

Bowen Technique *(p. 138)* This therapy is designed to stimulate and relax muscles and tendons. Although it has not been extensively researched, in one 2002 UK study review, 20 patients with frozen shoulder found it gentle, relaxing and helpful.

See also Back and neck pain, Bursitis and tendonitis

See your doctor

The first stage of frozen shoulder is often the most painful, while the second stage, when the shoulder becomes increasingly immobile, can be the most disabling. Early diagnosis may minimize its duration. You may need steroid injections and numbing medications. In a few cases, surgery is required.

Quick fix Applying an ice pack (see Cold therapy, *p. 161*) or a heat pad (see Heat therapy, *p. 204*) to your shoulder can reduce the early pain, as can a hot bath.

FUNGAL INFECTIONS

COMMON SITES OF FUNGAL INFECTIONS include feet, nails, mouth, groin, vagina and under pendulous breasts and bellies. Tinea infections cause athlete's foot, nail problems and ringworm, while candida infections are responsible for oral and vaginal thrush, and a certain type of diaper rash. Symptoms include irritation, redness, stinging, itching and sometimes a discharge and unpleasant odor. The infections usually respond well to antifungal treatments, including natural remedies.

Suggested remedies

Lifestyle factors If you have athlete's foot, wash your feet thoroughly, especially between the toes, dry well, use talcum powder to reduce sweating and change socks or tights frequently. To prevent fungal infections from spreading, don't share footwear or towels and avoid going barefoot in public changing rooms. Bleach-clean your bath or shower, and launder clothes and bedclothes regularly to remove fungus.

Dietary measures Fungal skin infections have been linked to uncontrolled diabetes, so it is important to keep your blood glucose under control by following a healthy diet. Some alternative therapists suggest avoiding simple sugars, yeast, alcohol and processed foods to combat candida infections. Practitioners also recommend probiotics *(p. 261)* to colonize the gut and vagina with "friendly bacteria." A recent Indian study suggests that several strains are effective against antibiotic-induced candida infections.

Garlic (p. 191) Eating a clove a day, or taking a garlic supplement, may help prevent candida infections. Garlic's antifungal properties are legendary: It is said that Romans on the march put cloves between their toes to prevent athlete's foot.

Propolis (p. 263) Created by bees from tree buds and sap, propolis has proven antifungal properties and combats oral thrush.

Essential oils Topical applications of tea tree *(p. 293)* and eucalyptus *(p. 173)* show some promise for fighting tinea infections; both have a proven antifungal activity.

See your doctor

Seek medical advice if:

❖ you've never had the problem before or get it repeatedly

❖ itching is severe

❖ the area is blistered

❖ the infection has spread.

Also seek medical advice if you have a fungal foot infection and diabetes or a suppressed immune system as it can quickly lead to unwanted secondary bacterial infections.

Quick fix Fungal infections don't clear instantly but tea tree oil *(p. 293)* acts (relatively) fast. In one Australian study, athlete's foot was cured within four weeks in nearly two-thirds of those using a 50 percent solution, compared to less than a third in the control group.

See also Diabetes and insulin resistance, Nail problems

GALL BLADDER PROBLEMS

LOCATED JUST BELOW THE LIVER, the gall bladder's main function is to store, concentrate and release bile, which helps to break down fats. Problems can arise if the constituents of bile, including cholesterol and calcium salts, thicken and bind together forming stones, which can block a duct, causing inflammation and pain, and lead to infection.

Risk factors include being overweight, or losing weight then regaining weight rapidly. A temporary blockage may cause only minor, occasional bouts of pain—often after eating fatty foods and usually felt below the right rib cage and radiating up to the shoulder. You will need the assistance of your doctor, though natural remedies may help prevent stones from forming and keep your gall bladder healthy.

Suggested remedies

Lifestyle factors Lose weight, if necessary, but do so gradually, getting plenty of exercise *(p. 175)*.

Dietary measures Fatty, sugary foods encourage the liver to produce excess cholesterol; replacing them with a low-fat, high-fiber diet will help prevent stones forming.

***Coffee** (p. 158)* In one US population study, men who drank several cups a day had a reduced risk of gall bladder problems.

***Turmeric** (p. 298)* Curcumin, the spice's active constituent, increases the production of bile and thins its consistency, which helps prevent the formation of stones.

***Milk thistle** (p. 238)* Extracts containing silymarin may help to thin bile and reduce its cholesterol content, according to Italian laboratory research.

See also Cholesterol, high

See your doctor

See your doctor immediately if you experience intense, lasting pain, a high temperature with chills, nausea or signs of jaundice (yellowing of the skin and eyes). An inflamed, blocked gall bladder could rupture. Troublesome gall bladders are usually removed, often by keyhole surgery, a procedure that appears to have no long-term consequences.

Quick fix Enteric-coated peppermint oil capsules may help dissolve small gallstones; research suggests peppermint *(p. 255)* and other essential oils have a beneficial effect.

GASTROENTERITIS

WHETHER THE CAUSE IS A VIRUS or contaminated food, gastroenteritis is painful and debilitating. Vomiting and diarrhea are common symptoms as the stomach lining becomes inflamed and the infection stops fluids from being absorbed from the intestines. Both symptoms can quickly lead to dehydration, so it is important to drink plenty of clear fluids. Most types of gastroenteritis are infectious so careful hygiene is essential to prevent its spread. Get plenty of bed rest and use a heating pad or hot-water bottle for stomach pain.

Suggested remedies

Hydration (p. 209) Sip constantly on homemade or proprietary rehydration drinks or water to ensure the regular passing of clear or pale straw-colored urine.

Calming teas Sipping mild herbal teas such as chamomile with honey added to taste helps to maintain hydration and may help to ease cramping.

Dietary measures When you start eating again, try bland foods such as toast, bananas, rice or chicken. Avoid dairy foods, caffeine, alcohol and fatty, spicy foods. When traveling, taking **probiotics** *(p. 261)* before and during a trip will help you maintain healthy gut bacteria to fight off potential infections.

Black raspberry (p. 134) Korean research shows that black raspberry may be highly effective at combating the norovirus, which causes 90 percent of infectious gastroenteritis outbreaks around the world.

Cinnamon (p. 155) This herbal remedy may help soothe and repair damage to the stomach lining, according to recent Korean laboratory research.

Meadowsweet (p. 232) An infusion of meadowsweet can effectively relieve the nausea and stomach acidity that usually accompanies bouts of gastroenteritis.

Milk thistle (p. 238) If gastroenteritis has been caused by fungal poisoning, milk thistle may be the best treatment.

Quick fix You may not be able to keep anything down, so try sucking on small chips of ice to replenish lost fluids. Clear broths and warm herbal teas may sometimes be better tolerated than sweet drinks. Avoid caffeinated drinks.

See your doctor

Infants, elderly people and those with weakened immunity should see a doctor if:

- there is severe pain
- they appear dehydrated (sunken eyes, dry mouth, listless, passing little or concentrated urine)
- the condition does not improve after a day.

Otherwise healthy adults should seek assistance if the symptoms are very severe or last more than a few days.

See also Diarrhea, Nausea and vomiting

WATCH OUT!

Infection can easily spread so disinfect the toilet area after bouts of diarrhea or vomiting. Wash hands after going to the toilet and before eating or preparing food. Clean chopping boards and surfaces regularly, keeping raw and cooked foods apart. Ensure foods are thoroughly cooked.

GOUT

GOUT STRIKES YOUR JOINTS WITH SUDDEN severe pain, redness and tenderness. Often felt at the base of the big toe, gout is a form of arthritis that erupts when too much uric acid accumulates in the blood. The uric acid leaks out of the blood and forms spiky crystals that jab at joints and soft tissue, triggering an inflammatory attack that can last up to 10 days. Natural remedies can help soothe or prevent these flare-ups.

Suggested remedies

Lifestyle factors Maintaining a healthy body weight by engaging in regular exercise *(p. 175)* and lowering your intake of dietary fats and avoiding sugary drinks can help prevent attacks. Sugar-sweetened soft drinks and fructose (including high fructose corn syrup) are strongly associated with an increased risk of gout in men as is alcohol consumption. Substitute plenty of water, which helps flush uric acid from the blood (see Hydration, *p. 209*).

Dietary measures Avoid purine-rich foods. All of our cells are partly composed of purines, which form uric acid when they break down. Meat with a high purine content, such as beef, goose and offal, as well as mussels, anchovies, herring and mackerel, can aggravate gout. However, purine-rich dairy products (such as milk or yogurt) may help prevent it.

Cherries (p. 149) A study published in the *Journal of Arthritis and Rheumatism* found that patients with gout who ate tart cherries or drank cherry extract for two days had a 35–45 percent lower chance for gout attack.

Celery seed (p. 149) Celery seed oil has long been used to help treat inflammatory conditions such as gout or rheumatism.

Bromelain A natural blood thinner and anti-inflammatory, bromelain is an enzyme derived from the stem of a pineapple. Supplementing with bromelain may stimulate circulation and help drain swollen tissues. (See Enzymes, *p. 172*.)

See your doctor

If you experience sudden, intense joint pain, see a doctor. If your gout goes untreated, the pain can become debilitating and the condition can cause permanent damage. Head to the doctor immediately if you develop a fever or if the joint is swollen and hot.

Quick fix If you have gout pain, think RICE: rest, ice, compression and elevation. If the pain will allow you to do so, use an ice pack (see Cold therapy, *p. 161*) and raise the joint above the level of your heart. Ice the affected area several times a day for 20–30 minutes.

HEMORRHOIDS

DESPITE THE ITCHING, ACHING AND BURNING pain that hemorrhoids cause, some people are too embarrassed to seek help and treat this common problem. It occurs when veins in or around the rectum become swollen, inflamed and sometimes bleed. The bleeding from hemorrhoids is usually painless and can be distinguished from anal fissures, which are small tears that usually cause painful bleeding. Eating little fiber, being constipated, overweight or sedentary, and lifting heavy objects make you more susceptible; hemorrhoids may also occur during pregnancy. While surgery might be recommended for extreme cases, usually a combination of dietary measures and natural remedies can effectively treat the symptoms and the cause.

Suggested remedies

Lifestyle factors To minimize everyday irritation, wear loose clothing and cotton underwear. Avoid straining, if possible.

Dietary measures Chronic constipation is a common cause of hemorrhoids. Getting more fiber *(p. 184)* into your diet, taking regular exercise *(p. 175)* and drinking plenty of fluids (see Hydration, *p. 209*) all help prevent and treat constipation. Probiotics *(p. 261)*, such as live yogurt, containing "friendly" gut bacteria, also help by treating and preventing constipation.

Flavonoids (p. 187) French and other research suggests that two citrus flavonoids—hesperidin and diosmin (Daflon)—can be especially helpful for treating the symptoms of hemorrhoids and reducing their size. The flavonoid rutin may also be effective; studies show that oxerutins, chemicals derived from it, alleviate hemorrhoid symptoms.

Horse chestnut (p. 207) Aescin, the active ingredient in horse chestnut, is thought to help by reducing inflammation and strengthening veins. In one Italian study, aescin eased pain, swelling and bleeding within a week.

Psyllium (p. 264) Taking a fiber supplement and drinking plenty of water helps to soften stools and make them easier to pass.

Witch hazel (p. 315) Apply a pad soaked in witch hazel or a small ice pack to reduce the swelling.

See your doctor

If your hemorrhoids persist and are very painful, your doctor may suggest treatments to shrink the hemorrhoids or surgery to remove them.

Quick fix To relieve the agony, hydrotherapy *(p. 210)* might be worth a try. Sit in a warm bath or special sitz bath for about 20 minutes after a bowel movement and several more times a day to relieve itching and pain, and to relax the anal sphincter muscle. After bathing, always pat the area dry or use the cool setting on a hair dryer.

See also Constipation

HAIR LOSS

A NUMBER OF DIFFERENT FACTORS CAN CAUSE hair loss including genetics, poor nutrition, hormonal changes, severe illness, skin disorders and chemotherapy. Check with your doctor for the underlying cause. So-called male- and female-pattern hair loss is usually inherited and difficult to reverse.

Suggested remedies

Dietary measures Follow a healthy diet and don't crash diet. Weight loss of more than about 15 pounds (7 kg), too little protein and low iron levels can all cause hair to fall out, as can an excess of vitamin A (from supplements or medicines). People with eating disorders often experience hair loss.

Zinc *(p. 319)* Taking zinc sulfate can reverse hair loss in adults with alopecia areata—an auto-immune disorder that causes patches of baldness in people of all ages. In a recent Iraqi study of 100 patients, more than 60 percent using zinc sulfate experienced complete hair regrowth, compared to 10 percent in the placebo group.

Saw palmetto *(p. 278)* Like the hair-loss drug finasteride, saw palmetto is used to treat both prostate enlargement and hereditary hair loss; the two substances may work in a similar way. In a small US study of men aged between 23 and 64 years, six out of 10 experienced hair regrowth after treatment with saw palmetto extract and beta-sitosterol, a plant sterol. Unlike finasteride, saw palmetto can also be used by women.

Biotin *(p. 131)* Sometimes known as vitamin B_7, biotin has been used alone and in combination with zinc aspartate and a topical corticosteroid to successfully treat alopecia in children. However, it may only be effective in those with a biotin deficiency.

Silica *(p. 280)* The supplement can help by strengthening hair that has been overexposed to sunlight, according to a 2005 Belgian study. Women with photo-damaged skin who took silica for 20 weeks experienced a marked improvement in the appearance of their skin and the brittleness of their hair and nails.

Aromatherapy *(p. 122)* Essential oils can help hair to grow back. Scottish researchers massaged 43 of 86 patients daily with a blend of thyme, rosemary, lavender and cedarwood in jojoba and grape seed carrier oils. Nineteen of them experienced significant hair regrowth, compared to just six in the control group.

See your doctor

If hair loss is sudden, patchy and distressing, a doctor should be able to diagnose the cause. If it is alopecia areata you may be prescribed a steroid topical ointment or steroid injections to attempt to suppress the local immune reaction that has caused the problem.

DID YOU KNOW?

No treatment for hair loss is particularly effective. While treatments may prevent further hair loss and sometimes lead to some short-term regrowth, most men are not satisfied with baldness cures.

HAY FEVER

POLLEN ALLERGIES ARE ANNOYING—and can be dangerous. Beyond the sneezing, itching, congestion and watery eyes, hay fever can trigger an asthma attack or worsen a breathing problem. Natural remedies can ease symptoms, often enough to lessen the need for allergy medications.

Suggested remedies

***Nasal irrigation** (p. 242)* Rinsing your nose with a saline solution removes pollen and can thin mucus. In an Italian study of 20 children with hay fever, nasal irrigation worked so well they needed less allergy medicine.

***Nettle** (p. 244)* Capsules of freeze-dried nettles eased allergy symptoms for 55 percent of people with hay fever in one study, according to a report in *Alternative Medicine Review.*

***Probiotics** (p. 261)* Some beneficial bacteria-including *Lactobacillus acidophilus, L. paracasei and Bifidobacterium longum*-are showing promise for easing allergy symptoms, Swiss scientists say in a 2013 report.

***Acupuncture** (p. 112)* This traditional Chinese treatment reduced symptoms and lessened the need for allergy medications in a recent study from Germany's Charité University Medical Center.

Tinospora cordifolia *(p. 296)* In a 2005 study of 75 allergy sufferers from India's Indira Gandhi Medical College, this herb cleared up sneezing for 83 percent and congestion for 69 percent.

***Perilla** (p. 256)* Rosmarinic acid in this herb, also called Chinese basil, appears to soothe allergy symptoms by reducing inflammation, say researchers from South Korea's Institute of Oriental Medicine in a 2011 study.

***Nigella** (p. 246)* When 66 hay fever sufferers took this herb as part of a recent Iranian study, they found it reduced nasal congestion, itching and sneezing.

***Horseradish** (p. 208)* Applied as a nasal spray, the potent, pungent mustard oil glycosides in horseradish thin mucus for easy drainage and relief.

See your doctor

See your doctor if:

❖ you have sinus pain and a greenish-yellow discharge
❖ symptoms don't improve or get worse
❖ your allergy is interfering with your quality of life.

Quick fix Compounds found in butterbur *(p. 139)* decrease the production of congestion-causing histamines and leukotrienes. In a small study from Scotland, it worked as well as a prescription allergy medicine to dry up runny noses.

DID YOU KNOW?

You can make your bedroom a "no-sneeze zone," and so get a good night's sleep, with some simple steps. Take a shower and wash your hair before bed; shut windows and doors; use an air conditioning unit or air filter; vacuum regularly; change your clothes outside your bedroom when pollen counts are high; keep pets out.

See also Allergies, Asthma

HEADACHES

HEADACHES CAN BE CAUSED BY MANY factors, including muscle tension, emotional stress, skeletal misalignment, dehydration and the adverse effects of drugs and alcohol. Headaches may also be symptoms of other health problems, from injuries to minor infections and rare but serious conditions such as brain tumors or meningitis. If you suffer from headaches, using natural therapies while improving your diet and lifestyle may reduce their frequency and intensity. But if headaches persist, you should see your doctor.

Suggested remedies

Lifestyle factors Many headaches are due to some form of physical or mental stress such as long work hours, insufficient sleep, or living in an environment that is noisy, poorly ventilated, or exposes you to toxic or irritating substances. Taking steps to address these issues may help relieve your headaches.

Dietary measures Headaches (especially migraines) are sometimes triggered by sensitivities to certain foods or chemicals within foods (such as monosodium glutamate, gluten and sulfites). An elimination diet *(p. 171)* may help you identify the culprit. Other contributing factors can include dehydration and caffeine withdrawal. Make sure you have adequate hydration *(p. 209)*, and work with your doctor to determine whether changing your diet could help you to manage your headaches.

Relaxation (p. 269) Progressive relaxation is an effective way to reduce headaches, and is often recommended in combination with other interventions.

White willow bark (p. 312) A traditional remedy that remains useful, white willow bark contains salicin, which acts in a similar way to aspirin to relieve headaches.

Ginger (p. 192) The anti-inflammatory and analgesic (pain-relieving) actions of ginger mean it may be helpful in relieving headaches and migraines.

Musculoskeletal manipulation Some (but not all) studies suggest that chiropractic *(p. 152)* and osteopathy *(p. 251)* may be beneficial for headaches, especially those arising from musculoskeletal issues in the head and neck.

5-HTP (p. 186) In a small study published in the journal *Headache*, tension headache sufferers who took 5-HTP were able to reduce their consumption of painkillers.

See your doctor

Occasionally, headaches are symptoms of serious illness. Seek urgent medical attention if you experience:

- sudden, severe headache
- headache with double vision, seizures, fever, numbness, difficulty speaking, loss of consciousness, severe nausea and/or vomiting, stiff neck, rash or shortness of breath
- headache following an injury
- a headache that worsens when you cough, move suddenly or exert yourself.

Quick fix Got a headache? Try massaging your forehead and temples with peppermint oil *(p. 255)* or Tiger Balm *(p. 295)*. Clinical studies have found that both are effective remedies for headaches with similar pain-relieving effects to those of paracetamol.

See also Back and neck pain, Migraines

HEART AND CIRCULATORY HEALTH

LIKE CANCER, CARDIOVASCULAR DISEASE is one of the world's leading killers. Chronic ailments of the heart and circulatory system are often caused by arteriosclerosis, a condition in which the arteries throughout the body start to stiffen and collect plaque. These blockages or narrowing in the blood vessels can result in peripheral arterial disease (poor circulation in extremities), angina (chest pain), stroke or heart attack.

Cardiovascular disease is more common in people who smoke, have diabetes, or are overweight and/or inactive, or those with an unhealthy diet as well as those who are socially isolated or depressed. But while heart disease was traditionally blamed on an excess of cholesterol-rich foods, many scientists now believe arterial plaque accumulates as a result of chronic inflammation throughout the body created by a diet high in sugar, refined carbohydrates and other processed foods (as well as unhealthy lifestyle habits).

Your heart sends oxygen- and nutrient-rich blood to every cell in your body, so when you encourage healthy circulation, decrease blood pressure, increase oxygen intake and cool inflammation, you protect not only your heart, but the health of your entire body.

Key defense strategies

Up to 80 percent of heart disease is caused by lifestyle factors, which means you can choose plenty of lifestyle strategies that will reduce your risks. These interventions can be summarized by the SENSE approach (Stress management, Exercise, Nutrition, Social and spiritual interaction and Education). This holistic approach offers a way to optimize health in general as well as to reduce or reverse heart disease.

Using techniques from deep breathing to guided imagery, **relaxation** *(p. 269)* can help relieve stress and tension. Not only does relaxation help to calm your mind and lower your blood pressure, it may have a physiological effect by reducing the ravages of stress hormones such as cortisol. These hormones can cause inflammation in the body, which encourages the deposit of cholesterol-rich plaque in your blood vessels. **Meditation** *(p. 234)* is another proven stress-busting remedy, highly recommended by the American Heart Association.

You should also find a form of **exercise** *(p. 175)* you enjoy and do it regularly. Start gently and build up gradually. US researchers found that heart attack patients who participated in a formal exercise program reduced their risk of death by up to 25 percent. Pair regular exercise with a healthy diet that replaces saturated fats with healthier fats like **olive oil** *(p. 249)*, and you will be able to achieve and maintain a healthy weight, manage diabetes and keep cholesterol in check—all factors that have an impact on heart and circulatory health.

In addition to exercise, stress reduction and good nutrition, there are natural remedies that have been shown to help the cardiovascular system and these are discussed on the following page.

CAUTION: If you have a heart problem, you need to be under careful medical management. Please consult your doctor before making any changes to your program.

continued on page 66

Suggested remedies

***Omega-3 fatty acids** (p. 250)* Oily fish are rich in omega-3s and by eating them once or twice a week, you could reduce the risk of fatal heart attack by at least 33 percent. You may also benefit from taking omega-3 supplements.

***Garlic** (p. 191)* This has been trusted as a heart tonic for over 5,000 years; one clove a day can lower total cholesterol levels by 9 percent and decrease blood pressure by 5.5 percent.

Walnuts Packed with vegetarian omega-3s, walnuts boast large amounts of the amino acid L-arginine, which converts to nitric oxide that dilates the blood vessels, increasing blood flow and lowering blood pressure. (See Nuts, *p. 247.*)

***Psyllium** (p. 264)* The husks' soluble fiber stirred into a smoothie can help reduce cholesterol and help manage high blood glucose levels that can lead to excess inflammation.

***Ginger** (p. 192)* The potent anti-inflammatory qualities of ginger are well established. It contains gingerol, a compound believed to relieve pain, stimulate blood flow and relax blood vessels, bringing down blood pressure.

***Coenzyme Q_{10}** (p. 157)* This supplement may help prevent heart disease by soothing and protecting the mitochondria in cells from stress and the effects of aging.

***Hawthorn** (p. 203)* Preliminary research indicates that hawthorn, a traditional heart tonic, may work by lowering high blood pressure. More research will be required, however, before its effects are fully understood.

***Meditation** (p. 234)* Regular meditation—transcendental meditation in particular—has been shown in numerous studies to reduce blood pressure, most likely by reducing stress. Yoga *(p. 316)* may also have a beneficial effect on blood pressure.

***Sauna** (p. 277)* Research has shown that having regular saunas can be beneficial for the heart and circulation.

Quick fix The amino acid *(p. 118)* L-carnitine was shown in a Mayo Clinic review of 13 controlled trials to reduce the risk of death, soothe abnormal heart rhythms and reduce angina in people experiencing a heart attack.

See your doctor

Certain heart and circulatory health symptoms require immediate medical attention. Call emergency services if you or a loved one experiences:

Symptoms of a heart attack
Many heart attacks occur without any symptoms at all, but pain or heaviness in the chest, neck, shoulder, arm or jaw needs to be taken seriously, especially when associated with shortness of breath, nausea, dizziness or sweating.

Symptoms of a stroke
Get emergency help without delay if you or a loved one has any of these warning signs: drooping or numbness on one side of the face; weakness or numbness in one arm; sudden difficulty speaking.

DID YOU KNOW?

Eggs, because of the cholesterol they contain, were long thought to contribute to heart disease, but more recent research suggests that eggs may have a beneficial effect. It seems that eggs may help change the LDL cholesterol molecules into a less dangerous form.

See also Tooth and gum disorders

HERPES

SEVERAL TYPES OF HERPES VIRUS CAN affect humans. For example, *Herpes simplex* virus type 1 (HSV-1) causes cold sores, and *Herpes simplex* virus type 2 (HSV-2) causes genital herpes. Cold sores start with a tingling sensation around the lips that is followed by the appearance of painful, water-filled blisters. After the blisters burst, a crust forms over the lesion, and takes a few days to heal. The initial lesions of genital herpes are also blister-like, and then develop into small ulcers.

Even when no lesions are present, the herpes virus persists in the nerves of the affected area in a dormant state, ready to cause an outbreak of cold sores or genital herpes when reactivated. Common triggers include emotional and physical stress, minor infections (such as colds), menstruation and sunburn. Natural therapies can relieve symptoms, promote healing and reduce the frequency of outbreaks.

Suggested remedies

Lifestyle factors Stay well hydrated, keep your lips moisturized and protect your lips from UV exposure. Dry, cracked or sunburned lips may trigger a bout of cold sores. Stress may also trigger an attack so help keep stress levels down with regular exercise *(p. 175)*, relaxation *(p. 269)*, meditation *(p. 234)* or yoga *(p. 316)*.

Dietary measures Monitor your diet to see whether it affects your cold sores, as some herpes outbreaks are triggered by the consumption of certain foods (chocolate, for example). Following a healthy diet will help you keep your immune system strong and so minimize your risk of developing the minor infections that can trigger an attack. During an attack, avoid acidic or salty foods, which can aggravate a cold sore.

Amino acids (p. 118) In a study involving more than 1,500 participants, 92 percent of people affected by cold sores and 81 percent of those with genital herpes rated lysine supplements as either "very effective" or "effective." Participants reported improvements in the recurrence and healing time of outbreaks.

Lemon balm (p. 221) Topical ointments containing lemon balm may relieve symptoms of cold sores and speed up healing, as well as inhibiting the spread of infection.

Aloe vera *(p. 117)* Applying *Aloe vera* cream to genital herpes lesions may enhance healing.

See also Colds and flu, Frequent illness

See your doctor

See your doctor if you:

- ❖ think you have genital herpes or have been exposed to it
- ❖ have been diagnosed with genital herpes and have become pregnant
- ❖ have either genital herpes or cold sores, and are affected by an immune system disorder
- ❖ have outbreaks that are frequent or protracted
- ❖ experience herpes symptoms in or near your eyes.

Quick fix Applying a hot Earl Grey tea bag at the first sign of a cold sore is said to reduce swelling and aid healing. There's no research to prove whether this works, but recent laboratory studies show that compounds in black tea can reduce the infectivity of the HSV-1 virus. Also bergamot *(p. 129)*, the agent used to flavor Earl Grey tea, has long been used by aromatherapists to treat cold sores. So the tea bags might just be worth a try!

INCONTINENCE

URINARY INCONTINENCE IS THE LOSS OF voluntary control over the bladder. It can vary in severity from minor leakage brought on by laughing or coughing (known as stress incontinence) to a complete inability to control urination.

Causes include hormonal changes (for example after menopause), pregnancy (due to a combination of hormonal change and weight gain), childbirth (which can weaken pelvic floor muscles), urinary tract infections and constipation. Additionally, incontinence is sometimes caused by other health conditions, including prostate disease and neurological diseases such as multiple sclerosis.

Depending on the cause and severity of your incontinence, your doctor may recommend a combination of medical interventions and natural therapies to help manage the problem.

Suggested remedies

Lifestyle factors Being overweight increases the likelihood of developing incontinence, and losing weight may improve bladder control. Ensure you empty your bladder completely before traveling or sleeping; try repeat emptying by standing up after urinating and then sitting down again while compressing your lower abdomen to ensure that the bladder is completely empty.

Journaling (p. 215) Keeping a record of your "accidents" for a few days will help you define the type of incontinence you have and identify any triggers.

Pelvic floor exercises (p. 253) Up to 80 percent of women with mild stress incontinence experience improved bladder control after performing pelvic floor exercises (also known as Kegel exercises), usually over several months. Pelvic floor exercises may also be beneficial for men with incontinence, including those who become incontinent following prostate surgery.

Acupuncture (p. 112) Some studies suggest that acupuncture helps stress incontinence; however, more research will be required before its effects are completely understood.

Vitamin D (p. 305) Research shows that people with low vitamin D levels are more prone to incontinence than those with adequate levels of vitamin D, but it is not yet known whether taking vitamin D supplements improves bladder control.

See your doctor

Seek medical assistance if urinary incontinence develops very suddenly, is accompanied by symptoms indicative of urinary tract infection, prostate problems or diabetes, or if you suspect your prescribed medicines may be contributing to your bladder-control issues.

DID YOU KNOW?

Cranberry supplements or juice are sometimes employed in nursing home environments to help reduce urinary odor. Although there's no scientific research to support the practice, anecdotal reports suggest it may help.

See also Diabetes and insulin resistance, Menopausal symptoms, Prostate problems, Urinary tract infections

INDIGESTION

INDIGESTION (DYSPEPSIA) IS PAIN OR DISCOMFORT in the upper abdomen (often a burning sensation deep in the chest referred to as heartburn), which may be accompanied by symptoms such as belching, nausea, bloating, an acid taste in the mouth, regurgitation and/or sensations of being overly full.

In most cases there is no medical cause for dyspepsia. However, it is sometimes a symptom of an underlying health problem, such as gastroesophageal reflux disease (GERD), in which stomach acid enters the esophagus causing burning pain, regurgitation of food, and sometimes coughing and hoarseness, or peptic ulcer disease. Less commonly, it may be caused by a more serious condition such as gastric cancer. Natural remedies may help to relieve or prevent your symptoms.

Suggested remedies

Lifestyle factors Your doctor may advise you to stop smoking and/or lose weight. Avoid sleeping flat on your back and raise the head of your bed to help prevent reflux during the night.

Dietary measures Foods that are prone to causing indigestion, and so should be avoided or eaten only in moderation, include fatty foods, spices, alcohol, coffee and fizzy drinks. Swallowing excessive amounts of air may also contribute, so take the time to eat slowly and chew your food well. Avoid eating meals that are overly large or eating too close to bedtime.

Carminative herbs (p. 142) Many herbs aid digestion when taken after a meal. Replacing the after-meal coffee with peppermint *(p. 255)*, chamomile *(p. 147)* or ginger *(p. 192)* tea, or taking up the Indian custom of chewing on a few seeds of fennel, dill, anise and caraway may help relieve symptoms of indigestion.

Globe artichoke (p. 195) In clinical studies, globe artichoke extract has been shown to relieve a wide variety of dyspepsia symptoms including nausea, bloating and abdominal pain.

Iberogast (p. 213) Several clinical studies have shown that a combination of nine herbal extracts that includes peppermint, caraway seed, chamomile, licorice and milk thistle helps relieve symptoms of dyspepsia with no underlying medical cause.

Bicarbonate of soda (p. 130) A teaspoonful in a glass of water may give temporary relief of heartburn or gastroesophageal reflux disease (GERD).

See your doctor

Your doctor should investigate severe, recurrent or persistent indigestion symptoms to see if there is a medical cause. See a doctor immediately if you have:

- ❖ indigestion pain that radiates to the jaw, arm, shoulder or neck—this may be a symptom of a heart attack so call for an ambulance immediately
- ❖ severe pain in the abdominal region
- ❖ vomiting of blood or presence of blood in the feces
- ❖ unexplained weight loss.

Quick fix Did you know that the antacid chews you buy at your pharmacy or supermarket are actually a natural remedy? They're often made from calcium carbonate *(p. 140)*, and are widely used to provide effective relief from indigestion symptoms. (Many natural therapists recommend avoiding those that contain aluminum.)

See also Flatulence

INFLAMMATORY BOWEL DISEASE

INFLAMMATORY BOWEL DISEASE (IBD) is caused by inflammation deep in the intestinal lining that produces pain, diarrhea, weight loss and nutritional deficiencies as well as bleeding, blockages and ulcers. There are two types. Crohn's disease may strike anywhere in your digestive system but is usually restricted to the lower small intestine, called the ileum. Ulcerative colitis attacks the colon and rectum.

It's important to work with a health practitioner to diagnose your IBD and select the best prescription medications to keep it in remission. During a flare-up, you may also need prescription medications to control intestinal spasms and diarrhea. That said, natural remedies can be powerful add-ons proven by research to help calm inflammation, lengthen the time between flare-ups, ease pain and reduce the stress that can trigger a relapse.

Suggested remedies

Lifestyle factors By reducing stress, gentle **exercise** *(p. 175)* routines improve symptoms and cut the risk of flare-ups, according to Canadian research.

Dietary measures Smart dietary steps could help you steer clear of IBD flare-ups for longer. Eat regular small meals and cut back on red meat, dairy products, alcohol and fruit juice. Skip cola and other fizzy drinks, as well as chocolate. Indulging in these treats could double risk for a flare-up, Dutch researchers say. Consider taking a **multivitamin** *(p. 240)* and **vitamin D** *(p. 305)*. These supplements may reduce IBD risk by strengthening immunity. Research shows that **probiotics** *(p. 261)* soothe inflammation and may work as well as some prescription medicines to keep colitis in remission. Good-for-you lactobacillus bacteria in yogurt help by crowding out the bad bugs that boost inflammation.

Relaxation (p. 269) By easing inflammation-boosting stress, progressive muscle relaxation eases pain and prolongs remission, according to a small Spanish study of people with Crohn's disease who were given eight relaxation sessions.

Hypnotherapy (p. 211) Gut-directed hypnotherapy, which harnesses the power of your mind to calm your digestive system, can soothe pain and help reduce the risk of a flare-up.

Acupuncture (p. 112) German research suggests regular acupuncture treatments may reduce Crohn's symptoms.

See your doctor

Seek medical assistance immediately if you:

- ❖ have severe gastrointestinal symptoms—including diarrhea, abdominal pain, cramping or rectal bleeding—that aren't eased by over-the-counter remedies
- ❖ lose a large amount of blood
- ❖ have diarrhea that leaves you dehydrated
- ❖ feel dizzy or faint or have intense abdominal pain
- ❖ experience extended nausea and vomiting or a sudden fever over 102°F (39°C).

Quick fix A low-fiber, low-residue diet will give your intestinal tract a break during a flare-up. Cut out whole grains, nuts and seeds, raw produce, tough cuts of meat, fruit juice and milk as well as cooked vegetables and fruits containing seeds, stringy fibers or lots of roughage (such as corn).

INSECT BITES AND STINGS

MOST INSECT BITES AND STINGS PRODUCE minor, temporary symptoms, often characterized by localized swelling, inflammation, itchiness and irritation. However, bites by some types of spiders and scorpions may cause more severe symptoms, including generalized weakness, breathing difficulties, nausea, fever, destruction of the tissues in the area around the bite, coma and even death. An allergic reaction to an insect bite or sting can also have serious consequences. For example, some people experience life-threatening anaphylactic reactions to bee stings or mosquito bites.

While serious bites and stings require prompt medical treatment, topical applications of natural remedies may aid the management of minor problems.

Suggested remedies

***Neem** (p. 243)* Topical applications of neem oil have traditionally been used as insect repellents to prevent bites and stings. Studies suggest that neem oil is effective against a wide range of insects and other organisms, including mosquitoes, bedbugs, head lice and dust mites.

***Tea tree** (p. 293)* Products containing tea tree oil (sometimes in conjunction with lavender oil) can be applied directly to bites and have also been shown to effectively kill head lice.

***Cold therapy** (p. 161)* Application of an ice pack to a bite will help reduce swelling and inflammation. Itching may also be reduced by applying a paste of baking soda, banana peel, *Aloe vera* gel and even toothpaste.

***Sublingual immunotherapy** (p. 289)* This therapy lowers the risk of life-threatening reactions in people who are allergic to certain insect stings.

Quick fix A fast-working traditional remedy to relieve the pain of insect bites is a dab of lavender *(p. 218)* essential oil. Animal studies and *in vitro* research suggest that it works by inhibiting swelling and allergic reactions.

See also Allergies, Skin rashes

See your doctor

Seek emergency medical care if you suspect that you have been bitten by a venomous insect or are experiencing an allergic reaction. Signs include:

- dizziness
- swollen tongue or throat
- breathing problems
- hives (urticaria) or rash
- diarrhea
- any severe and/or rapidly developing symptoms after an insect bite or sting.

See your doctor, too, if you develop a bull's-eye rash around a bite site or have been in a region where malaria is common and you experience malaria symptoms such as fever and/or chills.

DID YOU KNOW?

If you're one of those people mosquitoes find particularly tasty, you've probably heard it said that taking high doses of vitamin B_1 helps protect you from being bitten. Unfortunately, research suggests that this is an old wives' tale and isn't a worthwhile remedy.

IRRITABLE BOWEL SYNDROME

IN IRRITABLE BOWEL SYNDROME (IBS), altered bowel habits (constipation, diarrhea or a combination of the two) are accompanied by abdominal pain and distension. The cause of IBS has not been determined; one theory is that changes in serotonin levels affect nerves in the bowel, interfering with normal function. Individual IBS episodes may be triggered by stress, food intolerances, or deviations from your regular routine (among other factors). Several natural therapies have been clinically proven to relieve the symptoms.

Suggested remedies

Dietary measures Try an elimination diet *(p. 171)* to detect any intolerances to foods such as dairy, citrus, wheat or spices. It is also wise to avoid alcohol, coffee and sweetened (including sugar-free) beverages, and to drink plenty of water. (See Hydration, *p. 209.*)

Low-FODMAP diet (p. 224) Consuming a diet that is low in a group of carbohydrate compounds collectively referred to as FODMAPs—fermentable oligosaccharides, disaccharides, monosaccharides and polyols—may relieve IBS symptoms of bloating, gas and abdominal pain.

Gluten-free diet (p. 198) Cutting out foods containing gluten helps some people with IBS, and in particular may help reduce the number of daily bowel movements experienced by those with diarrhea-predominant symptoms.

Peppermint (p. 255) Research shows that taking enteric-coated peppermint oil capsules helps relieve IBS symptoms such as diarrhea, constipation, abdominal pain and bloating.

Iberogast (p. 213) Several clinical studies have shown that a combination of nine herbal extracts, including peppermint, caraway seed, chamomile, licorice and milk thistle, helps relieve symptoms of IBS.

Globe artichoke (p. 195) In at least two studies, taking globe artichoke has led to improvements not only in IBS symptoms, but also in sufferers' quality of life.

Psyllium (p. 264) Psyllium may help improve bowel habits in constipation-dominant IBS. However, research suggests it does not reduce abdominal pain or bloating.

See your doctor

If you're concerned you may have IBS, see your doctor, who can investigate and diagnose your condition. Visit your doctor if you've been diagnosed with IBS and have worsening symptoms that interfere with daily life. You should also seek help if you observe blood in your feces or have unexplained weight loss, extreme fatigue, fever or severe abdominal pain.

See also Diarrhea, Flatulence, Inflammatory bowel disease

JAW PAIN

WHEN NOT CAUSED BY DENTAL PROBLEMS (such as a tooth abscess), pain in the jaw and surrounding tissues is often due to issues involving the temporomandibular joint (TMJ), which sits in front of the ear and enables the jaw to move up, down and sideways. Symptoms may include impaired jaw movement, headaches, neck pain and clicking or grinding sensations when the jaw is moved. The jaw and/or surrounding muscles may also be tender or painful to touch. TMJ symptoms may be aggravated by periods of stress or emotional upheaval, especially in those with chronic pain.

While surgery may occasionally be necessary, most TMJ problems are initially treated with noninvasive methods such as the use of dental splints to enhance alignment of the teeth. Natural therapies may play a valuable role in treatment.

Suggested remedies

Lifestyle factors Dealing with stressful issues and engaging in activities that will help you relax, such as **yoga** *(p. 316)*, **meditation** *(p. 234)* and hobbies, along with adequate **sleep** *(p. 281)* and **exercise** *(p. 175)*, can assist in reducing teeth grinding and muscle tension in the jaw. Relax the jaw muscles by placing the tongue behind the bottom teeth and moving the jaw up and down.

Laser treatment (p. 216) Based on analysis of 14 studies, a review published in the *Journal of Applied Oral Science* concluded that low-level laser therapy reduces pain and muscle tension in TMJ patients.

Acupuncture and acupressure (p. 112) Applying needles or finger pressure to sensitive trigger points around the jaw can help relieve jaw pain.

Musculoskeletal manipulation Interventions such as **chiropractic** *(p. 152)* and **osteopathy** *(p. 251)* that combine manipulation of the affected joint by a suitably qualified practitioner and specific exercises to enhance mobility may help.

Alexander Technique (p. 115) Treatments that promote improved posture may help relieve TMJ symptoms. The effect is gradual and the Alexander Technique usually involves ongoing treatment over a number of months.

See your doctor

See your doctor or dentist if you are having problems opening or closing your jaw, or are experiencing pain or other symptoms of TMJ dysfunction.

Quick fix In a survey published in the *Clinical Journal of Pain* that involved more than 1,500 people with TMJ disorders, hot and cold **compresses** *(p. 163)* were voted more effective at reducing symptoms than any other medical or natural treatment, bringing relief to 74 percent of those who tried them.

See also Back and neck pain, Headaches, Rheumatoid arthritis

JET LAG

UNDER NORMAL CIRCUMSTANCES, YOUR BODY and mind move through a daily cycle of sleepiness and wakefulness that's synchronized with the world around you. Due to these "circadian rhythms" you naturally become progressively more tired as the day winds down, then sleep through the night, and wake up again as the new day starts. However, when you travel across multiple time zones, your internal clock is disrupted, resulting in jet lag.

People with jet lag experience difficulties sleeping at night and feel excessively sleepy during the day. They may also experience concentration problems, mood swings and gastrointestinal disturbances. The symptoms persist until the circadian rhythms reset themselves and resynchronize with the new environment—a process that can take one day for every hour of time difference. Natural therapies for jet lag are aimed at helping your body to adapt to the time zone at your destination.

Suggested remedies

Adjust your body clock Your body clock is set by the timing of exposure to light, exercise, eating, socializing and sleeping. If you are going to be traveling west, delay your clock for a few days before you travel by exposing yourself to bright light for a couple of hours longer than normal in the evening and going to bed later. If traveling east, early morning light exposure will shift your body clock forward. Periods of increased darkness at the opposite end of the day assist the process.

Fly well While you are in the air it is best to avoid alcohol and maintain good **hydration** *(p. 209)*. Avoid eating or exposure to bright light if you arrive during the nighttime at your destination.

Sleeping strategies (p. 282) Simple steps can help get your body ready for sleep, including **relaxation** *(p. 269)*, using an eye mask and neck pillow when traveling, keeping the bedroom at a constant temperature and having a hot bath once you arrive.

Melatonin (p. 237) Among other functions, the hormone melatonin helps induce sleep and regulate our adaptation to dark and light. Numerous studies have shown that melatonin supplements help minimize jet lag when taken before bedtime in the destination time zone for several days prior to travel.

Quick fix Lying in bed trying vainly to drift off can be extremely frustrating! Rather than turning to prescription medicines, try a herbal sedative. Research suggests that a combination of **valerian** *(p. 300)* and **hops** *(p. 206)* helps reduce the amount of time it takes to fall asleep, and may also improve sleep quality.

See your doctor

If you travel frequently or tend to take a long time to recover from jet lag, ask your doctor to help you devise some sleeping strategies that suit your needs.

WATCH OUT!

Tempted to turn to coffee to help you stay awake when you're jet-lagged? While caffeine may assist daytime alertness, it can interfere with your sleeping patterns, and could actually prolong the amount of time it takes to adapt to your new time zone.

See also Sleeping problems

KIDNEY STONE PREVENTION

KIDNEY STONES DEVELOP WHEN MINERALS in the urine crystallize to form solid clumps or clusters. Many are able to move through the urinary tract without causing any symptoms, but in other cases they can be extremely painful to pass, sometimes because they've become lodged in the ureter.

Symptoms may include pain when urinating; a sharp pain in the lower abdomen, back, side or groin; blood in the urine; fever and chills; and nausea and vomiting. People who have experienced a kidney stone are more likely to develop another one, and are also at increased risk of kidney disease, making prevention an integral part of treatment.

Depending on the type of kidney stone you have and the presence of any other health issues or risk factors, your doctor may prescribe medicines and/or recommend specific nutritional strategies to help prevent recurrence.

Suggested remedies

Dietary measures If you have a history of kidney stones it is important to follow the general recommendation to drink at least 2 pints (1.2 L) of water daily and ensure that you regularly pass clear or pale straw-colored urine **(see Hydration, *p 209*)**. Your doctor may also recommend that you increase your consumption of fruits, vegetables and calcium-rich foods, and decrease your intake of salt, animal protein, and food and beverages high in oxalate (such as rhubarb and wheat bran). It is also wise to follow the general recommendation to curtail your intake of processed sugary foods and drinks.

Potassium (p. 260) In a study published in the *Journal of Urology*, taking potassium-magnesium citrate daily for up to three years reduced the risk of calcium oxalate stone recurrence by 85 percent compared to taking a placebo.

See your doctor

Seek medical assistance immediately if you experience kidney stone symptoms such as blood in the urine, severe pain in the abdomen, side, back or groin, nausea, vomiting, fever and/or chills.

DID YOU KNOW?

Made from the stringy, fibrous material found outside corn cobs, **corn silk** *(p. 164)* tea has traditionally been used to soothe urinary inflammation and address kidney stones. In a study published in the *International Journal of Health and Nutrition* in 2012, researchers found that drinking a couple of cups per day didn't promote the breakdown of kidney stones, but did make them easier to pass. (Ask your doctor whether corn silk is suitable for you before using it.)

MEMORY PROBLEMS

OUR MEMORY TAKES A HIT AS WE AGE, but it needn't mean dementia. Misplacing your car keys or struggling to recall an acquaintance's name, while irritating, does not mean you are losing your mind. Difficulty remembering things often happens at times of stress, whether it is emotional or work-related. Women entering menopause sometimes complain of being "scatterbrained," a malady that rights itself after menopause. For these minor memory lapses, there are several natural remedies that may help.

Suggested remedies

Lifestyle factors Take steps to reduce your stress levels if you can. **Yoga** *(p. 316)*, **meditation** *(p. 234)*, **massage** *(p. 230)* and other stress-relieving activities can help. Take regular **exercise** *(p. 175)*, too. The American Psychological Association credits regular exercise with enhanced cognition, academic achievement and better psychosocial outcomes, although **dancing** *(p. 165)* is the only physical activity associated with a lower risk of dementia.

Dietary measures Following a healthy diet with plenty of variety should help your brain to function at its best. You might want to add berries to your breakfast cereal-a Harvard study of over 16,000 women found that eating greater quantities of blueberries and strawberries protected memory and delayed cognitive decline by up to two and a half years.

Cognitive challenge *(p. 160)* A UK review found 23 studies in which neurofeedback (also known as brain training) showed a beneficial impact in several kinds of memory tests.

Holy basil *(p. 205)* This herb is used traditionally to enhance mental function and animal studies now confirm its ability to improve memory and reduce age-induced memory problems.

Rosemary *(p. 272)* In a UK study people in rosemary-scented rooms were better able to recall future appointments as well as tasks on their to-do list.

Ginseng *(p. 194)* American ginseng may protect against chronic stress-induced memory decline.

Ginkgo *(p. 193)* An Australian study found that 14 days of taking *Ginkgo biloba* improved participants' working memory, probably due to more efficient processing in the frontal lobe of the brain.

Sage *(p. 273)* Research is now backing up this traditional memory enhancer. In various studies a dose of sage improved word recall.

See your doctor

When you get lost on familiar routes, experience trouble with simple directions or use incorrect words ("hand clock" instead of "watch"), a doctor's visit is warranted. Seek immediate medical attention if you lose your memory after a fall or a knock to the head.

Quick fix If you need to remember something, pop in a stick of gum. A *British Journal of Psychology* study found that gum-chewing shortened reaction times and helped people remember a sequence of numbers within a 30-minute audio recording.

See also Menopausal symptoms

MENOPAUSAL SYMPTOMS

MOST WOMEN EXPERIENCE MENOPAUSE sometime between their midforties and midfifties. During this time, the ovaries stop producing estrogen and progesterone, and ovulation ceases. Although menopause is a natural time in a woman's life, it is sometimes associated with uncomfortable symptoms, which may include: irregular periods, hot flashes and night sweats, sleeping difficulties, mood swings, depression, weight gain, difficulties with concentration and memory, lowered libido and changes to hair, skin and genital tissue (e.g., vaginal thinning and dryness).

Additionally, the hormonal changes that occur during menopause increase the risk of developing heart disease and osteoporosis in subsequent years. A number of natural remedies may help you manage your symptoms and maintain your heart and bone health.

Suggested remedies

Lifestyle factors Recommendations that may help you cope with hot flashes include staying cool (for example by wearing light, cotton clothes and avoiding alcohol, coffee and hot or spicy foods and drinks) and stopping smoking. Losing excess weight and getting at least 20 minutes a day of aerobic **exercise** *(p. 175)* can help improve mood, sleep and hormonal balance. Regular exercise, especially weight-bearing forms of exercise such as **walking** *(p. 309)*, is also important for maintaining bone health after menopause and helping to reduce your risk of osteoporosis.

Dietary measures Maintaining a healthy diet can help ease your transition through menopause. Including **soy** *(p. 285)* foods or taking soy isoflavone supplements may relieve menopausal symptoms and prevent postmenopausal bone loss.

Flaxseed (p. 188) The seeds contain estrogen-like compounds, called lignans, that may have a number of health benefits for post-menopausal women such as reducing LDL cholesterol levels.

Black cohosh (p. 133) A favorite of herbalists, black cohosh has been the subject of numerous randomized, controlled clinical trials, many of which found it to be an effective treatment for menopause, improving symptoms such as hot flashes, mood changes and vaginal thinning.

Sage (p. 273) In a preliminary study involving 71 menopausal women experiencing at least five hot flashes per day, taking sage tablets led to improvements in both the frequency and intensity of hot flashes. Benefits for other menopausal symptoms (including psychological symptoms) were also noted.

See your doctor

Consult your doctor if you are less than 40 years old and think you may be going through menopause or you experience unusual bleeding (frequent periods, heavy bleeding, bleeding between periods or after intercourse, or bleeding after menopause).

See also Menstrual problems, Osteoporosis, Sexual problems, Sleeping problems

MENSTRUAL PROBLEMS

PROBLEMS THAT CAN AFFECT WOMEN'S menstrual cycles include premenstrual syndrome (PMS), dysmenorrhea (period pain) and polycystic ovary syndrome (PCOS). PMS occurs prior to menstruation, and can include an extensive array of symptoms that are relieved with the onset of menstrual bleeding (including irritability, depressed moods, headaches and bloating).

In dysmenorrhea, pain is experienced in the abdomen, back and/or legs around the time the period starts. In PCOS, ovarian dysfunction and hormonal imbalances mean proper ovulation rarely occurs and fertility is compromised. Symptoms of PCOS can include menstrual irregularity, excessive body and facial hair, mood swings, obesity and blood glucose problems. Though the more serious problems will require medical intervention, herbal and nutritional supplements can be of benefit for many minor menstrual problems.

Suggested remedies

Dietary measures Many doctors and natural therapists recommend that women who suffer from menstrual difficulties reduce their intake of sugar, refined carbohydrates, salt and caffeine. Adopting a low-glycemic index diet may be beneficial for those affected by PCOS. Drink plenty of water as dehydration can increase the likelihood of cramping **(see Hydration, *p. 209*).**

Herbal teas Drinking herbal teas made with **ginger** *(p. 192)*, fennel, **cinnamon** *(p. 155)* or **peppermint** *(p. 255)* can help relieve cramping.

Heat therapy (p. 204) A hot-water bottle or wheat pack can be used to help relieve abdominal cramps or back pain.

Chasteberry (p. 148) The herb *Vitex agnus-castus* relieves many premenstrual symptoms, including irritability, emotional instability, headaches and breast tenderness.

Calcium (p. 140) Taking daily calcium supplements over several cycles may help reduce symptoms of PMS.

Vitamin B_6 (p. 302) Vitamin B_6 has been shown to reduce PMS symptoms such as mood problems, insomnia and acne. It is sometimes taken with magnesium, which improves dysmenorrhea (period pain). **Dark chocolate** *(p. 167)* is high in magnesium and contains substances that boost levels of mood-elevating brain chemicals. Eating a few squares before a period may help to reduce some premenstrual symptoms.

See your doctor

See your doctor if you experience severe menstrual irregularities, your PMS symptoms don't abate after your period starts, or you experience severe mood problems or feelings of being out of control.

Quick fix To relieve period pain and other premenstrual symptoms try **acupressure** *(p. 112)*. Press your thumb as firmly as you can on the Sanyinjiao point. This can be found behind your shin bone on the inside of your leg, four finger-widths above the top of the ankle bone. Pressure should be applied in cycles of six seconds of pressure and two seconds of rest for 20 minutes in all (two sessions of five minutes on each leg).

See also Diabetes and insulin resistance, Headaches

MIGRAINES

AROUND 10 PERCENT OF THE POPULATION suffer from migraines, which affect about three times as many women as men and are often related to menstruation and stress. Attacks vary in their frequency and can severely impair a person's quality of life.

In order to be classified as a migraine, a headache must last for four to 72 hours, and have at least two of the following symptoms: moderate to severe headache; throbbing pain; symptoms on one side of the head; symptoms exacerbated by movement. In addition, nausea, vomiting and/or sensitivity to light or noise must accompany these symptoms. Some people also experience a migraine "aura" that precedes the headache (typically involving visual disturbances). Although no natural remedies have been proven to halt a migraine attack once it's taken hold, some remedies may be able to help reduce migraine frequency and intensity.

Suggested remedies

Lifestyle factors Many migraine sufferers find their headaches occur following exposure to certain dietary and/or environmental triggers such as stress, chocolate, alcohol, bright light and interrupted sleep. Take steps to identify and avoid the factors that can trigger your attacks. An **elimination diet** *(p. 171)* and **journaling** *(p. 215)* may help with this. Adaptogens such as **holy basil** *(p. 205)* and **ashwagandha** *(p. 124)* may be helpful in coping with stress.

Butterbur (p. 139) Research suggests that butterbur *(Petasites hybridus)* may decrease the frequency of attacks by up to 60 percent and improve symptoms for at least half of all migraine sufferers.

Feverfew (p. 183) Feverfew has been the subject of numerous scientific studies, many of which support its long-held reputation for preventing migraine.

Acupuncture (p. 112) A 2009 *Cochrane Review* found that acupuncture reduces the frequency of migraines, and that when it is combined with pharmaceutical medicines that prevent migraine, sufferers report greater improvement and fewer side effects from their drug therapy.

Chiropractic (p. 152) According to an article published in the *Journal of Headache Pain* in 2011, regular spinal manipulation by a chiropractor may be as effective as some pharmaceutical medicines for the prevention of migraine.

See also Headaches, Nausea and vomiting

See your doctor

If you suspect you are experiencing migraines, talk to your doctor. Seek immediate medical assistance if you experience:

- ❖ severe headache that comes on very suddenly
- ❖ double vision, seizures, fever, numbness, difficulty speaking, loss of consciousness, or uncontrollable vomiting
- ❖ headache following an injury
- ❖ long-lasting headache that worsens when you cough, move suddenly, or exert yourself
- ❖ a migraine that lasts longer than 72 hours.

Quick fix Some migraine sufferers find that a strong cup of **coffee** *(p. 158)* at the start of a migraine can lessen the severity and even ward off an attack. The effect is thought to be due to caffeine, though scientists are still debating exactly how the chemical works to alleviate pain.

MOUTH ULCERS

THOUGH SMALL, MOUTH ULCERS CAN CAUSE misery. Defined as areas of erosion or loss of tissue on the mucous membranes inside the mouth, they can occur singly or in groups, are usually circular, with raised red tissue around the edges, and are very tender. Recurrent mouth ulcers may be referred to by the medical term aphthous stomatitis.

Mouth ulcers often arise after injury or irritation of the mucous membrane. They may also be a symptom of an underlying health problem such as a deficiency of certain nutrients, including iron, zinc, folic acid and vitamins B_6 and B_{12}; infections; food allergies or an adverse reaction to certain prescribed medicines.

After identifying and addressing any underlying health problems, your doctor may recommend you try a number of natural therapies.

Suggested remedies

Lifestyle factors Some experts believe mouth ulcers are more likely to occur during times of stress and fatigue, so get plenty of rest, and take steps to address your stress levels. Maintain good oral hygiene and rinse your mouth regularly with warm salted water or a herbal tea such as holy basil or licorice.

Dietary measures Depleted immunity may contribute to the development of mouth ulcers, so support your immune system by following a healthy diet.

Holy basil (p. 205) This herb has broad spectrum antibacterial activity along with anti-inflammatory and antioxidant activity that makes it an effective mouthwash to treat and prevent mouth ulcers, bad breath and gum disease.

Vitamin B_{12} (p. 303) High doses of vitamin B_{12} may help reduce outbreaks of aphthous stomatitis and the associated pain, regardless of the sufferer's initial vitamin B_{12} levels.

Propolis (p. 263) In a pilot study published in 2007, patients with aphthous stomatitis who took propolis capsules experienced fewer ulcer outbreaks than those who took placebo capsules.

See also Allergies, Frequent illness, Fungal infections, Herpes, Inflammatory bowel disease

See your doctor

Consult your doctor if your mouth ulcers:

❖ are large—about ½ inch (1 cm) across
❖ take a long time to resolve
❖ recur frequently
❖ interfere with your ability to eat properly.

Also seek medical assistance if you are concerned that an ulcer has become infected or may be symptomatic of an underlying health problem.

Quick fix In two small studies, daily applications of licorice *(p. 222)* extract in the form of a dissolving patch that adheres to the inside of the mouth reduced the size and pain of recurrent mouth ulcers. If licorice patches aren't available where you live, try making a strong cup of licorice tea and using it as a mouthwash several times per day.

NAIL PROBLEMS

MANY DIFFERENT ISSUES CAN AFFECT THE HEALTH and condition of the fingernails and toenails. The most common problems include:

- fungal infections that can cause the nails to thicken and deform; these infections can be difficult to treat
- bacterial infections of the tissue around the nail, which are often caused by the bacterium *Staphylococcus aureus* and cause the skin in the area to become painful, swollen and red
- psoriasis, which sometimes causes nails to become pitted, thickened and lift from the nail bed.

In addition, nails that are weak, brittle, prone to splitting or crumbling, or have horizontal or vertical ridges are sometimes (but not always) due to poor nutritional status. When problems occur, natural therapies may help restore your nail health.

Suggested remedies

Lifestyle factors Keep your feet clean and dry, change your socks regularly and avoid synthetic socks. Use gloves when you wash dishes and avoid using products like nail polish and artificial nails, which can cause damage and discoloration. Avoid cutting your cuticles or picking or tearing hangnails.

Dietary measures Nourish your nails by eating a healthy diet with a variety of fresh produce and lean sources of protein.

Biotin (p. 131) Taking biotin supplements may help strengthen and thicken brittle nails, and may prevent splitting.

Silica (p. 280) Preliminary research suggests that taking silica supplements in the form of orthosilicic acid improves the condition of brittle nails. Horsetail and nettle are good sources of silica and can be taken as a tea.

Tea tree (p. 293) Topical applications of tea tree oil have been shown to improve fungal nail infections. Laboratory studies suggest that it may also be effective against some bacterial infections, including *Staphylococcus aureus*.

See also Fungal infections, Psoriasis

See your doctor

Certain chronic health problems, such as rheumatoid arthritis, heart disease and lung disease, can cause deformation of the nails, so your doctor should investigate any abnormalities—especially if changes develop quickly.

Quick fix Want smooth hands and soft cuticles in a flash? Put about a tablespoonful (15 ml) of brown sugar into your cupped palm, add a similar quantity of lemon juice, then rub your hands together for a few moments (taking care to avoid any areas of broken skin). Gently work the mixture into your cuticles to moisturize and soften them. When you're done, rinse off under running water.

NATURAL FERTILITY MANAGEMENT

HAVING CHILDREN SEEMS LIKE THE most natural thing in the world, yet around one in six people of both sexes encounters difficulties—as a result of medical problems or, more frequently, due to less specific low or "sub" fertility. It can be incredibly stressful, but there are steps you can take to make sure you are giving yourself the best chance. A healthy diet and some lifestyle changes can make all the difference. A few natural remedies may also help.

Suggested remedies

Lifestyle factors Quit smoking and cut down on, or better still cut out, alcohol. Lose any excess weight, since being overweight is linked to poor sperm quality in men, and lower fertility and miscarriage in women. Reduce exposure to industrial chemicals, excessive dust and air pollution, X-rays and heavy metals as they can all reduce fertility. Take steps to relax and relieve stress, with therapies such as **aromatherapy** *(p. 122)* and **massage** *(p. 230)*.

Dietary measures For men, cutting back on animal protein and fat, and eating more carbohydrates and foods rich in fiber, folic acid and lycopene, including fruit and vegetables for their antioxidants, can improve sperm health. In women, reducing caffeine intake, consuming less animal protein and more pulses and grains, fewer trans fats and more monounsaturated fats, such as olive oil, can help boost fertility. It is also important to identify any food allergies or intolerances and to consume mostly organic food as pesticides have been shown to reduce sperm quality.

Propolis (p. 263) In one small Egyptian study, 60 percent of women who took propolis daily became pregnant compared to 20 percent in the placebo group.

Chasteberry (p. 148) Just over a quarter of women taking a nutritional supplement containing chasteberry, green tea, L-arginine, vitamins and minerals became pregnant in a US study published in 2006, compared to a tenth in the control group.

Black cohosh (p. 133) When women taking the fertility drug clomiphene combined it with black cohosh, many more became pregnant than those who took clomiphene alone.

Zinc (p. 319) Combined with folic acid (but not alone), zinc helps to increase sperm concentration. In one Dutch study, the combination boosted the sperm count of subfertile men by 74 percent. **Folic acid** *(p. 189)* supplements are recommended for women who are trying to conceive to lessen the risk of birth defects.

See your doctor

If you've been trying for a child for a year or more (or less if the woman is aged over 35), see your doctor to help identify potential fertility problems.

Quick fix Relax and have sex with your partner as often as you can, preferably in the traditional "missionary" position, which offers the deepest penetration, delivering sperm close to the uterus.

See also Overweight and obesity, Sexual problems

NAUSEA AND VOMITING

NAUSEA IS THE FEELING OF UNEASE THAT you have in your stomach that makes you feel as though you want to vomit. Nausea and vomiting are not conditions within themselves, they're symptoms of other conditions such as gut infections, food allergies, cancer treatment, migraines, seasickness, severe pain or early pregnancy. Indeed, pregnant women have been the subject of much research about natural nausea remedies.

Suggested remedies

Dietary measures If you're able to eat, choose bland foods–nothing spicy or greasy. Pay attention to **hydration** *(p. 209)*, too. Choose clear liquids such as water and rehydration drinks, or herbal teas (hot or cold) made with herbs such as ginger, mint, cloves, cinnamon, fennel, aniseed and lemon or a combination that can be sweetened with honey. Sip small amounts and give children liquids by teaspoon or syringe to prevent repeated vomiting.

Ginger *(p. 192)* In Chinese medicine, ginger has been a favored remedy for stomach upsets, diarrhea and nausea for more than 2,000 years. In a randomized, placebo-controlled study of pregnant Thai mothers, 88 percent of those given ginger had improved nausea symptoms compared to 29 percent taking the placebo.

Vitamin B_6 *(p. 302)* A randomized, double-blind, placebo-controlled study on pregnant mothers in *Obstetrics and Gynecology* looked at the effectiveness of 25 mg of vitamin B_6 given every eight hours to control vomiting. After three days, only 26 percent of patients in the vitamin B_6 group vomited, compared to 54 percent of the placebo group.

Cold therapy *(p. 161)* A cold compress placed on the forehead will soothe feelings of nausea, especially if the symptoms are associated with a migraine.

See also Gastroenteritis

See your doctor

Go directly to the emergency room if you think the vomiting is related to poisoning or you notice blood or coffee-colored material in your vomit. Call your doctor if:

- ❖ you vomit more than three times in a day or if the vomiting lasts for longer than 24 hours
- ❖ you are unable to keep any fluids down for 12 hours
- ❖ you have a stiff neck or severe belly pain.

Quick fix Pressure on the sixth point on the Pericardium pathway in Chinese medicine, the exact point targeted by a motion sickness bracelet, quickly calms an upset stomach. (See Acupuncture and acupressure, *p. 112*.) Gently press your middle and index finger on the point about 2 inches (5 cm) above your wrist crease on the palm side, right in between the two tendons.

NEURALGIA

NEURALGIA IS THE MEDICAL TERM FOR nerve pain, which is often described as sharp, burning, cold or like an electric shock, and is sometimes accompanied by numbness, itching or tingling. The pain varies in severity from mild to excruciating, and tends to be localized to a specific area. It may be constant or sporadic, and although often temporary, it affects some people for many years.

Neuralgia is triggered by inflammation of the affected nerve, which can be due to many different causes, including pressure on a nerve (such as sciatica, trigeminal neuralgia and carpal tunnel syndrome), nerve injury or infection (such as shingles). Treatment varies according to its cause and severity, and may involve making changes to your lifestyle to relieve pressure on affected nerves, as well as taking medication to relieve pain. Different natural therapies may also bring some relief.

Suggested remedies

Musculoskeletal manipulation Therapies such as **chiropractic** *(p. 152)* and **osteopathy** *(p. 251)* may help restore nerve function and improve joint mobility in carpal tunnel syndrome. Some research suggests that spinal manipulation may also be beneficial for sciatica.

Acupuncture (p. 112) Acupuncture may relieve symptoms of carpal tunnel syndrome and trigeminal neuralgia.

TENS and electro-acupuncture (p. 294) These work in a similar way to acupuncture but can be performed at home using small electronic devices that deliver electrical impulses to affected areas. Some neuralgia sufferers find they offer relief.

Relaxation (p. 269) Methods of calming the mind, including deep breathing, **meditation** *(p. 234)* and **hypnotherapy** *(p. 211)*, may help you to cope with the pain of intractable neuralgia and lessen its impact on your daily life.

Quick fix In some countries, neuralgia is treated with high-strength patches containing capsaicin (see Cayenne, *p. 145*). A single application may provide long-term pain relief, but needs to be applied by a doctor (often using local anesthetic as the process is painful). Capsaicin creams are also available, but are not as potent or long lasting as the patches, and need to be used more regularly.

See your doctor

It is important that the cause of neuralgia is investigated and addressed as quickly as possible. Severe pain, muscle weakness, numbness or loss of control of the limbs, bladder or bowel all warrant immediate medical attention.

WATCH OUT!

Deficiency of vitamin B_6 has been associated with carpal tunnel syndrome, and high doses of vitamin B_6 have been used to treat the condition. However, current research suggests the remedy is not effective.

See also Back and neck pain, Chronic pain, Shingles

OSTEOARTHRITIS

OSTEOARTHRITIS OCCURS WHEN THE cartilage lining of a joint deteriorates or is damaged and can no longer perform its normal functions of acting as a shock absorber and enabling the bones of the joint to glide smoothly against each other. Symptoms include joint pain, stiffness, inflammation and reduced mobility. The muscles, ligaments and tendons around the affected joint may weaken, and the joints may develop bony growths on them called spurs. The joints most commonly affected are in the knees, hips, spine and hands. There are natural remedies that may help to relieve your symptoms.

Suggested remedies

Lifestyle factors Management strategies often include weight loss to help relieve the pressure on weight-bearing joints and light **exercise** *(p. 175)* to help maintain joint mobility and improve muscle strength. **Tai chi** *(p. 290)* is particularly recommended.

Glucosamine (p. 196) Many clinical studies have shown that glucosamine and chondroitin supplements relieve osteoarthritis pain, reduce joint swelling and improve mobility.

SAMe (p. 276) S-adenosyl-L-methionine (SAMe) has been the focus of numerous clinical trials, some of which have shown it to be as effective as pharmaceutical drugs for treating osteoarthritis.

Boswellia (p. 136) Research suggests that in osteoarthritis, this Ayurvedic remedy relieves pain, tenderness, swelling, stiffness and creaking of the joints, and makes movement less painful.

Rose hips (p. 271) Rose hips contain galactolipids, which have anti-inflammatory properties and may help relieve osteoarthritis pain.

Celery seed (p. 146) Australian research found that celery seed extract, taken over several weeks, helped reduce painful joints in people with long-standing arthritic pain.

Green-lipped mussels (p. 201) In recent clinical trials, green-lipped mussel extract has shown promise in reducing osteoarthritis pain and improving mobility.

Devil's claw (p. 168) Some research suggests that this herb may be as effective as commercial painkillers at relieving arthritic pain.

Ginger (p. 192) The anti-inflammatory properties of ginger account for its ability to alleviate arthritic pain.

Stretching (p. 286) A tailored program of stretches can help ease the joint pain associated with osteoarthritis.

See your doctor

Many different conditions can cause joint pain, so see your doctor for investigation and diagnosis. Seek medical attention if your joint pain:

❖ is accompanied by a fever or rash, or sensations of heat or warmth in the affected area
❖ starts or worsens suddenly or progresses to additional joints
❖ prevents you using your joint properly.

Quick fix At least five clinical trials have found the topical use of capsaicin gel to be effective for relieving joint pain and other symptoms of osteoarthritis (see Cayenne, *p. 145*). However, some patients experience adverse effects such as burning sensations and redness—which is not surprising given that capsaicin is the compound that makes cayenne peppers hot!

See also Chronic pain, Overweight and obesity, Rheumatoid arthritis

OSTEOPOROSIS

OSTEOPOROSIS IS A CONDITION IN WHICH the bones become progressively more brittle and easily fractured. These changes occur when calcium (which the skeleton needs for its strength and structure) is lost from the bones more rapidly than the body can replace it, leading to an ongoing decline in bone mineral density and mass.

Osteoporosis is often symptom-free, and sufferers may be unaware they're affected until a fracture occurs, commonly in the bones of the hips, spine, ribs or arms. Osteoporosis becomes more prevalent in both sexes with age. Women's risk of developing the condition increases markedly after menopause due to declining estrogen levels.

It's never too early or too late to take steps to reduce your risk for osteoporosis and improve your bone health.

Suggested remedies

Lifestyle factors There are steps you can take to help prevent osteoporosis such as maintaining a healthy body weight and getting regular **exercise** *(p. 175)*. Resistive or weight-bearing forms of exercise such as **walking** *(p. 309)* and lifting weights are best, unless advised otherwise by your doctor. Smoking increases the risk of developing osteoporosis, and should be avoided.

Dietary measures Make sure your diet includes plenty of foods rich in **calcium** *(p. 140)* and **magnesium** *(p. 227)*. Avoid excessive consumption of alcohol, caffeinated beverages or soft drinks.

Calcium (p. 140) Calcium is vital for the prevention of osteoporosis and maintenance of bone density; however, many people don't get enough from their diets and need to take supplements. Many people also have low levels of **vitamin D** *(p 305)*, which helps absorb calcium and, in older people, may help prevent falls and fractures.

Minerals Other nutrients that may help maintain bone health and prevent osteoporosis include boron, copper, **zinc** *(p. 319)*, manganese and **silica** *(p. 280)*.

Soy (p. 285) Eating soy foods or taking soy isoflavone supplements may help prevent postmenopausal bone loss.

See your doctor

Seek emergency medical care if you think you may have a fracture. You should also see your doctor if you've become unsteady on your feet and prone to falling.

Quick fix While there's no quick fix for osteoporosis, you can reduce your risk of fracturing a bone in a matter of hours by eliminating hazards around your home that could cause you to trip or fall. Simple tips include removing floor rugs and keeping thoroughfares clear of obstacles.

See also Fall prevention, Menopausal symptoms, Rheumatoid arthritis

OVERWEIGHT AND OBESITY

FOR MOST PEOPLE, BEING OVERWEIGHT is defined as having a body mass index (BMI) greater than 25. A BMI greater than 30 is classified as obese. To calculate your BMI, enter your height and weight—English and metric versions—at the Mayo Clinic's BMI Calculator page on their website (www.mayoclinic.org).

Being overweight or obese increases your risk of health problems such as heart disease, diabetes and arthritis. Some of these risks are elevated in those who carry their excess weight around their belly. Weight issues are usually due to a poor diet (consuming excessive quantities of foods that are high in calories, fat or sugar) and/or low levels of physical activity. Other contributing factors can include genetics, hormonal imbalances, stress and the use of certain prescribed medicines.

The core of any weight-loss program involves changing your diet and exercising more. While there's no magic pill that can make you lose weight, there are some natural therapies available that can support your efforts.

Suggested remedies

Dietary measures Find a sensible diet you can stick to for life that includes plenty of vegetables and fruits and healthy fats rather than a short-term weight-loss diet. Expect to lose weight gradually—no more than about 2 pounds (1 kg) per week—rather than in a rapid burst, which is likely to result in rebound weight gain. A 2007 *Cochrane Review* concluded that low-glycemic index diets lead to greater reductions in body weight, BMI, body fat and cholesterol than other diets, and may be easier to stick to.

Exercise (p. 175) Combining dietary changes with increased exercise results in greater weight loss than diet alone. Find something you enjoy and do it regularly.

Garcinia (p. 190) This herb, and in particular a compound it contains called hydroxycitric acid (HCA), may aid weight loss by increasing sensations of fullness and inhibiting the conversion of carbohydrates into fat.

Coffee (p. 158) In recent research trials, overweight people who took green coffee extracts standardized for their chlorogenic acid content experienced greater reductions in body weight, body fat and BMI than those who took placebo supplements.

See your doctor

See your doctor if you are concerned your weight is impacting your health. Sudden, unexplained weight gain or loss warrants immediate medical investigation.

DID YOU KNOW?

There are no quick fixes for losing weight, but here are some tips for keeping the weight off. Research shows that people who lose significant amounts of weight and successfully keep it off over the long term are those who are very physically active, monitor their weight regularly, don't skip breakfast, and don't deviate from their healthy, low-fat diet—even on the weekend!

See also Diabetes and insulin resistance, Menopausal symptoms

PHOBIAS

FROM SPIDERS AND HEIGHTS TO INJECTIONS and dental checkups, almost anything that can trigger fear and panic can become a phobia. Some of these anxieties are scary inconveniences but others–such as a fear of injections or of driving over tall bridges–can get in the way of good health, work and even relationships. Nondrug approaches are often a cornerstone of care for overcoming a phobia.

Suggested remedies

Lifestyle factors Take your troubles down to the gym as part of a regular **exercise** *(p. 175)* regime. In a recent US study, a vigorous workout eased tension for people with "high anxiety sensitivity"–an intense fear of the nausea, dizziness and racing heart that come with panic.

Dietary measures Reducing your intake of sugar, caffeine and alcohol can help you feel less anxious; at the same time follow a healthy diet. Check for food intolerances, too, and eliminate culprits. An **elimination diet** *(p. 171)* may help with this.

Cognitive behavioral therapy (p. 159) In 12–16 sessions, CBT may gently help to replace phobic fears with more realistic attitudes and expectations according to the Anxiety and Depression Association of America.

Hypnotherapy (p. 211) Many mental health professionals recommend hypnotherapy to help ease the worry, nervousness and panic associated with phobias. In a Dutch study, hypnotherapy helped 55 percent of people with dental phobias stay on track with recommended dental appointments.

Relaxation (p. 269) In a 2008 review of 27 studies, researchers at Italy's San Giuseppe Hospital concluded that all sorts of relaxation techniques can ease the anxiety that comes with a phobia. In a US study, brain scans of 16 people with social anxiety disorder showed that mindfulness-based stress reduction (see **Meditation**, *p. 234*) helped by reducing activity in a part of the brain that processes negative emotions.

Acupuncture (p. 112) Ear acupuncture has been shown to help people deal with dental anxiety and receive dental treatment they would have otherwise avoided.

Yoga (p. 316) In a recent small US study, yoga increased gamma-aminobutyric acid (GABA), a calming brain chemical. Yoga breathing has also been shown to tame tension.

See your doctor

If a phobia is interfering with your well-being, it's time to seek help. Many of the natural strategies listed here will require help from a therapist.

Quick fix During a phobia-induced panic attack, rapid breathing may reduce the levels of carbon dioxide in your bloodstream—further contributing to panic symptoms. Calm, slow, deep breathing is a better alternative, while rebreathing into a paper bag will help raise carbon dioxide levels.

DID YOU KNOW?
Slowly getting used to a phobia trigger, with the help of a therapist, can reduce feelings of distress and panic. In one 2008 Norwegian study of 375 people with social anxiety, exposure therapy worked better than an antidepressant.

See also Anxiety, Food intolerances

PROSTATE PROBLEMS

MANY OLDER MEN EXPERIENCE PROSTATE problems, particularly benign prostatic hyperplasia (BPH), a condition where enlargement of the prostate gland puts pressure on the urethra, interfering with normal urination. Scientists are not sure what causes BPH. One theory is that it's a consequence of the hormonal changes that occur as men age, which include reduced levels of testosterone and increased levels of dihydrotestosterone (DHT) and estrogen in prostate tissue. Genetic factors may also play a role.

Symptoms of BPH include needing to get up at night to urinate (nocturia), difficulty starting to urinate, intermittent urinary flow, incontinence, the sensation that the bladder has not completely emptied, and recurrent urinary tract infections. Similar symptoms are also associated with prostate cancer and prostatitis (inflammation of the prostate, often caused by infection), so you should never ignore them.

In addition to lifestyle and dietary changes, there are herbal medicines that may aid the management of BPH and relieve its symptoms.

Suggested remedies

Lifestyle factors Steps you can take to look after your prostate include maintaining a healthy body weight and getting regular exercise *(p. 175)*.

Dietary measures Avoid high-fat foods (especially high-fat dairy products), limit your intake of red meat (especially processed meats such as sausages) and eat plenty of fruit and vegetables as part of a healthy diet.

Saw palmetto (p. 278) Saw palmetto has been investigated in numerous clinical trials, many of which indicate that it can improve urinary function in BPH.

Pygeum (p. 265) A 2011 *Cochrane Review* concluded that pygeum provides moderate relief from BPH symptoms.

Nettle (p. 244) Research indicates that stinging nettle may relieve BPH symptoms when taken alone or in combination with saw palmetto or pygeum.

DID YOU KNOW?

Tomatoes contain an antioxidant called lycopene, which is particularly beneficial for the prostate. Population studies have shown that men who consume large quantities of lycopene in their diets have a reduced risk of prostate cancer. Tomato paste *(p. 297)* and tomato sauce offer a concentrated supply, and when consumed with olive oil, the lycopene becomes more available.

See your doctor

Your doctor should investigate all prostate symptoms so that their cause can be determined. Annual screening for prostate cancer is recommended for all men over 50 years old and from 40 years old for those with a family history of the condition. Seek prompt medical attention if you experience:

- ❖ blood or pus in the urine
- ❖ a complete inability to urinate
- ❖ pain in your lower back (beneath your rib cage)
- ❖ a fever or chills in conjunction with urinary symptoms.

See also Incontinence, Urinary tract infections

PSORIASIS

SYMPTOMS OF THIS CONDITION INCLUDE raised red patches of itchy, flaky skin that are covered with thick, silvery scales. These plaques appear on the elbows, knees and scalp. Sometimes the nails are also affected, appearing as though they've been pricked with a pin. Around a third of sufferers experience psoriatic arthritis, with pain, swelling and tenderness of one or more joints accompanying the skin symptoms.

The causes of psoriasis are not fully understood though it is thought to be associated with immune system dysfunction. It is sometimes triggered by stress, illness or medication use.

People with psoriasis have an increased risk of some other health conditions (including heart disease, diabetes and depression), so it's vital you keep an eye on your general health. Natural therapies may help you manage your symptoms.

Suggested remedies

Lifestyle factors Keep your skin clean to prevent infection but avoid harsh soaps. Try not to scratch your skin lesions, as this may worsen them, and use moisturizer to prevent your skin drying out. Take regular exercise *(p. 175)* and stop smoking. Try to avoid skin trauma and sunburn, which can aggravate the condition.

Dietary measures Follow a healthy diet (as discussed in the introduction). Some people benefit from a gluten-free diet *(p. 198)*.

Omega-3 fatty acids (p. 250) Taking omega-3s while using standard topical treatment for psoriasis reduces itching, redness and skin scaling, and improves quality of life. It may be helpful to simultaneously avoid "bad fats" such as those found in red meat and processed foods.

Vitamin D (p. 305) Topical treatment with creams containing natural or synthetic versions of vitamin D can relieve psoriasis, but may cause side effects. Ask your doctor for more information.

Aloe vera *(p. 117)* *Aloe vera* cream or lotion and/or apple cider vinegar *(p. 120)* may be beneficial for psoriasis, although research has so far yielded mixed results.

Light therapy (p. 223) Harnessing the therapeutic effects of ultraviolet (UV) rays, specialists sometimes treat psoriasis with light therapy. Your doctor will refer you to a dermatologist for this.

See your doctor

See your doctor if you're concerned you may have psoriasis or psoriatic arthritis, or if you've been diagnosed with psoriasis and experience:

❖ symptoms of infection, including pain, swelling, heat, fever or pus

❖ plaques that are more extensive, inflamed or painful than usual

❖ symptoms that may be side effects of your prescribed medicines.

Quick fix Many psoriasis sufferers swear by an old-fashioned oatmeal bath to soothe itchy skin and loosen plaques. Place 2 tablespoons (30 ml) of fine oatmeal in some clean pantyhose or muslin and tie it into a ball. Place the ball in the bath while you fill it with warm water then use it to gently sponge your skin.

See also Depression, Diabetes and insulin resistance, Heart and circulatory health

RAYNAUD'S DISEASE

RAYNAUD'S DISEASE (RD) IS A CONDITION in which the blood vessels of the extremities periodically constrict in response to stress or cold temperatures, dramatically restricting circulation to the fingers and toes (and sometimes the nose and ears). During an attack, the skin first turns white as the blood vessels spasm, then blue due to a lack of oxygenated blood, and finally red as blood flow to the affected area is restored. The extremities may feel cold or numb, and then start to throb or tingle when blood flow recommences.

In most cases, no underlying disease is responsible. Less frequently, it may be a symptom of a health problem (where it is referred to as Raynaud's phenomenon) such as the autoimmune conditions rheumatoid arthritis and scleroderma. Natural therapies that help maintain healthy circulation may reduce the number and intensity of Raynaud's attacks.

Suggested remedies

Lifestyle factors Keeping yourself warm is vital to managing Raynaud's and minimizing its impact on your life. Regular exercise *(p. 175)* may help by encouraging circulation. Reduce your caffeine intake and stop smoking cigarettes as they contribute to blood vessel constriction. Protect your hands and feet from injury and avoid the use of constricting rings or footwear. Also avoid the use of vibrating power tools as vibrations can trigger an attack.

Ginkgo (p. 193) In a study published in the journal *Vascular Medicine* in 2002, a standardized *Ginkgo biloba* preparation reduced the number of Raynaud's attacks experienced per day by 56 percent.

Vitamin D (p. 305) A study published in the journal *Rheumatology International* in 2013 suggests that a large proportion of people affected by Raynaud's have low levels of vitamin D, and that monthly megadoses of vitamin D may help reduce symptoms.

Acupuncture (p. 112) Acupuncture may help reduce the frequency, duration and severity of Raynaud's episodes.

See your doctor

See your doctor if you suspect you have RD; it is important that any underlying cause is identified and treated. If you have been diagnosed with RD, seek medical attention if ulcers or sores develop on your fingers or toes, or if attacks only affect one side of your body.

Quick fix If you experience a Raynaud's attack, using heat therapy *(p. 204)* to warm yourself helps limit its duration. You can expect it to take 15 minutes for your blood flow to return to normal after you've warmed up.

See also Heart and circulatory health

RHEUMATOID ARTHRITIS

RHEUMATOID ARTHRITIS (RA) IS AN autoimmune disease that causes inflammation and swelling of the joints. It affects multiple joints on both sides of the body (often in the hands and feet)–making them stiff, tender, hot, swollen and painful to move–as well as affecting internal organs. The damage to the joints and cartilage leads to deformities, and can affect nearby muscles, tendons and ligaments. Fatigue, mood problems and lumpy growths beneath the skin called rheumatoid nodules are other common symptoms.

The cause of RA has not been determined, but genetic factors are strongly involved, and smoking is a known risk factor. The onset of RA is often triggered by stress or infection. In addition to adjustments to your lifestyle and diet, your doctor may also recommend certain natural therapies to ameliorate the symptoms.

Suggested remedies

Lifestyle factors Try to lower your stress levels and get regular exercise *(p. 175)*, tailored to your capability. These factors can help manage your RA and reduce the associated increased risk of other health problems such as heart disease and osteoporosis.

Dietary measures Work with your doctor to determine whether changing your diet affects your RA; common approaches include Mediterranean, gluten-free and vegan diets rich in antioxidants and healthy fats. You may need to follow an elimination diet *(p. 171)* aimed at identifying foods that exacerbate your condition.

Omega-3 fatty acids (p. 250) The fatty acids in fish oil reduce RA pain, the number of tender joints, and the duration of morning stiffness. High doses may be required, under the supervision of your doctor, and it may take three months or more before improvements are noticeable. Fish oil is sometimes taken with evening primrose *(p. 174)* oil, which has also been shown to improve the symptoms of RA.

Rose hips (p. 271) The fruit of the dog rose is rich in phytonutrients including a galactolipid that has potent anti-inflammatory activity. Preliminary clinical studies suggest a standardized preparation can assist RA sufferers.

Vitamin D (p. 305) Having inadequate vitamin D appears to increase the risk of developing RA, and may be linked to the severity of the disease. It is not yet known whether increasing vitamin D levels improves symptoms.

Celery seed (p. 146) Celery seed extract is a traditional treatment for relieving the joint pain associated with RA.

See your doctor

Early diagnosis and treatment can help minimize joint and tissue damage. See your doctor if your joint pain:

- affects more than one joint at a time
- makes your joints swollen, tender or hot
- is accompanied by fever or morning stiffness.

Quick fix You can obtain rapid relief from arthritis through heat therapy *(p. 204)* and cold therapy *(p. 161)*, which may even temporarily raise your pain threshold. Many RA sufferers report feeling better after exercising in a warm water hydrotherapy *(p. 210)* pool than after land-based forms of exercise, as the water relaxes muscles and supports the weight of the body.

See also Chronic pain, Fatigue, Osteoarthritis

SCALP AND HAIR PROBLEMS

HAIR CAN FALL ON EITHER END OF THE greasy/dry continuum, based on factors such as genetics, hygiene, hormones and nutrition. Oily hair is often the result of overactive hormones (due to puberty, pregnancy, menopause or certain medicines). It can also be caused by deficiencies in vitamin B_2, riboflavin or essential fatty acids. Dry hair is usually associated with general aging or from damage caused by excess sun, heat or chemicals. Dandruff can occur with oily or dry hair; or may be due to an underlying condition such as psoriasis, fungal infection or eczema. Fortunately all minor problems respond to natural remedies and there are several to try.

Suggested remedies

Dietary measures For shiny, healthy hair, make sure you are eating a healthy diet that provides a good variety of fresh produce and plenty of vitamins and minerals.

Tea tree (p. 293) The antimicrobial properties of tea tree oil make it a first-line treatment for dandruff. Find a mild shampoo that contains 5 percent tea tree oil.

Apple cider vinegar (p. 120) Vinegar can act as conditioner, shine-enhancer, dandruff-fighter and frizz tamer. Add a tablespoon to your hair after washing to condition it; rinse well in the shower.

Avocados (p. 126) Mash up an overripe avocado, spread it on your hair, and leave it in for an hour to encourage speedier hair growth. Rinse well with warm water.

Tea (p. 292) Oily hair may respond to a tea rinse. The tannic acid in tea acts as an astringent, helping your hair release any excess oil.

Lemon (p. 220) The juice of one lemon mixed with 1 cup (250 ml) of water makes a rinse to control dandruff and get rid of shampoo buildup that weighs hair down.

Olive oil (p. 249) Relieve an itchy dry scalp by rubbing in some warm oil to which you can also add a few drops of tea tree *(p. 293)* essential oil. After you rub it on, cover your hair with a cap and leave it on overnight, then shampoo and rinse the oil out in the morning. Coconut oil can be used instead of olive oil.

Quick fix All kinds of hair benefit from bicarbonate of soda *(p. 130)*. It clarifies oily hair, makes dry hair shiny and helps get rid of dandruff. Start with wet or dry hair. Mix one part bicarbonate of soda with three parts water and work the paste from roots to ends. Leave for a few minutes, then rinse with warm water. Add an apple cider vinegar rinse for extra shine.

See also Eczema and dermatitis, Fungal infections, Psoriasis

SEASONAL AFFECTIVE DISORDER

THE SHORTER DAYS OF AUTUMN AND WINTER can trigger a syndrome known as seasonal affective disorder (SAD), marked by depression, fatigue, carbohydrate craving, weight gain, excess sleeping and loss of libido. When days shorten, the brain's pineal gland responds to darkness by releasing an excess of melatonin, wreaking havoc on sleep/wake rhythms and energy levels. Most SAD resolves itself in the spring, but natural remedies can help you through the winter months.

Suggested remedies

Dietary measures SAD often causes carbohydrate cravings, possibly due to the body's attempt to boost energy levels, but sugar and starches give a brief boost followed by a sugar crash after which the cravings intensify. Follow a healthy diet, particularly a diet that keeps your blood glucose steady, and try to avoid alcohol and caffeine, which can exacerbate mood swings. Increase foods containing tryptophan–such as turkey, eggs and dairy products–which helps your body generate more serotonin, a mood-calming brain chemical.

Melatonin *(p. 237)* The optimal interval between melatonin release and mid-sleep is six hours-but 71 percent of SAD sufferers have shorter intervals. Melatonin supplements in the afternoon can lengthen intervals and double improvement in depression scores.

Vitamin D *(p. 305)* Increased exposure to natural light decreases incidents of SAD, partly because the skin is producing mood-elevating vitamin D. Aim to get some gentle late afternoon sun on your skin each day.

Light therapy *(p. 223)* Our brain needs 5,000 lux of sunlight to operate correctly; the average office has 400. Use full spectrum lighting where possible and consider bright light therapy with a special lamp that is designed to mimic early morning full daylight (2,500–10,000 lux) without the harmful ultraviolet (UV) rays.

Sleeping strategies *(p. 281)* Help your struggling body clock retain its fragile rhythm by maintaining regular times for bed and rise-and-shine. Try a daily walk at dawn and dusk. It signals to your suprachiasmatic nucleus–your internal body clock–to adjust to the correct time.

Acupuncture *(p. 112)* Acupuncture can help regulate melatonin secretions, and improve your sleeping patterns.

See your doctor

SAD can lead to depression, which always requires medical attention. See your doctor if you experience intense sadness accompanied by feelings of helplessness or hopelessness, or trouble sleeping or eating. If you ever consider hurting yourself, call a help line such as The Samaritans or Lifeline.

Quick fix SAD is rarely found in countries within 30 degrees of the Equator, where there is sunshine all year round. The Canadian Mental Health Association recommends a winter vacation in a sunny destination for temporary relief of SAD symptoms. Symptoms usually recur after the return home, unfortunately.

See *also* Depression, Fatigue, Sexual problems, Sleeping problems

SEXUAL PROBLEMS

DON'T BE EMBARRASSED ABOUT YOUR SEXUAL concerns—these issues are very common and often respond well to treatment. Both men and women can experience problems that prevent them from fully enjoying sex, including: lack of desire; inability to become aroused or maintain arousal; pain during intercourse; and orgasm problems (either an inability to orgasm, or in men, premature ejaculation).

Underlying causes of sexual dysfunction may include psychological and emotional issues and a wide range of health problems including diabetes, cardiovascular disease and hormonal imbalances. Sexual dysfunction can also be an adverse effect of some prescribed medicines, including antidepressants. Your doctor can advise you on natural remedies and other treatments that can help.

Suggested remedies

Lifestyle factors Avoid alcohol as it can impair sexual function and quit smoking as it can lead to atherosclerosis and constricted blood vessels, and in turn reduced blood flow to the genitalia. Reduce performance anxiety by focusing on the moment rather than the endpoint and make sex fun. Engaging in nonsexual touch and learning to authentically share your feelings can create greater intimacy and lead to more fulfilling sex.

Ginseng (p. 194) Research has shown Korean ginseng root to be of benefit for erectile dysfunction and men's sexual desire and it may also enhance sexual arousal in menopausal women.

Maca (p. 226) Some (but not all) studies show that maca improves sexual functioning and desire in men and menopausal women. It may also improve erectile dysfunction, sperm health, mood problems and energy levels.

Acupuncture (p. 112) In a clinical trial published in the *Journal of Alternative and Complementary Medicine*, acupuncture improved antidepressant-induced sexual problems in both men and women.

WATCH OUT!

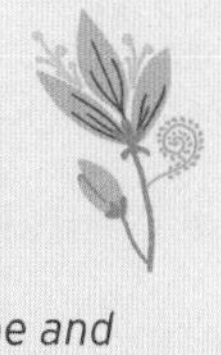

In some countries, yohimbine is available for the treatment of low libido and erectile dysfunction. It's derived from the bark of the yohimbe tree, which is a traditional male sexual tonic in parts of Africa. Despite their natural origins, yohimbe and yohimbine should be taken only under medical supervision. They can cause serious adverse effects, especially if taken to excess.

See your doctor

Seek medical advice if sexual problems are causing you or your partner pain or distress. Men should also seek immediate medical help if they:

❖ experience an erection lasting longer than three hours

❖ have taken prescription medicine for erectile dysfunction and are experiencing chest pain

❖ experience erection problems after an injury affecting any part of the lower body

❖ experience erection problems with symptoms of fever and abdominal or urinary tract pain.

Women should see their doctor if they experience pain or bleeding during intercourse.

See also Depression, Diabetes and insulin resistance, Heart and circulatory health, Menopausal symptoms

SHINGLES

SHINGLES IS A SKIN CONDITION CAUSED by the varicella zoster virus (VZV). The same virus is responsible for causing chicken pox, after which it remains dormant in the nerve cells, manifesting as shingles if it is reactivated—often at times when the patient's immune system is run down. Since VZV is present in nerve cells, the extremely painful, fluid-filled blisters that characterize shingles follow the path of the affected nerve, often forming a band around a specific part of the body. The skin lesions and pain usually resolve after four to six weeks, although some people continue to experience the nerve pain long after the skin lesions have healed—sometimes for months or years. This is called postherpetic neuralgia (PHN), and is most common in older people and those who have shingles near the eye or on other parts of the face.

There is no cure for shingles, but if you have had chicken pox, talk to your doctor or pharmacist about getting the shingles vaccine. If you do get shingles, natural therapies can play a valuable role in managing the condition.

Suggested remedies

Lifestyle factors Adequate sleep and regular exercise *(p. 175)* as well as a healthy diet will help support a healthy immune system and offer important protection against shingles.

Cold therapy (p. 161) Applying cold packs or compresses made with chamomile *(p. 147)* or other soothing teas can help relieve pain and reduce inflammation.

Acupuncture (p. 112) In one study, acupuncture was found to be as effective as standard treatments for acute shingles pain. Electrical stimulation (see TENS and electroacupuncture, *p. 294*) is sometimes used in conjunction with acupuncture, and may be beneficial for the prevention and treatment of PHN.

Vitamin C (p. 304) In a study of patients with acute shingles, administration of intravenous vitamin C in addition to regular treatment improved pain, fatigue and concentration and reduced the distribution and quantity of shingles lesions.

Multivitamins (p. 240) People with PHN may have low levels of calcium, zinc, vitamin C and other nutrients, so a good multivitamin supplement may be beneficial.

See also Chronic pain, Frequent illness, Neuralgia

See your doctor

If you're concerned that you may have shingles or PHN, see your doctor as quickly as possible. The earlier that treatment with antiviral medication is begun, the greater the likelihood of reducing the severity of an attack.

Quick fix Capsaicin relieves PHN when applied topically as a cream or patch (see Cayenne, *p. 145*). High-strength patches are particularly effective and provide rapid pain relief that is sustained for weeks at a time after being applied to the affected area for just an hour. Use of the patches can be painful, however, and they need to be applied by a doctor, sometimes after applying a local anesthetic.

SINUSITIS

SINUSITIS (MORE CORRECTLY KNOWN by the medical term rhinosinusitis) causes inflammation of the mucous membranes that line the sinus and nasal cavities, along with mucus congestion of the sinuses themselves, which are the hollow spaces in the bones of the face, nose and eyes. Additional symptoms can include headache, pain and fullness in the face, toothache, fatigue, fever (especially if infection is present), bouts of coughing and a reduced sense of smell.

Acute sinusitis is usually a symptom of an infection, the cause of which may be viral or bacterial. Chronic rhinosinusitis (CRS) is sinusitis that lasts for at least 12 weeks. It often involves persistent low-grade symptoms that may be intermittently worsened by acute episodes of infection. Contributing factors may include bone abnormalities, allergy, poor immunity and exposure to respiratory irritants. People with CRS also often experience hay fever and asthma. Natural therapies may help to clear congestion.

Suggested remedies

Lifestyle factors If you suffer from sinusitis, avoid exposure to cigarette smoke (including secondhand smoke), damp environments and airborne allergens (such as pet hair and pollen). Drink plenty of water, because staying hydrated will help keep the mucus thin (see Hydration, *p. 209*).

Steam inhalation Placing you head over a bowl of recently boiled water with a few drops of eucalyptus *(p. 173)* essential oil can help to reduce congestion and make breathing easier. Using a humidifier, or even going into a bathroom with a hot shower running may help, too.

Nasal irrigation (p. 242) Flushing the nasal passages with a saline solution softens mucus and helps to clear it from the nose. This may be of benefit in cases of chronic rhinosinusitis and frequent acute sinusitis.

Sublingual immunotherapy (p. 289) This therapy may decrease symptoms of allergic rhinitis (sneezing and a runny nose) in people who react to airborne allergens such as pollen or dust mites.

Bromelain In a 2005 study, children with acute sinusitis who took bromelain supplements recovered more quickly than those treated with standard medical therapy or a combination of bromelain and standard therapy. (See Enzymes, *p. 172*.)

See your doctor

Sinus infections can spread to other tissues if not addressed quickly. See your doctor if symptoms are severe, persist for more than seven days or recur frequently.

Quick fix Although there's little scientific evidence to support its use, horseradish *(p. 208)* is popularly taken to ease breathing and relieve congestion in sinusitis. It's believed that the sulfur-containing compounds within it are able to rapidly liquefy mucus, making it easier to clear from the sinus passages.

See also Allergies, Asthma, Colds and flu, Fever, Frequent illness, Hay fever, Headaches

SKIN RASHES

SKIN RASHES CAN BE CAUSED BY MANY medical conditions. The symptoms vary according to the cause, but can include skin that's dry, red, flaky and/or scaly, as well as spots, blisters, bumps and welts (weals), which may be present all over the body or in patches.

Rashes can be caused by: eczema and dermatitis; psoriasis; infections such as shingles, chicken pox and measles; systemic disorders such as rheumatoid arthritis; and insect bites and stings. In addition, urticaria (hives), which causes raised, itchy welts, are an inflammatory response to the body's release of histamine, and can be triggered by allergies, food intolerances and stress. Topical applications of herbal medicines can relieve the symptoms of some rashes. Your doctor may also recommend the use of other natural therapies.

Suggested remedies

Calendula *(p. 141)* A traditional salve for rashes, calendula has been clinically researched as useful for radiotherapy-induced dermatitis, bed sores and diaper rash.

Chamomile *(p. 147)* A soothing wash or compress can be made with chamomile tea.

Apple cider vinegar *(p. 120)* A few drops applied to a clean cloth and dabbed on the affected area can help relieve pain and itching.

Oats A warm bath containing a scoop of uncooked oats can provide soothing relief to inflamed skin.

Licorice *(p. 222)* In a study published in the *Journal of Dermatological Treatment*, a gel containing licorice root standardized for its content of glycyrrhizinic acid reduced atopic dermatitis symptoms such as itching, swelling and redness. You may need to ask a herbalist for a suitable formulation.

Elimination diet *(p. 171)* To determine the cause of hives and other allergies, you may need to undergo an elimination diet or other allergy tests under the supervision of your doctor.

Vitamin C *(p. 304)* Combined with quercetin and grape seed extract, vitamin C has been shown to have antihistamine properties that may be beneficial for allergies. However, more research is needed before its efficacy is fully known.

See your doctor

Call an ambulance if skin changes are accompanied by breathing difficulties, a swollen tongue or throat, low blood pressure or loss of consciousness—these symptoms may indicate a life-threatening anaphylactic reaction.

See your doctor if your rash:

❖ persists for longer than 14 days

❖ is accompanied by symptoms of fever, fatigue, swollen lymph nodes or any indication that an open sore or blister has become infected.

Quick fix Creams and gels made from chickweed *(p. 151)* have traditionally been valued for their cooling properties and ability to relieve itchiness and other symptoms of rashes.

See also Allergies, Eczema and dermatitis, Insect bites and stings, Psoriasis, Rheumatoid arthritis, Shingles

SLEEPING PROBLEMS

CAN'T GET TO SLEEP OR STAY ASLEEP? You're not alone. Nearly half of all adults report difficulty sleeping sometimes—and for one in four it's a nightly struggle. Natural remedies are an effective, safe alternative to over-the-counter and prescription sleeping pills—and research shows that many work better!

Suggested remedies

Sleeping strategies (p. 281) Simple steps prime body and mind for restful sleep, experts say. **Relaxation** *(p. 269)* may help.

Exercise (p. 175) A physical workout helps you feel relaxed and ready for sleep. In a US study of 66 people, regular exercise helped them fall asleep sooner and sleep more deeply.

Yoga (p. 316) Regular yoga practice that includes yogic relaxation (yoga nidra) has been shown to be effective in improving sleep length and quality in elderly people with insomnia.

Tai chi (p. 290) This gentle exercise routine helped people fall asleep 18 minutes faster and get 48 minutes more nightly sleep in a 2004 Oregon Research Institute study.

Melatonin (p. 237) When experts from Israel's Hadassah Medical Center reviewed 17 melatonin studies, they concluded that this supplement can help you fall asleep slightly faster (by about four minutes) and increase sleep time by 13 minutes.

Passionflower (p. 252) A cup of this herbal tea nightly improved sleep quality in a recent study from Australia's Monash University. Herbalists also recommend a cup of **chamomile** *(p. 147)* before bed.

Valerian (p. 300) This herbal soother helped 30 percent of menopausal and postmenopausal women get better sleep in a recent study from Iran. Store-bought sleeping aids often pair valerian with **hops** *(p. 206)*, another calming herb.

Cognitive behavioral therapy (p. 159) CBT can retrain your body and mind for faster, deeper sleep. In a landmark Harvard University study of 63 insomniacs, CBT was more effective than prescription sleeping pills, cutting the time it took to fall asleep in half and improving sleep quality by 17 percent.

Light therapy (p. 223) Bright light resets your body clock for better sleep. Daily use of light-therapy lamps helped insomniacs fall asleep faster and sleep longer in a 2004 US study. Going outdoors around noon could help, too.

See your doctor

See your doctor if insomnia lasts more than four weeks or is affecting your quality of life.

Quick fix Set your bedroom CD player or iPod on a timer and nod off as your favorite soothing melodies play. **Music** *(p. 241)* helped 60 problem sleepers drift off faster and sleep more soundly in a 2005 study from Taiwan's Buddhist Tzu-Chi General Hospital.

See also Chronic pain, Fatigue, Menopausal symptoms

SNORING

UP TO HALF OF ALL ADULTS SNORE occasionally. That loud, rasping sound originates in the soft palate tissue at the back of the mouth that vibrates as air moves in and out during sleep. Natural remedies can help by shrinking or strengthening this tissue or making it less prone to wiggling and therefore less noisy.

Suggested remedies

Lifestyle factors By shrinking flabby throat tissue, shedding excess weight could silence snoring. In one study of 690 people, 26 percent of those with sleep apnea who lost 10 percent of their weight cleared up this noisy problem. Follow a sensible weight-loss diet such as the low-glycemic index diet. You should avoid alcohol before sleeping, as it will reduce the muscle tone in your throat, and quit smoking as cigarettes irritate the throat lining, causing swelling. A Swedish study of 15,000 people found that 24 percent of smokers were loud snorers compared to 14 percent of non-smokers.

Raise your head Raising the head of your bed about 4 inches (10 cm) may help reduce snoring, according to the Mayo Clinic. This keeps flabby tissue in your throat from collapsing into your airways and vibrating. Use sturdy blocks of wood or purchase bed-raising supports. Or tuck a foam wedge under your pillow.

Nasal strips In a Swiss study of 35 snorers, their bed partners reported that adhesive strips quieted their mates' nighttime noises. The strips hold nasal passages open wider.

Hydration (p. 209) Staying hydrated thins nasal mucus, relieving congestion so you breathe easier and more quietly.

Nasal irrigation (p. 242) Rinsing your nasal passages with a simple saline solution can ease congestion and reduce snoring according to the British Snoring and Sleep Apnea Association.

Quick fix People commonly snore when sleeping on their back as this position makes tissues in the throat vibrate. Sew a tennis ball into the back of your pajamas or try a brush, pillow or other device to discourage you from sleeping on your back.

See your doctor

Loud snoring can be a sign of obstructive sleep apnea, a serious condition in which breathing stops briefly through the night. See your doctor if:

- ❖ you feel fatigued after a full night's sleep
- ❖ your partner says you seem to stop breathing, snort or snore extremely loudly at night
- ❖ you are excessively sleepy during the day.

DID YOU KNOW?

Singing or playing a wind instrument such as the clarinet, flute or tuba could significantly pipe down your snoring, say studies from England and Switzerland. Both activities strengthen the muscles that support the soft palate, so that it doesn't vibrate during sleep.

See also Sleeping problems

STRAINS AND SPRAINS

STRAINS HAPPEN WHEN MUSCLES or tendons (which connect muscle to bone) are stretched or torn. Sprains occur when ligaments—the tissue that supports joints like your ankles, knees and wrists—meet the same fate. Mild injuries will respond well to natural treatments (often with the addition of an over-the-counter painkiller).

Suggested remedies

***Exercise** (p. 175)* A conditioning routine can build muscle strength to protect against future strains. Daily **stretching** *(p. 286)* can help, too, according to the American Academy of Orthopedic Surgeons.

***Arnica** (p. 121)* In gel form, arnica eased muscle soreness in a 2003 Norwegian study of 82 marathon runners. Derivatives of thymol in arnica's roots may explain its anti-inflammatory benefits.

***Horse chestnut** (p. 207)* Used as a gel, horse chestnut may reduce swelling due to the saponins it contains.

***White willow bark** (p. 312)* Salicin in white willow bark acts in a similar way to aspirin and can help ease pain.

***Turmeric** (p. 298)* The yellow spice contains over two dozen anti-inflammatory compounds that support healing.

***Massage** (p. 230)* The benefits of massage include suppressing inflammation-boosting chemicals in the tissues and stimulating repair, according to a 2012 study from Canada. The use of massage oils containing a few drops of wintergreen, marjoram, basil, cypress or other oils may further aid healing.

***Acupuncture** (p. 112)* This therapy can reduce swelling and pain and promote healing by boosting the circulation.

***Chiropractic** (p. 152)* In a 2010 study of 59 Australian Rules football players, chiropractic care led to fewer injuries and faster recovery, say researchers from Macquarie University.

***Comfrey** (p. 162)* Comfrey ointment can reduce the pain and swelling of sprained ankles, while improving joint mobility.

***Tiger Balm** (p. 295)* The clove bud oil, mint oil and menthol in this aromatic rub have a pain-relieving effect on strained muscles.

See your doctor

See your doctor if you have severe pain, cannot use the injured muscle or joint or simply have concerns about your injury.

Quick fix Within 10 minutes of a muscle strain, ease pain and discourage swelling with cold therapy *(p. 161)*. Apply ice, wrapped in a towel, for 20–30 minutes every few hours. Rest the injury, wrapped with an elastic bandage and elevated above the level of your heart.

DID YOU KNOW?

A few days after your muscle strain, think MICE (movement, ice, compression and elevation) for better healing. Experts now recommend activity three to seven days after an injury instead of continued bed rest.

See also Bursitis and tendonitis, Cramps, muscle, Frozen shoulder

STROKE PREVENTION

A TINY BLOOD CLOT OR MICROSCOPIC TEAR in a blood vessel is all it takes to trigger a stroke—the disabling brain attack that happens to 15 million people worldwide each year. The aftermath? Strokes kill 5 million and disable another 5 million each year. The good news is that you have the power to significantly lessen your risk of stroke. Work with your doctor to control your blood pressure and cholesterol. The natural strategies here may help.

Suggested remedies

Lifestyle factors Stop smoking—a pack-a-day habit boosts your stroke risk six-fold, say UK stroke experts. Lose any excess weight, as being overweight raises your odds for a stroke by 22–64 percent, Italian researchers found. And find time for **relaxation** *(p. 269)*—chronic stress doubled stroke risk in a recent Spanish study of 450 people. Make **exercise** *(p. 175)* part of your life (keeping within your limits, of course). Physical activity four times a week cut stroke risk by 20 percent in a recent large Australian study.

Dietary measures A key strategy in reducing the risk of stroke (and a whole host of other ailments) is a healthy diet. In a US study of 71,768 women, eating plenty of fresh produce, whole grains and fish reduced their risk of stroke by 26 percent. It works for men, too. Studies have also shown that replacing butter with heart-friendly **olive oil** *(p. 249)* can cut stroke risk by 41 percent. Fiber helps, too: every extra 1/4 ounces (7 g) of daily **fiber** *(p. 184)* lowers risk by 7 percent, says a 2013 report from the UK's Leeds University. And eating plenty of produce rich in **vitamin C** *(p. 304)* could reduce the risk by a third, another UK study suggests.

Tea (p. 292) Sipping three cups of green or black tea a day could reduce your odds for a stroke by 21 percent, say US researchers. Prefer coffee? One or more daily mugs of **coffee** *(p 158)* could lower risk by 20 percent, Japanese researchers have found.

Holy basil (p. 205) Regular consumption of holy basil tea may help prevent stroke through its beneficial effects on blood pressure, glucose metabolism and cholesterol and its protective antioxidant and anti-inflammatory actions. Animal studies have also shown the herb can even prevent brain injury after an experimentally induced stroke.

Garlic (p. 191) Having one fresh clove a day somewhere in your diet could help discourage blood clotting, a 1995 study from Kuwait found. Meanwhile, garlic supplements may help keep arteries flexible, a small 1997 German study suggests.

See your doctor

Get emergency help without delay if you or a loved one has any of these warning signs:

❖ drooping or numbness on one side of the face

❖ weakness or numbness in one arm

❖ difficulty speaking.

Quick fix Keep your blood pressure in check. Lowering your systolic blood pressure (the top number in a blood pressure reading) by 10 points or your diastolic pressure (the bottom number) by 5 points can reduce your risk of stroke by 41 percent, say UK researchers.

See also Blood pressure, high, Cholesterol, high, Heart and circulatory health

TINNITUS

CHARACTERIZED BY A LOW-LEVEL RINGING in the ears, tinnitus strikes one in five people. It may be in one or both ears, constant or intermittent. As sound waves travel through the ear, damaged hair cells in the inner ear have trouble translating the signals to the auditory cortex. The brain never receives the expected signals, and generates a "fake" sound: the ringing, buzzing, roaring or humming. Tinnitus can be difficult to budge and is a quality-of-life issue that can worsen with age. But there are natural remedies that may help.

Suggested remedies

Dietary measures Avoid caffeine, tobacco, salt and alcohol, which can all aggravate tinnitus by impacting blood pressure. For example, alcohol dilates the blood vessels, increasing blood flow to the inner ear area, making tinnitus more pronounced.

Olive oil *(p. 249)* Three or four drops of olive oil in the ear two or three times a day for one to two weeks loosens ear wax that can aggravate tinnitus.

Relaxation *(p. 269)* Biofeedback can help by tackling the stress associated with the condition. By capturing biological data (such as the heartbeat and skin temperature), biofeedback helps people to see how thoughts and feelings impact their current body state, so they can make changes that will help reduce tinnitus flare-ups.

Acupuncture *(p. 112)* A Brazilian study of 76 tinnitus sufferers found that acupuncture treatments made a significant difference in the experience of tinnitus.

Coenzyme Q_{10} *(p. 157)* A small German study found that in patients with low levels of CoQ_{10} in the blood, taking a CoQ_{10} supplement may decrease tinnitus expression.

Ginkgo *(p. 193)* Evidence from multiple clinical trials suggests a standardized *Ginkgo biloba* extract can be effective in relieving the symptoms of tinnitus.

See your doctor
Check in with your doctor if your tinnitus comes on suddenly without apparent cause, or if you simultaneously feel dizzy or lose your hearing.

WATCH OUT!
No matter how bad your tinnitus, do not be tempted to use ear candling to relieve pressure in your ear. It supposedly works by the "chimney effect." A cone of wax paper is placed in the ear and lit on fire, creating a vacuum that draws wax out of the ear. Repeated studies have shown that ear candling fails to remove wax from the ear. Reports of dropped cones and burned ear drums make this a very dangerous (and ineffective) practice.

Quick fix White noise can be used to provide temporary relief from tinnitus in an otherwise quiet setting. You can buy white noise generators or an application for a smart phone. Some websites (such as www.simplynoise.com) offer white noise and other sounds.

TOOTH AND GUM DISORDERS

PROTECTING YOUR DAZZLING SMILE begins at home. Regular brushing and flossing are crucial for reducing your risk for gum disease and cavities. There are some natural remedies that can help, too. Treat any cavities or signs of infection promptly—chronic inflammation has been linked to numerous illnesses including heart disease.

Suggested remedies

Lifestyle factors Kicking the smoking habit could cut your risk for oral health problems in half, suggests a 2012 report from the US Centers for Disease Control and Prevention. And start doing some regular exercise *(p. 175)*—it could reduce gum disease risk by 54 percent, says a 2005 report in the *Journal of Dentistry*.

Dietary measures Sip water to combat a dry mouth; saliva helps protect teeth and gums. If you have diabetes, keep it under control—high blood glucose can boost the risk for gum disease. Cut down on sugary snacks between meals as the bacteria in plaque feast on sugar. Skip the fizzy drinks, too, as the acids in sodas can damage tooth enamel. If you have sore gums, try eating probiotics *(p. 261)*. Milk with added *Lactobacillus reuteri* soothed inflammation and reduced bleeding linked with gum disease in a 2009 study from the University of Leipzig.

Holy basil (p. 205) Drinking and/or rinsing the mouth with holy basil tea after a meal can effectively reduce oral bacteria including *Streptococcus mutans*, which is responsible for tooth decay.

Calcium (p. 140) Skimping on calcium (from supplements or food) could increase the risk for severe gum disease by as much as 54 percent, Japanese scientists report in a 2000 study. Make sure you are getting enough.

Vitamin D (p. 305) Get some vitamin D with your calcium. The combination improved gum health in a year-long Saint Louis University study of 51 people with signs of early gum disease.

Green tea Sipping a cup or more of green tea per day reduced the signs of gum disease in 940 men in a 2009 study from Japan's Kyushu University. It is thought that catechins in green tea may help by reducing inflammation. (See Tea, *p. 292*.)

Neem (p. 243) This herbal remedy, available in toothpastes and mouth rinses, has antiseptic properties. In a 2012 Indian study of 45 people with early gum disease, those who used a mouthwash containing neem had less bleeding and less plaque after 21 days.

See your dentist

Regular checkups will keep your teeth and gums healthy. See your dentist if you have any of the following signs as they could indicate an abscess:

❖ pain when eating or pressing on a tooth
❖ redness or swelling of the gums
❖ a bad taste and/or odor in your mouth.

Quick fix The traditional remedy for toothache, cloves *(p. 156)*, is now backed up by science. In a 2006 study at Kuwait University, clove oil numbed participants' gums as effectively as the anesthetic benzocaine.

DID YOU KNOW?

If you love chewing gum, why not choose one with natural products that love your teeth and gums, too? Propolis *(p. 263)* was shown in studies to reduce plaque and help fight gum disease; the sweetener xylitol reduced cavities in a 1995 University of Michigan study; and in 2002 another study from the US showed that the bark extract of maritime pine *(p. 229)* reduced gum bleeding.

URINARY TRACT INFECTIONS

A BURNING SENSATION WHEN YOU URINATE, frequent trips to the bathroom, belly pain, cloudy or odd-smelling urine, even a fever—these signs mean you may have a urinary tract infection (UTI). The culprit? Most UTIs are caused by the *E. coli* bacterium found in the human digestive tract. Natural remedies can help prevent UTIs, which is good news if you're prone to them. When you develop one, however, it's wise to consult a doctor. An untreated UTI can cause kidney damage.

Suggested remedies

Lifestyle factors Simple measures to help prevent UTIs include: avoiding synthetic underwear and urinating frequently (don't hold it in for long periods). Women should empty the bladder after sexual activity and wipe from front to back after urinating.

Vitamin C (p. 304) Women who took 100 mg of vitamin C daily for three months had 50 percent fewer UTIs than those who did not, says a 2007 study from Mexico.

Bicarbonate of soda (p. 130) Drinking a glass of water with a teaspoon of baking soda will help alkaline the urine and reduce irritation and discomfort caused from infected urine.

Probiotics (p. 261) Probiotic vaginal suppositories cut the number of UTIs in half in a 2011 University of Washington study of 100 women with recurring bladder infections. The probiotic used in the study was *Lactobacillus crispatus* CTV-05.

Uva-ursi (p. 299) This traditional herbal remedy was used for UTIs before the development of antibiotics. Research now suggests that, used sparingly, it may help mild infections.

Acupuncture (p. 112) In a 2002 Swedish study of 100 women with recurrent UTIs, 73 percent of those who had four weeks of acupuncture treatments were UTI-free for six months compared to 52 percent of women who did not receive acupuncture.

Horseradish (p. 208) This folk remedy for UTIs has been shown to be effective in German studies, when combined with nasturtium.

Corn silk (p. 164) Though there is little evidence to support it, corn silk has long been used to relieve the symptoms of cystitis.

Celery seed (p. 146) Another traditional remedy, celery seed extract has a diuretic effect and is mildly antiseptic, making it useful for the treatment of cystitis and other UTIs.

See your doctor

Visit your doctor if you have symptoms of a UTI.

Quick fix At the first sign of a UTI, make sure you are drinking enough water (see Hydration, *p. 209*). You need at least 2 pints (1.2 L) a day, according to the US National Institutes of Health. The water will help to flush bacteria out of your bladder.

DID YOU KNOW?

A recent UK review of 24 studies concluded that cranberry juice may not be as effective against UTIs as is widely believed. However, it may have a small benefit for women who suffer repeated bladder infections. It is thought to prevent bacteria from adhering to the bladder wall. Drinking a couple of glasses a day seems to help.

VARICOSE VEINS

THE ROPY, SWOLLEN VEINS THAT APPEAR just under the skin's surface, usually on your legs, are known as varicose veins. Veins bring blood back to the heart, working against gravity, and sometimes their valves get weak or "flappy" and allow blood to flow backward, producing the unsightly bulging appearance. Varicose veins are mostly harmless, yet they can be uncomfortable and there are natural remedies that can help.

Suggested remedies

Lifestyle factors As a preventive measure, lose any excess weight to give your veins an easier job. Exercise *(p. 175)* that includes flexing and extending the ankles will help to keep the blood moving through your veins and improve muscle tone. If you have varicose veins, avoid tight clothes, and spend time with your feet raised above your heart every day.

Dietary measures Cutting back on salt helps reduce water retention and swelling and so may help to ease some of the discomfort of varicose veins.

Avoid prolonged standing or sitting Standing causes blood to pool in the lower legs while prolonged sitting slows blood return. Sitting with crossed legs may also slow blood flow from the legs.

Ginkgo (p. 193) The herb *Ginkgo biloba* is a tonic for the circulatory system, strengthening your veins and encouraging increased blood flow.

Grape seed extract (p. 200) Flavonoids found in grape seeds reduce leakage in veins and swelling in the legs. Work with your doctor as grape seed extract may raise the risk of bleeding if paired with blood-thinning medications.

Horse chestnut (p. 207) A *Cochrane Review* of seven placebo-controlled studies found that horse chestnut extract is a safe and effective short-term treatment for chronic venous insufficiency, a condition that can lead to varicose veins.

Hydrotherapy (p. 210) Alternating the application of hot and cold water can help decrease swelling and improve circulation.

Witch hazel (p. 315) The astringent tannins of *Hamamelis virginiana* may help reduce topical swelling.

Laser treatment (p. 216) The precise application of laser light to the varicose veins means the veins simply fade away. Ask your doctor for a referral.

See your doctor

If you have pain, burning, or sudden swelling linked to your varicose veins, see your doctor right away.

Quick fix Compression stockings provide immediate relief by supporting varicose veins and encouraging blood flow back up the leg. Find them over the counter in any pharmacy, or you can order prescription-grade stockings from a medical supply store. When you remain stationary for a long time, such as on a flight, use them to prevent blood from pooling in the lower legs.

VERTIGO

VERTIGO IS THE ILLUSION OF MOVEMENT and disturbed balance that usually originates from the inner ear or central nervous system and while it is associated with dizziness, it should be distinguished from faints, fits and funny turns that may be due to cardiovascular problems. You can become imbalanced and dizzy or experience room-spinning vertigo when either the function of your inner ear is off or there's a problem with your central nervous system's ability to process sensory information. You may have Meniere's disease, a common inner ear problem, a viral infection in the inner ear, or benign paroxysmal positional vertigo (BPPV), caused by the misplacement of gravity-sensing crystals into the spinning motion sensors of the ear. Once diagnosed, work with your doctor to find the best strategy for managing your vertigo.

Suggested remedies

Lifestyle factors Quit smoking as nicotine can aggravate symptoms by constricting blood vessels and limiting blood flow to the inner ear. Try raising the head of your bed. In BPPV, sleeping with your head elevated at night can prevent the gravity-sensing crystals in the inner ear from slipping back.

Dietary measures Fluid balance is key to vertigo. To avoid being dizzy, cut down on fluid-retaining salt and drink plenty of water, especially during hot weather (see Hydration, *p. 209*). Limit caffeine (which aggravates vertigo) and alcohol (which tampers with the volume and composition of fluid in the inner ear).

Computer games The Nintendo Wii game console has been used by physical and occupational therapists to treat vertigo. Patients stand on the WiiFit balance board and sensors record the movements of their feet and legs, allowing them to challenge themselves to further develop their balance.

Head movements BPPV can be eased with a specific set of doctor-prescribed head movements to move the gravity-sensing crystals back into the correct areas. (But avoid postures in which you put your head upside down.)

See your doctor

Go to an emergency room if you are dizzy and have:

- a head injury
- a very stiff neck
- seizures
- a fever
- chest pain
- your heart skipping beats
- an inability to move an arm or leg
- a change of vision or speech
- feelings of faintness or you lose alertness for more than a few minutes.

Quick fix During an attack of dizziness or vertigo, sit down right away so you don't fall, and don't make any sudden movements or changes in position. Avoid bright lights, TV and reading. Slowly increase activity as the vertigo recedes. Rise slowly from a seated position, to allow your blood pressure time to adjust.

WARTS

CAUSED BY STRAINS OF THE HUMAN papillomavirus, warts on your skin normally go away by themselves. Their ugly medical name—verruca vulgaris—matches the unappealing appearance of these rough-textured skin eruptions. (Another type, plantar warts, occurs on the soles of the feet.) Natural remedies can help you speed a wart's departure by giving your immune system a hand in fighting the virus that causes them or by attacking the wart directly.

Suggested remedies

Lifestyle factors Recurrent eruptions of warts could be a sign of impaired immunity. Follow a healthy diet; make regular **exercise** *(p. 175)* a part of your life; take steps to tackle stress and make sure you are getting enough rest **(see Sleeping strategies,** *p. 281***)**. With a healthy immune system, most warts disappear on their own. Warts are contagious and it is important not to scratch or pick at them. Keep them dry and always wash your hands after touching them.

Hypnotherapy (p. 211) A traditional cure for warts is to "wish them away." The power of suggestion can be a powerful healing tool that may be effective in treating warts in some people, especially children.

Antiviral herbs Alternative-medicine practitioners sometimes suggest virus-fighting botanicals to help your body vanquish the culprit that causes warts. Top recommendations include: **cat's claw** *(p. 144)*, **medicinal mushrooms** *(p. 233)* and **holy basil** *(p. 205)*.

Garlic (p. 191) Eaten in food, garlic boosts the immune system. It has been shown to have antiviral properties, which backs up its traditional use as a treatment for warts, either rubbed on the wart or crushed and applied as a poultice.

Laser treatment (p. 216) For this treatment, a dermatologist uses a beam of laser light to destroy the wart. Laser therapy is often performed when warts don't respond to other treatments, are large, or occur during pregnancy. In a 2009 study from Korea's Chung-Ang University, laser therapy cleared up 77 percent of skin warts and 44 percent of plantar warts in one treatment; just 3 percent returned.

See your doctor

See your doctor if you have genital warts or a wart elsewhere on your body that is painful, interferes with everyday activities, won't go away or keeps returning.

Quick fix It may sound odd, but covering a wart with a piece of banana peel can speed healing, say natural-medicine experts. For this home remedy, use a piece of peel slightly larger than the wart and tape in place, with the inner side of peel in contact with the wart. Repeat for several days.

See also Frequent illness, Skin rashes

WOUND HEALING

WOUNDS HAPPEN WITH ANY BREAK in the skin, from a cut, scrape, puncture or burn, to a surgical incision or pressure ulcer (bedsore). From the minor abrasion to the complex suture, the speed at which a wound heals depends on its size and type. It also depends on the status of your immune system. Diet and lifestyle strategies can assist this and there are natural remedies that can help your body to heal and keep infections at bay.

Suggested remedies

Lifestyle factors Keep blood moving around the body with gentle exercise *(p. 175)*. Change position regularly to avoid pressure ulcers: in a chair, every 15 minutes; in bed, every two hours. Keep skin clean and dry. Change wound dressings frequently.

Dietary measures You can boost your immune system and hasten healing by making sure you eat a healthy diet rich in nutrients such as zinc *(p. 319)* and vitamin C *(p. 304)*. These nutrients help your body to repair itself and fight infection.

Gotu kola (p. 199) Long used for minor burns, psoriasis, preventing surgical scars and preventing or reducing stretch marks, gotu kola has chemicals called triterpenoids, which strengthen skin and increase blood supply.

Horse chestnut (p. 207) In an Australian triple-blind randomized placebo-controlled trial, 54 people with venous leg ulcers found horse chestnut increased their wounds' self-moisturizing properties and reduced the need for new bandages.

Seaweed Wound-care research suggests that infected or exudating wounds are best treated by keeping them moist and that this can be best accomplished with alginate wound dressings–pads made from seaweed that form a moist gel.

Holy basil (p. 205) A unique combination of antioxidant, anti-inflammatory, analgesic and antimicrobial activity makes holy basil tea, either sipped or cooled and applied topically, particularly effective in dealing with wounds and assisting in healing.

Laser treatment (p. 216) Low-level laser treatment may help to encourage wound healing and tissue regeneration. Ask your doctor for a referral to a clinic.

See your doctor

Seek immediate help if there is fever, weakness and confusion. Call the doctor if the wound:

- has a foul odor
- exudes pus
- is red, tender or warm to the touch
- is accompanied by swollen lymph nodes.

Quick fix Speed wound healing with a little honey. Slow-healing wounds have an alkaline environment, but the acidic pH of manuka honey *(p. 228)* makes them heal faster. Manuka honey reduces tissue breakdown and increases the body's cell-building activity while its broad-spectrum antimicrobial activity keeps infections at bay.

REMEDIES

ACUPUNCTURE AND ACUPRESSURE

use for ✓ ***Back and neck pain*** ✓ ***Bursitis and tendonitis*** ✓ ***Cancer support*** ✓ ***Chronic pain*** ✓ ***Eye infections*** ✓ ***Frequent illness*** ✓ ***Frozen shoulder*** ✓ ***Hay fever*** ✓ ***Incontinence*** ✓ ***Inflammatory bowel disease*** ✓ ***Menstrual problems*** ✓ ***Migraines*** ✓ ***Nausea and vomiting*** ✓ ***Neuralgia*** ✓ ***Phobias*** ✓ ***Raynaud's disease*** ✓ ***Seasonal affective disorder*** ✓ ***Sexual problems*** ✓ ***Shingles*** ✓ ***Strains and sprains*** ✓ ***Tinnitus*** ✓ ***Urinary tract infections***

THE PRACTICE OF BOTH ACUPUNCTURE and acupressure (the application of pressure, rather than needles) is rooted in antiquity. The oldest surviving acupuncture needles were discovered in the tomb of a Chinese prince, buried in 113 BC, but the therapy may date back centuries if not millennia earlier in the Far East—and possibly much farther afield. When researchers examined the 5,000-year-old mummified body of Ötzi the Iceman, found in the Austrian Alps in 1991, they noticed a number of tattoos on his body, which were located strikingly close to classical acupuncture points.

How they work

One remarkable feature of acupuncture and acupressure is that 21st-century science cannot fully explain them. Acupuncture needles are known to stimulate specific nerve fibers that modify pain transmission in the spinal cord as well as stimulating the secretion of pain-relieving endorphins and other neurotransmitters in the brain. Acupuncture points have also been found to correspond to myofascial trigger points—regions of heightened pain sensitivity.

Practitioners of traditional Chinese medicine (TCM) explain their methods quite differently. According to the holistic principles of TCM, ill health is due to an imbalance or blockage in the flow of *qi* or vital energy along energy pathways known as meridians. Stimulating certain points with needles or pressure helps to restore the flow through these pathways. The insertion and manipulation of an acupuncture needle can often lead to the sensation of *dechi*, which is a feeling of heaviness, soreness, numbness or fullness that travels along the meridians and is usually a sign of an effective treatment.

Effective and safe

Acupuncture has been shown to treat not only pain of many kinds, but also conjunctivitis, sexual dysfunction, tinnitus and even phobias. The World Health Organization lists 28 disorders for which acupuncture has proved effective, including some such as morning sickness for which conventional medicines might not be prescribed.

Similarly, acupressure may help patients manage pain during labor, and relieve nausea and vomiting induced by chemotherapy. The virtue of both practices is that they are safe, non-invasive, drug-free and holistic—treating the condition and its underlying causes. Some research shows that acupuncture boosts immune function, suggesting it has a preventive role, too.

continued on page 114

Energy pathways

According to traditional Chinese medicine, energy or *qi* continually flows through the body via a series of pathways, known as meridians. There are 14 major meridians that relate to different organs, tissue types, emotions and bodily functions. Physical, emotional and environmental factors may alter the flow of *qi*, resulting in a deficiency or excess of energy in different meridians. Using fine needles to stimulate particular points along the meridians, an acupuncturist aims to restore the normal flow of energy through the body, returning the body to health.

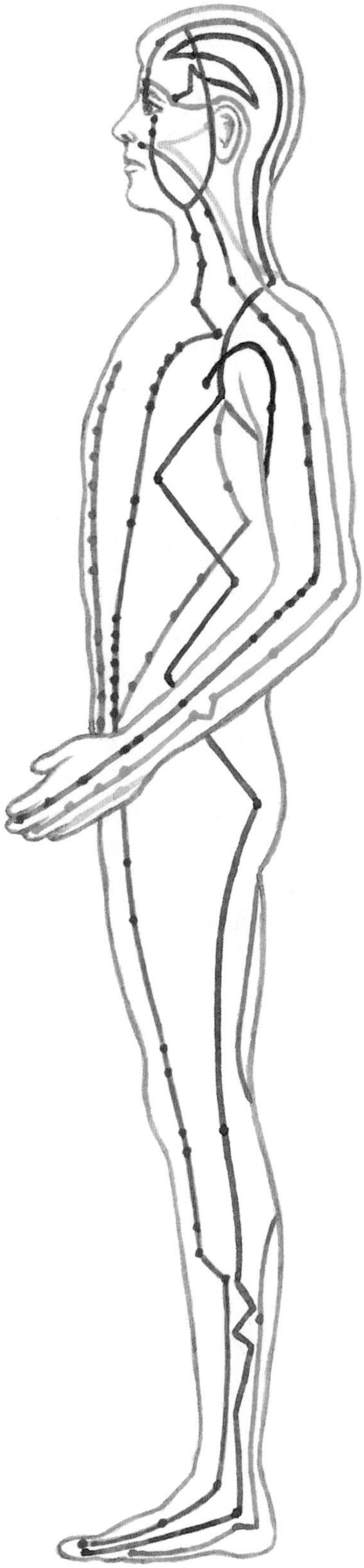

ACUPUNCTURE AND ACUPRESSURE *continued*

A visit to the practitioner

Acupuncture is practiced by many doctors as well as by TCM practitioners and each practitioner may have a slightly different approach. A practitioner will usually take a detailed medical history and he or she may also take your pulse, examine your tongue, study your skin or look for other physical signs that might have a bearing on your condition. For both acupuncture and acupressure treatments, patients lie on a padded couch or table, usually fully clothed but with sleeves or trousers rolled up to allow access to acupuncture points. Sessions vary in length from around 30 minutes to two hours, depending on the practitioner and the problem.

An acupressure practitioner will use deep-finger pressure at points along the meridian lines to reduce tension, relieve pain and treat a variety of disorders. During acupuncture, the practitioner inserts between three and 15 or more extremely fine needles at certain points along the appropriate meridian lines, gently twisting them as they go in. You may feel an initial twinge or *dechi*, which feels like a traveling fullness. Some practitioners may choose to connect the needles to an electrical stimulation device and adjust the intensity and frequency of an electric current between two needles. At the end of the session the needles are painlessly removed. The number of sessions required will depend on the condition and your response to the treatment.

Other TCM treatments

For certain disorders, including arthritis and digestive problems, the practitioner may use moxibustion—a practice as ancient as acupuncture. This involves holding a burning stick of moxa—Chinese mugwort *(Artemesia argyi* or *A. vulgaris)*—close to various acupuncture points, until the skin warms and reddens. Like the insertion of needles or application of pressure, this helps clear the meridian pathways.

"Cupping" may also be used to draw out harmful substances and improve the flow of *qi*. In this case, a flame is inserted into a glass cup to remove the air. This creates a vacuum, so that when the glass is placed over the skin, suction holds it in place.

Safety first *Make sure your acupuncturist uses only disposable needles. Both acupuncture and acupressure are safe and well tolerated but tell the practitioner if you are pregnant and mention any medical condition you have and other treatments or medicines you are taking.*

Where to find *Ask your doctor if he/she offers acupuncture or you can search for a certified TCM practitioner at the National Certification Commission for Acupuncture and Oriental Medicine (www.nccaom.org).*

ALEXANDER TECHNIQUE

use for ✓ ***Back and neck pain*** ✓ ***Jaw pain***

THIS THERAPY WAS DEVELOPED BY Frederick Matthias Alexander, an Australian-born actor, in the early 20th century. When working, he was irritated by bouts of hoarseness and was unable to obtain satisfactory medical advice. While watching himself in a mirror he found that his posture greatly affected his voice and that he often moved his head back and down and tensed his neck and throat, which impaired his breathing.

Alexander became interested in the effects of posture and developed his own method to "retrain" the head, neck, shoulders and torso to move correctly. Alexander called this process the "Primary Control," for he believed that all correct body movement would flow from correcting faults in the head and upper torso. In particular, he believed extended sitting or standing were problematic, as they compress the neck and spine. Alexander's clients included the actress Lily Langtry and the writer George Bernard Shaw.

How it works

The Alexander Technique focuses on self-awareness and encourages patients to observe and "unlearn" habitual responses that interfere with the body's natural movements. Typically, a patient is taught to sit, arise, stand and walk in new ways that are less stressful to the body. Patients are re-educated to correct faulty alignment, primarily of the upper parts of the body, and are shown exercises that will help to lengthen and free the neck and spine.

This gentle technique may be of assistance for people with scoliosis (spinal curvature), lordosis (swayback syndrome) or rounded shoulders. Arthritis, jaw pain and back and neck pain may also be improved, along with balance in the elderly. Breathing and digestive disorders may even be improved with the technique, since poor posture negatively affects the lungs and digestive system.

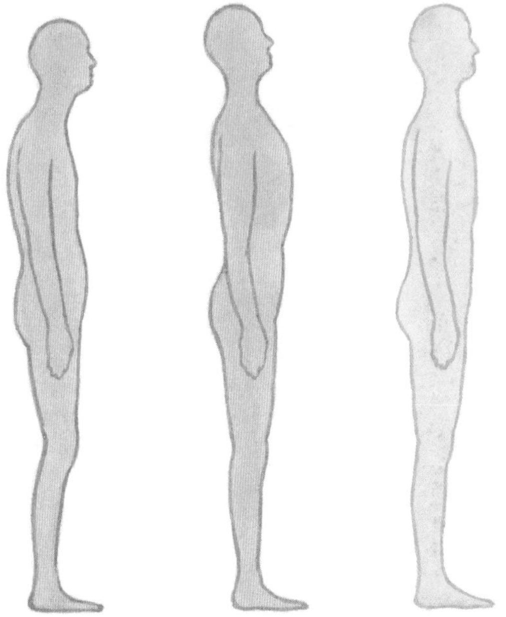

Slouched Overcorrected Correct

How to stand

Simply learning the right way to stand can put less strain on muscles and joints. Slouching is clearly an unnatural stance, but people often overcorrect this, standing extra upright and stiff, which is equally harmful. An Alexander Technique teacher will show you how to "stand tall" in a relaxed and balanced way.

continued on page 116

A visit to the Alexander Technique practitioner

You remain clothed throughout while the practitioner first observes your normal ways of sitting, standing and moving and then teaches you small, subtle changes to adopt that will restore balance and ease to the body. You may be taught in small classes or individually. The length of a course varies, from between 15 and 30 lessons: Changing the postural habits of a lifetime takes time and practice.

Safety first *Tell your practitioner if you are pregnant or affected by musculoskeletal injuries or chronic disease to ensure your program is tailored to your specific needs.*

Where to find *Find a local practitioner from the website: www.alexandertechnique.com.*

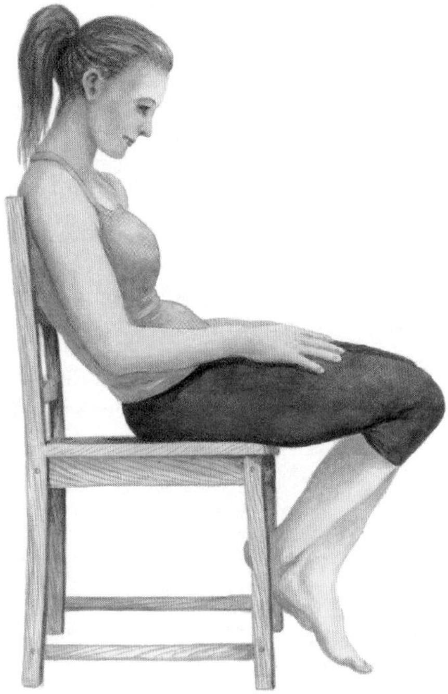

INCORRECT Sitting with your head down, shoulders rounded and stomach compressed results in restricted breathing. Crossing the legs restricts blood flow and twists the pelvis and spine.

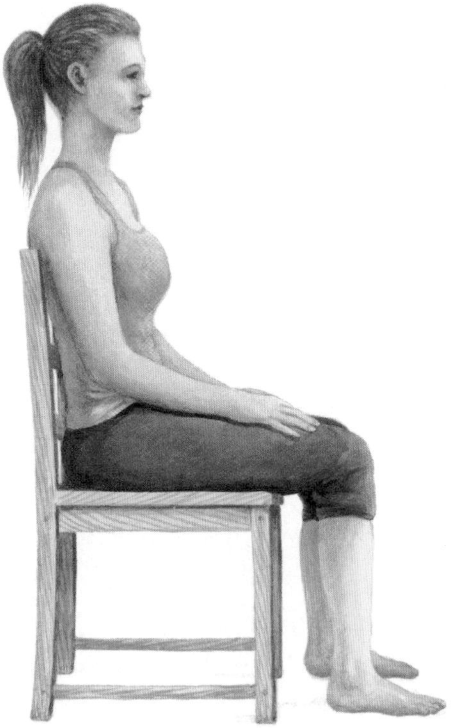

CORRECT Hold your head up and freely poised, with shoulders relaxed against the back of the chair. Keep the thighs supported on the chair with knees slightly apart. Feet should be firmly on the floor.

ALOE VERA *Aloe vera, A. barbadensis.* Also called: Bitter aloe

use for ✓ ***Burns*** ✓ ***Cuts and scrapes*** ✓ ***Herpes*** ✓ ***Psoriasis***

A MEMBER OF THE LILY FAMILY, *Aloe vera* has a striking flower, but is better known for its fleshy leaves that contain a soothing gel-like pulp. The pulp has long been used to alleviate skin problems. Aloe plants were well known to physicians in ancient Greece and Rome, and Cleopatra is said to have used the pulp to preserve her beauty.

How it works

Aloe's thick pulp has antiseptic, moisturizing, anti-inflammatory and soothing properties. It is useful for skin conditions that require soothing, cooling and astringing, like eczema, psoriasis, rashes, acne, herpes sores, sunburn, gingivitis, mouth ulcers, rosacea and varicose veins. It contains anthraquinones, which help promote the growth of healthy skin cells and therefore speed wound healing.

Safety first *Some forms of aloe, such as the concentrated tincture, have a strongly laxative effect and should only be taken internally under professional supervision. Internal use should be avoided by women during pregnancy or breastfeeding and by the elderly or anyone with kidney disease. If using the fresh gel topically, avoid the yellow sap at the base of the leaf as this may have an irritant effect.*

Where to find Aloe vera *is available in a range of personal care and first aid products in health food stores and pharmacies. Supplemental forms are available in health food stores or from a qualified herbalist.*

Fresh aloe pulp is a great first aid treatment for minor scalds, cuts, scrapes, burns or insect bites. Snap open a leaf, scoop out the gel and smooth onto the affected area.

Aloe vera also contains a bitter constituent called aloin, found in the yellow sap at the base of the leaf, which is responsible for its traditional use as a purgative, tonic and gall bladder stimulant, both for human and veterinary purposes. A natural therapist or herbalist may recommend the gel for internal use to treat peptic ulcers, colitis or irritable bowel syndrome; or a tincture or capsules to stimulate appetite or treat constipation.

How to use

Aloe vera is easy to grow as a houseplant or outdoors in temperate climates. The plants are farmed commercially and the pulp is available as a gel, freeze-dried powder, liquid extract or concentrate in personal care products like shampoos, moisturizers, wipes and sunscreens. It is also sold in supplements for internal use, which may be in tablet, capsule or liquid form. Follow label instructions or take as professionally prescribed.

AMINO ACIDS

Arginine, carnitine, glutamine, lysine, N-acetyl cysteine

use for ✓ ***Bronchitis*** ✓ ***Heart and circulatory health*** ✓ ***Herpes*** ✓ ***Wound healing***

USED BY OUR BODIES TO CREATE the thousands of different proteins we require to survive and function, amino acids are vital for our well-being. Of more than 500 that occur in nature, humans use 20, yet our bodies can manufacture only half of these. The others are considered "essential" amino acids and must come from the diet. While a healthy person eating a balanced diet can usually create or obtain all the necessary amino acids, supplementation can help treat certain disorders.

How they work

Supplemental amino acids may either remedy a deficit or boost a particular function. For instance, N-acetyl cysteine (NAC) helps the body make glutathione, an antioxidant that protects cells against damage by free radicals. Taking NAC regularly may have a protective effect, particularly against chronic bronchitis, though its precise mode of action is not known.

Similarly carnitine is used by cells to convert fat into energy and supplemental carnitine appears to boost energy production in tissues such as heart muscle, which has especially high energy requirements. It has been used to complement conventional angina treatment and may help prevent complications following a heart attack.

Lysine, an essential amino acid supplied by meat, cheeses and beans, helps the body create carnitine and also collagen, the main protein in connective tissue such as skin and cartilage. In supplement form, it appears to combat the herpes simplex virus, responsible for cold sores and genital herpes, by blocking the production of arginine, an amino acid that helps the virus to replicate.

While herpes sufferers should avoid supplemental arginine, people recovering from wounds may find it helpful. Injuries, burns and infections deplete the body's arginine supply, so hospitals sometimes prescribe the nutrient to speed recovery.

Safety first *Consult your doctor before taking supplemental amino acids, as (particularly at high doses) some may enhance the effects of your natural levels or react with medications.*

Where to find *Supplements are available in health food stores and pharmacies in liquid, powder, capsule and tablet form.*

Similarly, illness or injury raises levels of the stress hormone cortisol, which can reduce supplies of the normally abundant amino acid glutamine. Because glutamine plays a role in immune function, supplementation can help healing and recovery.

How to use

Most people are able to get enough amino acids from a healthy, balanced diet. However, if you think supplemental amino acids may help your particular condition, consult your doctor. He or she will be able to guide you on the most appropriate supplement and dosage for your needs.

ANDROGRAPHIS *Andrographis paniculata*

use for ✓ ***Colds and flu*** ✓ ***Fever***

ANDROGRAPHIS, ALSO KNOWN AS "the king of bitters," is an ancient medicinal herb with an extensive history of use in Asia, especially in the traditional medical system of India, Ayurveda. It has long been used to treat upper respiratory tract infections and fever. In Chinese medical philosophy it is classified as a bitter and cooling medicine, and is therefore used to treat conditions defined as "hot" and characterized by inflammation.

How it works

Andrographis has several active constituents that have antiviral, antimicrobial, antibacterial, anti-inflammatory and immune-stimulating properties. In particular, it contains andrographolides, compounds considered to be responsible for the herb's ability to ward off harmful bacteria and viruses. It is high in antioxidants, while also supporting liver and gall bladder function and increasing bile flow, thus speeding the removal of toxins from the body. It may be of assistance in treating or preventing a variety of respiratory tract infections, including the common cold, sore throat and flu, as well as ear, nose and throat infections such as tonsillitis and sinusitis.

Andrographis has been traditionally prescribed for digestive complaints, including poor appetite, diarrhea, bowel infections and inflammatory bowel disease, intestinal worms, dysentery, flatulence and liver and gall bladder problems. There has also been a small amount of clinical research undertaken into its possible use for treating HIV-positive patients.

How to use

In traditional Chinese medicine and Ayurveda, a cooling herb like andrographis may be prescribed in conjunction with a "warming" one such as ginger. A practitioner qualified in either modality may prepare a personalized formula for you. Dosages may vary depending on whether the herb is being taken during an infection or as a preventive—follow label instructions or take as professionally prescribed. Due to the herb's extremely bitter taste, some people may find it easier to take in capsule or tablet form.

Safety first *Avoid andrographis during pregnancy and while breastfeeding, or if you suffer from heartburn or have a gastric ulcer. In rare cases it may cause an allergic reaction, ranging from a rash to dizziness and headache. High doses may cause nausea and vomiting.*

Where to find *Andrographis is available in pharmacies and health food stores in tablet or capsule form, often combined with other immune-boosting ingredients like echinacea, holy basil and zinc. Andrographis may also be prescribed by a qualified herbalist as a tincture or in dried form.*

APPLE CIDER VINEGAR

use for ✓ ***Diabetes and insulin resistance*** ✓ ***Psoriasis***
✓ ***Scalp and hair problems***

A POPULAR FOLK REMEDY, apple cider vinegar (ACV) has played multiple roles over the centuries. It has been a wound-healing agent, preservative, condiment, tonic, deodorant, preventer of scurvy, disinfectant and even an elixir of youth. Today its use as a remedy centers on its ability to help certain skin and scalp disorders when applied topically. It is also being studied for its potential in taming blood glucose levels and its ability to promote weight loss.

How it works

The main constituent of ACV is acetic acid, which has antimicrobial properties. Acetic acid is used topically in conventional medicine to combat antibiotic-resistant bacteria that infect open wounds, and has proved effective against *Staphylococcus aureus* in patients with leg ulcers. ACV also contains other acids, mineral salts and amino acids, which may have a therapeutic role. The US National Psoriasis Foundation suggests that diluted ACV applied topically can relieve the itch that occurs with scalp psoriasis. Some sufferers report that mixing it with honey improves skin quality and reduces irritation in other areas and that drinking it with honey is also effective, though as yet there is no clinical evidence to support these uses. Elsewhere ACV has long been acclaimed as a hair-conditioning treatment, which produces shinier, less tangled and more manageable locks.

Like other vinegars, when ingested ACV may help lower blood glucose. One theory is that it does this by deactivating enzymes that break down carbohydrates into glucose, thus slowing the digestive process. A 2007 study of 11 people with type 2 diabetes found that taking 2 tablespoons (30 ml) of ACV in water at bedtime reduced waking glucose levels by 4–6 percent. Other research suggests that taking ACV might encourage weight loss.

Safety first *Drinking large quantities may deplete potassium and sodium levels. Diabetics should consult their doctor before taking ACV as it can affect insulin levels. Applied neat, topical vinegar may burn your skin.*

Where to find *Apple cider vinegar is available in supermarkets and health food stores. Cloudy, organic ACV, which still contains some "mother" of vinegar (the mixture of bacteria and yeast that produced it), is believed by naturopaths to be the most potent.*

How to use

ACV is sometimes taken with water and honey as a tonic: 2 tablespoons (30 ml) of ACV in 1 cup (250 ml) of water, taken with meals. To make a gargle for soothing a sore throat, add 1 teaspoon (5 ml) of ACV to 1/2 cup (125 ml) of water. Do not drink it undiluted or in large quantities as the acid may damage your tooth enamel. For topical use, ACV can be diluted, mixed with honey or added to bathwater to treat skin conditions.

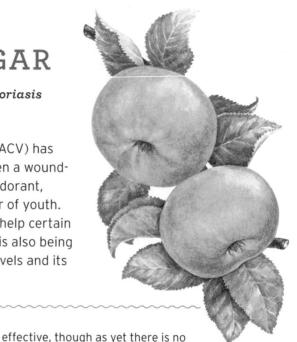

ARNICA *Arnica montana.* Also called: Mountain tobacco, Leopard's bane

use for ✓ ***Bruises*** ✓ ***Strains and sprains***

PREPARATIONS MADE FROM THE YELLOW flowers and root of *Arnica montana* have been used for centuries to treat bruises, sprains, muscle pain and other disorders. The German poet Johann Wolfgang von Goethe reputedly took arnica tea to cure chest pains. No modern practitioner would suggest that, as arnica can be poisonous and should not be taken by mouth, except in highly diluted homeopathic form.

How it works

The plant contains anti-inflammatory chemicals called sesquiterpene lactones, which help to reduce swelling, and flavonoids, which strengthen blood vessels reducing the leakage of blood under the skin that occurs with bruising. In German laboratory research, a tincture of arnica flowers was shown to suppress two enzymes in joint cartilage that contribute to the swelling and joint damage seen in osteoarthritis and rheumatoid arthritis.

Helenalin, the most powerful of the plant's sesquiterpene lactones, has also been studied in the laboratory for its antitumor effects and its potential to combat the bacterial infection *Staphylococcus aureus.*

Human research, although not always consistent, supports the plant's traditional role for treating bruises, strains and sprains. One 2010 study concluded that a 20 percent topical arnica preparation was more effective than a vitamin K formulation for reducing bruising. An earlier 2008 study found it as effective as ibuprofen gel for treating osteoarthritis of the hand.

For reasons that scientists find harder to explain, homeopathic arnica has been shown to reduce muscle soreness in marathon runners; in other research homeopathic arnica cream helped athletes with sports injuries recover faster. Taking homeopathic arnica has also proved effective for reducing postoperative swelling and bruising in patients undergoing cosmetic surgery.

How to use

Arnica gels, ointments and creams can be applied to the skin as directed, while tinctures can be used in compresses and poultices. Take homeopathic arnica as advised by your practitioner or according to the label instructions.

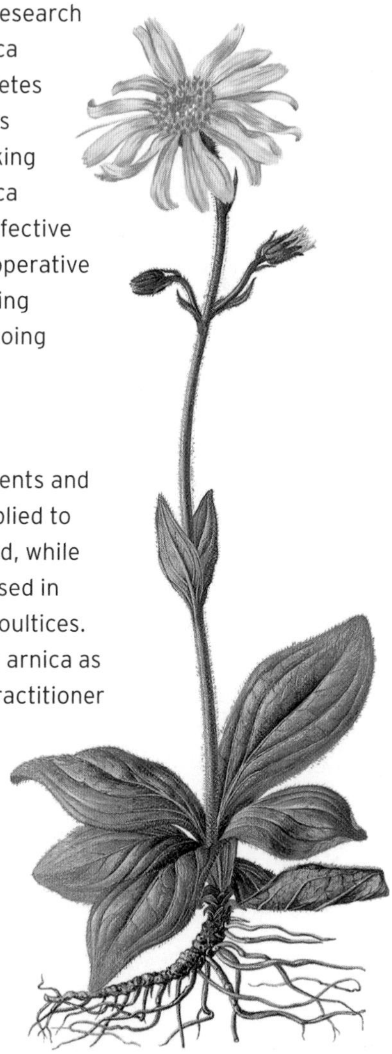

Safety first **Arnica should not be taken internally (except in homeopathic form).** *Don't use arnica on broken skin or on an open wound. Topical arnica may irritate the skin if used long term and can trigger allergies in susceptible people. If pregnant or breastfeeding, consult your doctor before using arnica in any form.*

Where to find Arnica preparations are available in health food stores and pharmacies or from a qualified homeopath.

AROMATHERAPY

use for ✓ ***Anxiety*** ✓ ***Bronchitis*** ✓ ***Concentration, improved*** ✓ ***Dementia*** ✓ ***Hair loss***

ANCIENT CIVILIZATIONS FROM EGYPT TO CHINA used essential oils ritually, medicinally and in cosmetics. The modern practice of aromatherapy owes much to an explosion in a French laboratory in 1910 that severely burnt chemist and perfumer René-Maurice Gattefossé. When his burns developed gangrene and failed to respond to conventional treatment, he applied an old Provençal remedy—essential oil of lavender—as a last resort and the wounds healed rapidly. Inspired by the experience, he began to analyze the chemical properties of lavender and other essential oils. As well as his own findings, he promoted the work of other scientists and summarized the research in *Aromathérapie*, published in 1937. Today in France and elsewhere in Europe, aromatherapy is a part of mainstream medicine and is gaining popularity worldwide.

How it works

Essential oils distilled from the leaves, roots, bark, flowers and other parts of the plant are used in inhalations, massages, topical ointments and medicines to treat a variety of mental and physical ailments. Their highly concentrated plant constituents have antiseptic, anti-inflammatory, antifungal and antibacterial properties, as many studies have confirmed. Some also have psychological effects, promoting relaxation or boosting cognitive performance.

Inhaling the oils is a key way to enjoy their psychological benefits. Smell bypasses the analytical part of the brain by acting on olfactory receptor cells in the nose that communicate directly with the limbic system, the part of the brain in charge of emotions and memory. This explains why a certain smell can trigger a vivid memory or inspire a particular feeling.

Research has shown that lavender oil, lemon balm, rose oil and orange oil all have a measurable calming effect on patients with dementia. In a UK study of dental patients, those who inhaled lavender oil experienced significantly reduced pretreatment anxiety. The benefits of aromatherapy are not necessarily dependent on the sense of smell. In one Japanese animal experiment, cedarwood oil had a tranquilizing effect on the brain even when the sense of smell was impaired.

Essential oils applied to the skin can also benefit mood. In another recent study, when lemon balm lotion was used on the face and arms of patients with advanced dementia, their behavior improved significantly compared to those who received only sunflower oil. Massage with essential oils has also been shown to alleviate anxiety and depression in cancer patients. This combination of active plant constituents plus the well-known therapeutic

Safety first **Never take essential oils by mouth unless prescribed by a qualified medical practitioner.** *Always dilute them before use on the skin as they can burn and may have a toxic effect if absorbed. If you have a nut allergy, tell your practitioner as almond oil, a popular carrier oil, could be harmful. In some people, the essential oils themselves may trigger an allergic reaction.*

Where to find *Seek out a qualified aromatherapist via your country's register of accredited practitioners. It may also be worth consulting your doctor to determine if aromatherapy is appropriate and suitable for your particular health problems.*

elements of touch and manipulation appears to treat both psychological problems and ailments as disparate as alopecia and arthritis.

Studies that examine the benefits of eucalyptus for treating respiratory ailments including bronchitis provide further evidence that essential oils work not only through inhalation but also permeate the skin. Whether inhaled or rubbed on the chest, the efficacy of eucalyptus oil as an antiviral agent and its safety make it an attractive alternative to pharmaceutical drugs. A standardised mixture of three essential oil constituents—cineole from eucalyptus, limonene from citrus fruits and alpha-pinene from pine—taken orally has also proved effective in studies.

How to use

You don't have to be unwell to enjoy essential oils. Their ability to soothe headaches, ease muscular pains and promote relaxation makes them a popular everyday choice. It is important to buy pure essential oils, not synthetic ones, and to use them sparingly. Pure oils are highly concentrated, so should never be applied neat to the skin.

Try the following:

- For a massage, add 4–6 drops of essential oil to 4 teaspoons (20 ml) of a vegetable-based carrier oil such as sweet almond or grape seed
- For a relaxing bath, add a few drops of essential oil to bath water
- For an inhalation, add 2–3 drops of essential oil to a bowl of hot water.

Different oils have different properties, so it is worth consulting a qualified aromatherapist who will help you understand which will work best for you.

A visit to the aromatherapist

A consultation will often start with questions about your medical history, diet and lifestyle as this is a holistic treatment. Most treatments involve a massage using one or more essential oils, so you will usually have to remove some clothes.

An initial treatment with preliminary questions may last up to two hours; subsequent sessions will probably be an hour or 90 minutes, as agreed. Your practitioner may also suggest inhalations and recommend specific oils that you can use at home.

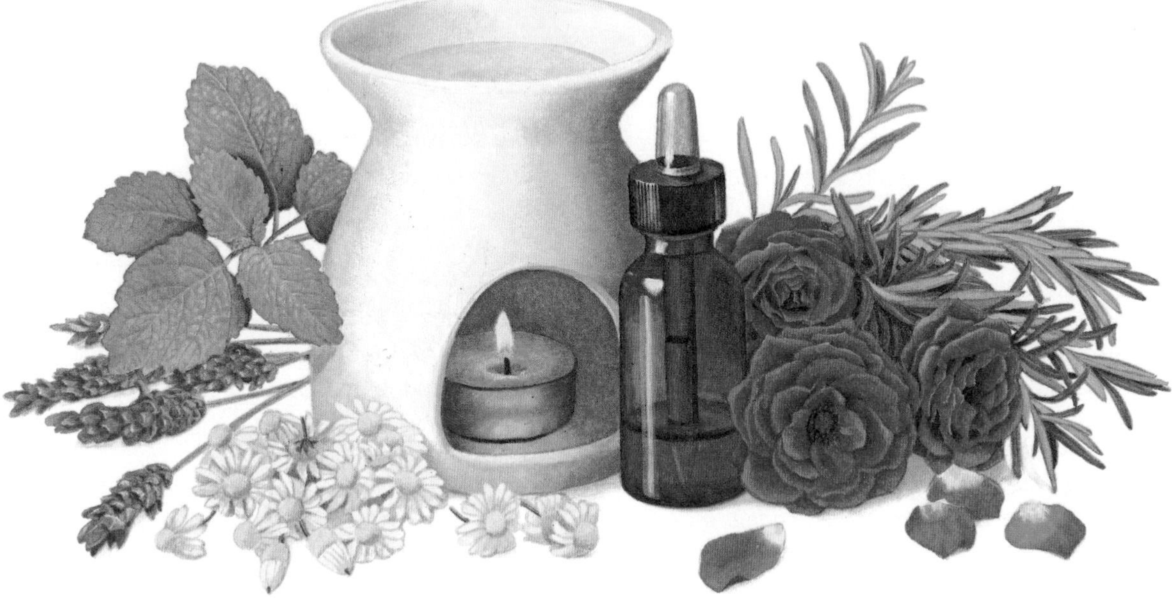

ASHWAGANDHA *Withania somnifera.*

Also called: Withania

use for ✓ ***Anxiety*** ✓ ***Frequent illness***

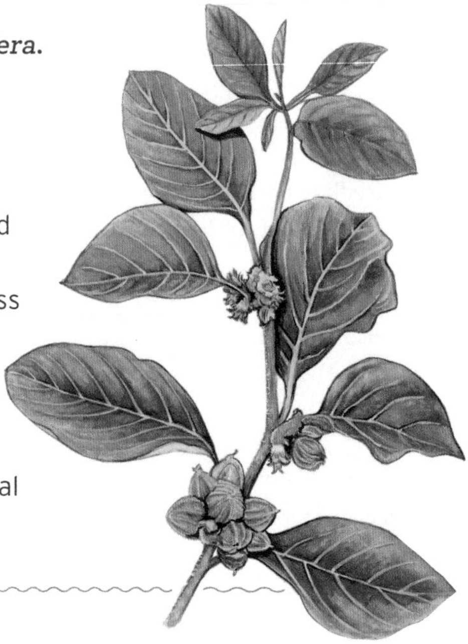

FOR MORE THAN 3,000 YEARS ashwagandha—a Sanskrit word describing the horse-like smell of the herb's root—has been an important ingredient in Ayurvedic medicine. It belongs to a class of Ayurvedic herbs known as adaptogens or vitalizers, which are prescribed to boost health and increase longevity. Its root has also been used traditionally to induce sleep, as its Latin name suggests. It can help combat stress and anxiety and its most abundant compound—Withaferin A (WA), a steroidal lactone—is being studied for its potential to fight cancer.

How it works

Alone and in combination with maitake (*Grifola fondosa*) extract (see Medicinal mushrooms, *p. 233*), ashwagandha appears to strengthen the immune system. A number of studies show that its active constituents, including alkaloids, steroidal lactones and withanolides, have natural antoxidant, antitumor, anti-inflammatory and tranquilizing effects. The herb is high in iron, too, and can help raise hemoglobin levels and red blood cell counts.

Safety first *Ashwagandha is considered safe but, because there are no formal safety studies, pregnant and nursing mothers, young children or anyone with severe kidney or liver disease should avoid it. It may also raise thyroid hormone levels so should not be taken by anyone with an overactive thyroid (hyperthyroidism). Check with your doctor if taking other sedatives as ashwagandha may enhance the effect.*

Where to find *Ashwagandha is available in health food stores, or may be prescribed by a qualified herbalist or Ayurvedic practitioner.*

Because stress and anxiety weaken the body's defenses, making people more susceptible to disease, ashwagandha's calming effect is significant. When a group of chronically stressed people received standardized ashwagandha leaf and root extract daily in a double-blind placebo-controlled study in India, all reported improved well-being and their stress levels were markedly lower than those receiving a placebo. In a recent Canadian study, naturopathic treatment that included ashwagandha was more effective than psychotherapy for relieving anxiety and improving quality of life. In two other recent studies, drinking tea fortified with Ayurvedic herbs including ashwagandha was found to provide significantly more protection against chronic coughs and colds than regular tea.

How to use

Traditionally, a small portion of the root is boiled in milk or water and taken as a tonic. Ashwagandha root extract is widely available in capsule, tablet and powder form. Follow label instructions or take as professionally prescribed.

ASTRAGALUS *Astragalus membranaceus, A. mongholicus*

use for ✓ ***Colds and flu*** ✓ ***Frequent illness***

THE DRIED ROOT OF A PEA-FAMILY PLANT native to northern and eastern China, astragalus has been a key ingredient in traditional Chinese medicine's immune-enhancing herbal tonics for more than 2,000 years. In this ancient healing practice, it is known as *Huang-qi* or "yellow leader"—describing this root's butter-yellow hue and its role in blends of herbs used to invigorate the body's vital energy and fend off disease. In the West astragalus is a relative newcomer, gaining popularity during the resurgence of interest in botanical medicine in the 1980s.

How it works

Herbalists classify astragalus as an adaptogen, able to help the body withstand physical, mental and emotional stress. Recent studies suggest that this root's immune-enhancing reputation may have some basis in science. For example, in laboratory studies certain chemicals found in astragalus have been shown to stimulate the activity of white blood cells (which attack invading bacteria and viruses). There is some evidence from a small, 2002 study from Taiwan that it reduces fatigue in athletes. In a 2009 study from Croatia's Clinical Hospital Dubrava, astragalus eased pollen-allergy symptoms when participants took the herb daily for six weeks.

How to use

Astragalus is most often taken as a tea in Chinese medicine and as a tea, tincture, capsule or tablet in the West. Since it is a tough, somewhat fibrous root, astragalus tea is usually made as a decoction. Some herbalists suggest boiling 1/2 teaspoon (2 ml) of dried root in 2 cups (500 ml) of water until the liquid is reduced to 1 cup (250 ml). When taking astragalus supplements, follow label instructions or take as professionally prescribed.

Safety first *Avoid astragalus if you take lithium, are undergoing chemotherapy or take immune-suppressing medications to reduce risk of rejection of a transplanted organ. Since astragalus may increase immune-system activity, avoid it if you have an autoimmune disease such as multiple sclerosis, lupus or rheumatoid arthritis. Astragalus has not been widely tested during pregnancy or breast-feeding and so it is best avoided or used only under medical supervision during these periods.*

Where to find *Buy the sliced root, whole root, capsules, tablets, teas and tinctures in health food stores or from a qualified herbalist.*

AVOCADOS

Persea americana

use for ✓ ***Scalp and hair problems***

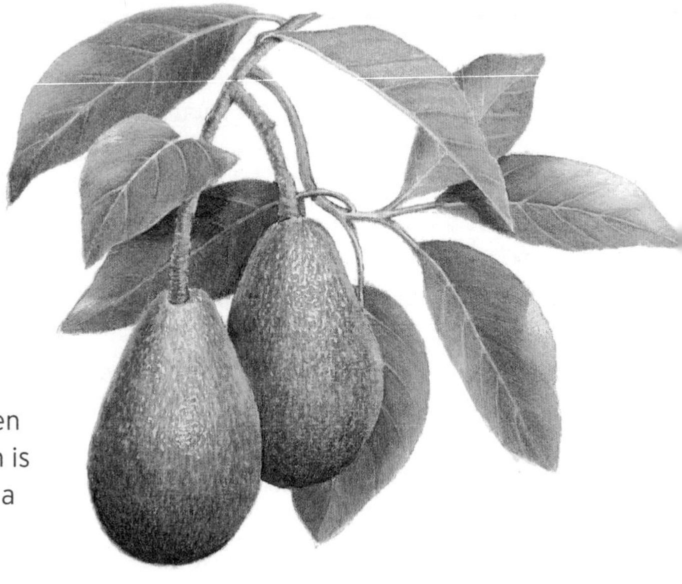

PACKED WITH NUTRIENTS, avocados were a mainstay of the Aztec and Inca diets for hundreds of years. In 1519 the Spanish historian Fernandez de Oviedo gave a description of this hitherto unreported plant: "In the center of the fruit is a seed like a peeled chestnut. And between this and the rind is the part which is eaten, which is abundant, and is a paste similar to butter and of a very good taste."

How they work

Unique among fruits, the avocado has high levels of fat, but it's "good" monounsaturated fat, similar to olive oil and helpful in the prevention and treatment of heart disease, skin problems, osteoarthritis and diabetes. One study showed that the monounsaturated fat in avocados reduced blood cholesterol levels while increasing protective HDL (high-density lipoprotein) levels. The assortment of beneficial essential oils in avocados are thought to assist in hair growth and are useful for dry scalp conditions. Avocados also contain good amounts of soluble fiber, vitamin E, folate, betacarotene and lutein *(p. 225)*, a substance that is believed to reduce the formation of cataracts and offer protection against age-related macular degeneration.

Safety first *Avocados are generally well tolerated and allergies are rare.*

Where to find *Supermarkets, greengrocers, farmers' markets.*

How to use

Avocados will mature but not ripen on the tree. This is due to a hormone produced by the leaves that inhibits the production of ethylene, the ripening chemical. Once picked, the hormone has no influence and the fruit will ripen within days. Best eaten raw, avocados contain tannins that become bitter when cooked. Due to their oil content, avocado flesh is susceptible to oxidation and will turn brown quickly unless you apply lime or lemon juice to the flesh directly after cutting it.

To treat a dry scalp, first wash and towel-dry your hair. Mash the flesh of an avocado with a tablespoon of coconut oil, an egg yolk and a tablespoon (15 ml) of honey. Apply to damp hair, rubbing into scalp. Cover with a shower cap and leave for 20 minutes. Rinse out thoroughly and wash hair again.

Avocado is an excellent, healthy substitute for butter, margarine or mayonnaise. It has roughly one-quarter the calories of those spreads, with many additional nutrients.

AYURVEDA

use for ✓ ***Acne*** ✓ ***Burns*** ✓ ***Frequent illness***

THIS MOST ANCIENT OF HEALING SYSTEMS has much appeal for the modern world. Practiced in India for thousands of years, Ayurveda takes a holistic and personalized approach, treating the whole person and providing a unique assessment of each individual. The goal of any treatment is to create a harmonious mental and physical balance, synonymous with health and well-being.

How it works

In Ayurvedic terminology, everyone has a unique combination of three *doshas* or energy types: *vata* (which controls movement), *pitta* (which controls digestion and metabolism) and *kapha* (which controls growth and maintenance). Anything such as stress or a poor diet that upsets the balance of the *doshas*, and a number of subcomponents, can have adverse physical and mental effects. Once the precise type of imbalance has been identified, the practitioner prescribes a tailor-made treatment.

While the nature of such a system challenges scientific evaluation, Western research supports individual components. Mainstays of Ayurveda, including lifestyle practices, yoga, meditation and certain dietary interventions, have been borrowed and adapted across the world. Studies of specific Ayurvedic herbs are revealing constituents that help explain their therapeutic powers. For example, compounds in **ashwagandha** *(p. 124)* and **holy basil** *(p. 205)*, known as adaptogens, are thought to balance and revitalize the body.

Similarly, research suggests that various enzymes, hormones and sugars in ***aloe vera*** *(p. 117)* help burns and other wounds heal faster; while the combination of aloe with two anti-inflammatory herbs—ashwagandha and **turmeric** *(p. 298)*—has been shown to treat acne. Studies of another ayurvedic herb, **andrographis** *(p. 119)*, suggest that certain bioactive constituents may hold the key to its ability to prevent and curtail the common cold.

Safety first *Tell the Ayurvedic practitioner if you are pregnant and mention any medical condition you have. Ensure that you inform your doctor of any Ayurvedic herbs you are taking and tell your Ayurvedic practitioner about any prescription medicines you are on.*

Where to find *To find a qualified Ayurvedic practitioner, visit the National Ayurvedic Medical Association (www.ayurvedanama.org) or ask your doctor for a referral.*

A visit to an Ayurvedic practitioner

At an initial treatment session, your practitioner will ask about your medical history, diet and lifestyle. He or she will conduct a short physical examination, taking your pulse, looking at your eyes, tongue and skin and even assessing your voice. Treatment will be designed to restore your personal *dosha* balance and may include lifestyle and dietary changes, mantras and meditation, as well as cleansing strategies and herbal medicines.

continued on page 128

AYURVEDA *continued*

Food as medicine

The diet is a key component of the Ayurvedic healing system and a practitioner will ask you closely about yours. He or she will recommend you eat more or less of certain types of food, herbs and spices—depending on your *dosha*—with the aim of bringing your body back into balance. When the body is well nourished and in balance, it is better able to fight off infection and ailments are less likely to arise. Common ingredients in Ayurvedic cooking are shown below such as (clockwise from the top) holy basil, ginger, fenugreek, garlic, gotu kola, turmeric and sesame seed oil. The dark substance in the silver dish is a kind of herbal jam known as Chyawanprash. There are various recipes, all containing more than 20 different herbs and spices, while the main ingredient is amla (Indian gooseberry). Chyawanprash is eaten on bread or in warmed milk as a general tonic.

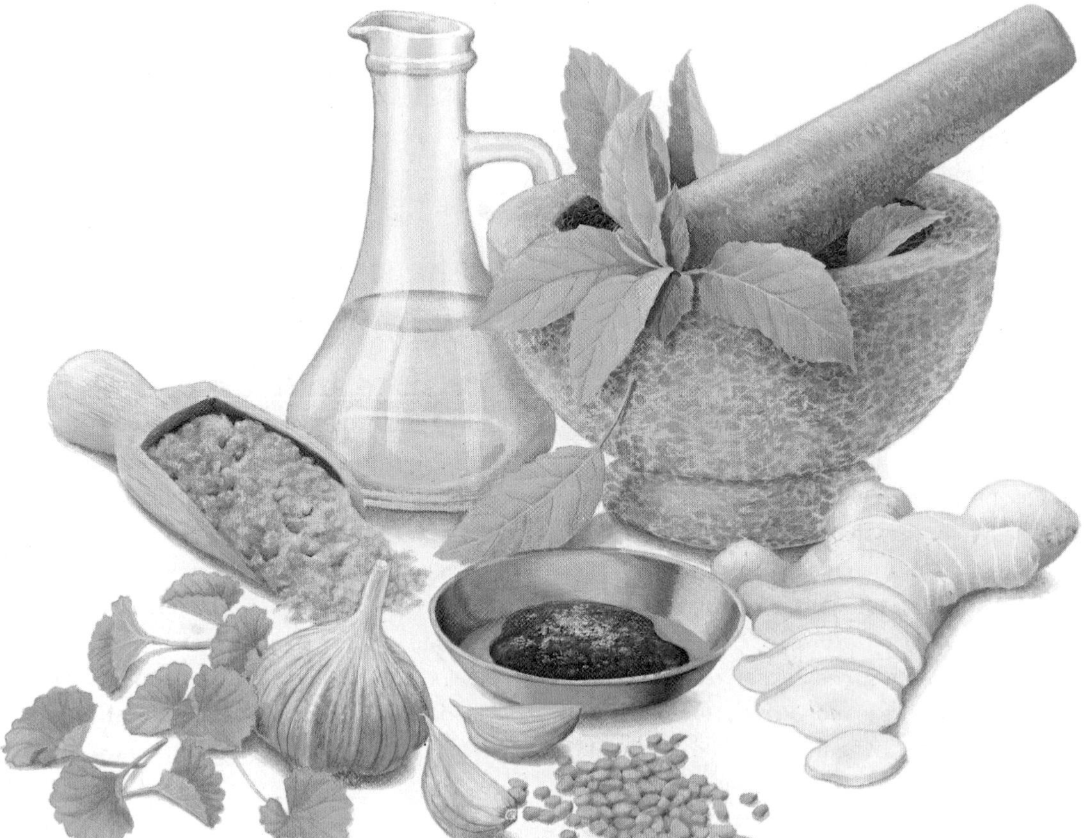

BERGAMOT *Citrus bergamia*

use for ✓ ***Anxiety*** ✓ ***Herpes***

BERGAMOT ESSENTIAL OIL IS PRODUCED from the rind of the fruit of the bergamot tree, a sour, inedible, citrus native to Calabria, Italy. It has a light, refreshing aroma and is an important ingredient in many perfumes including eau-de-cologne. Bergamot is also used to impart the signature aroma and flavor to Earl Grey tea.

How it works

Essential oils such as bergamot not only heal through the effect of smell, they also contain natural chemicals with beneficial actions, including linalool that has been found to have anti-anxiety and mildly sedating properties. With its gentle uplifting fragrance, bergamot is often recommended for helping those who suffer from anxiety and sleeping problems. Aromatherapists also use bergamot to treat a variety of conditions including eczema and psoriasis, the early stages of cystitis, and to reduce the effects of cold sores, chicken pox and shingles where it is often combined with tea tree and lavender essential oils. Bergamot oil is also used to relieve indigestion, where it is rubbed on the stomach.

How to use

For anxiety or to reduce stress, add 5–8 drops of bergamot oil to your bath. Or you can add some to a vaporizer and put it beside your bed at night. For topical application, bergamot oil can be added to a carrier oil, such as jojoba or olive oil, to create a massage blend that would be helpful for anxiety as well as digestive upsets.

Safety first **Bergamot essential oil should not be taken internally.** *Bergaptene, a natural chemical found in bergamot oil is phototoxic, so avoid exposure to direct sunlight after applying the oil in a bath or massage. Bergamot essential oil has not been widely tested during pregnancy or breastfeeding so it is best avoided or used only under medical supervision during these periods.*

Where to find *Bergamot oil can be found in health food stores and some pharmacies.*

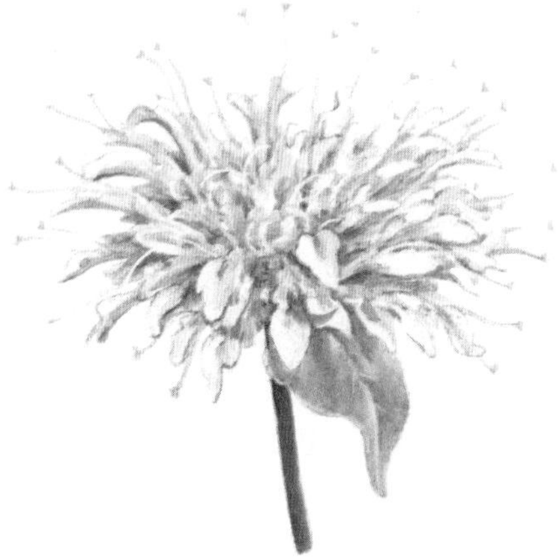

BICARBONATE OF SODA

use for ✓ ***Bad breath and body odor*** ✓ ***Indigestion*** ✓ ***Scalp and hair problems*** ✓ ***Urinary tract infections***

COMMONLY KNOWN AS BAKING SODA, bicarbonate of soda can do more than simply make your scones light and airy. It is often used as a "green" alternative to harsh chemical household cleaning products and there are also health benefits to be had from this pantry staple. It is derived from a naturally occurring mineral, nahcolite, comprised of sodium hydrogen carbonate ($NaHCO_3$). Nahcolite occurs in nature as a solid white crystal, while baking soda is sold as a fine white powder.

How it works

Bicarbonate of soda, containing carbonate (CO_3), has a buffering effect on the acid/alkaline balance in the body, rendering it useful for relieving the pain of heartburn, gastro-esophageal reflux disease (GERD) and stomach ulcers. It may also help reduce the burning sensation experienced during urinary tract infections. Bicarbonate of soda can be used as a breath freshener as well as an effective teeth whitener and toothpaste alternative. Bicarbonate of soda can help remove the buildup of hair products, assisting in keeping hair clean. Bicarbonate of soda can also be used as a deodorant, as it masks the odor of sweat, although it has no antiperspirant activity. Bicarbonate of soda will react with and neutralize strong odors in the refrigerator and can serve as a cleaning aid on hard surfaces.

Safety first *Bicarbonate of soda is generally considered safe. Use for short-term complaints of no more than two weeks duration, and see your doctor if symptoms persist. Avoid if you are on a low-sodium diet.*

Where to find *Bicarbonate of soda is found in supermarkets in the baking section.*

How to use

For temporary relief of heartburn or GERD, or to help soothe the pain of urinary tract infection, put 1 teaspoon of bicarbonate of soda in a glass of water and drink (do not take on a full stomach). To make toothpaste, mix six parts bicarbonate of soda with one part salt, make into a paste with a little water. Gently massage the paste onto your teeth and gums. Rinse after two to three minutes.

For a deodorant, pat some dry bicarbonate of soda under the arms or wherever required. For a mouthwash to combat bad breath, add 1/2 teaspoon (2 ml) of bicarbonate of soda and 1/2 teaspoon (2 ml) of salt to a small amount of water and gargle for up to 30 seconds then spit out. For cleaner hair, add a teaspoon of bicarbonate of soda to your shampoo.

BIOTIN

use for ✓ ***Hair loss*** ✓ ***Nail problems***

BIOTIN IS ONE OF THE B-COMPLEX GROUP of vitamins. It is found in a wide range of foods, including liver, eggs, sardines, whole grains, bananas, nuts and cauliflower, but is believed to be more readily absorbed from meat sources than from plant sources.

Since biotin is available in many foods, outright deficiency rarely occurs in developed countries. However, some researchers believe that many pregnant women are marginally deficient in biotin, and that this could increase their children's risk of genetic abnormalities or birth defects.

How it works

Biotin is essential for several of the enzymatic reactions involved in the breakdown of fats, proteins and other food components. When deficiency is present, signs and symptoms may include hair loss, dermatitis, developmental delays in babies and children, nervous system issues (including seizures), and eye and vision problems. Blood glucose problems (such as impaired glucose tolerance) may also occur.

Safety first *If you have diabetes, talk to your doctor before taking biotin supplements as they may affect your blood glucose levels and medication requirements. High-dose biotin supplements should only be taken under professional supervision.*

Where to find *Biotin supplements are available in health food stores and pharmacies.*

How to use

Health authorities in the US estimate an Adequate Intake (AI) of biotin for adult men (19+) is 30 mcg/day. Women need 30 mcg/day, 30 mcg/day during pregnancy and 35 mcg/day while breastfeeding. No upper intake level has been determined.

People with alopecia areata (a condition in which hair is lost from the scalp and other parts of the body in patches, leaving areas of baldness) may have low levels of the enzyme biotinidase, which is involved in the breakdown and utilization of biotin. Taking supplements containing high doses of biotin may promote new hair growth in affected people. Biotin supplements may also help make brittle fingernails firmer and prevent them from splitting.

High-dose biotin supplements are sometimes prescribed along with chromium picolinate for people with diabetes whose blood glucose levels are poorly controlled despite the use of antidiabetic medication.

BITTER MELON *Momordica charantia*

use for ✓ ***Diabetes and insulin resistance***

IN TROPICAL AREAS FROM CHINA, Asia and Africa to the Caribbean and South America, bitter melon is both a food and a medicine. Unripe, its fruit resembles a warty, green cucumber that gradually turns orange with bright red edible seeds as it matures. Despite an exceedingly bitter taste, the fruits and sometimes the leaves are widely used in a variety of ethnic dishes. Bitter melon is a major constituent of the Okinawan diet and, some say, is key to the renowned longevity of the Japanese island people. Modern research has largely focused on its potential for treating diabetes.

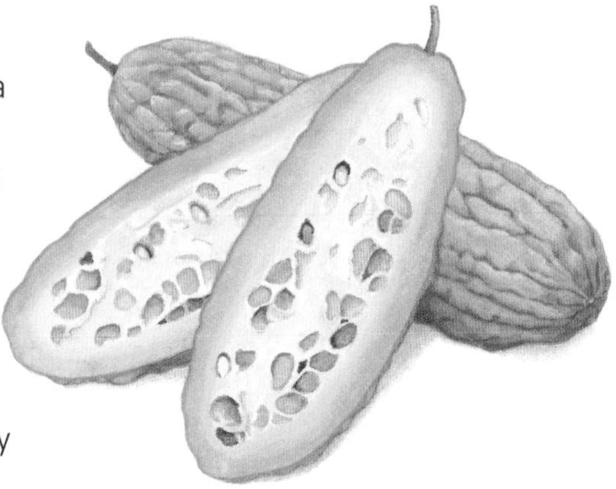

How it works

Although the human evidence is not yet strong, laboratory studies show that bitter melon has a hypoglycemic (blood glucose–lowering) action, and helps to control insulin levels. The constituents thought to be responsible for this action are charantin, plus alkaloids and peptides that mimic insulin. They may also trigger the production of a protein that encourages glucose uptake in the body.

In addition, charantin appears to stimulate the growth of pancreatic beta cells, which produce insulin. In type 1 diabetes, the immune system destroys beta cells; in other types of diabetes the functioning of beta cells is impaired.

Laboratory studies support other traditional uses of bitter melon, suggesting that different constituents have antiviral and antibacterial properties that might help to treat disorders including salmonella and *E. coli* infections, herpes and HIV viruses, malaria and parasitic worms. An extract of bitter melon proteins is claimed to inhibit prostate tumor growth and a number of in vitro studies suggest it may have potential for combating other cancers and leukemia.

Safety first *Take care if taking bitter melon with blood glucose–lowering medications as it can enhance their effect. It has a weak uterine stimulant activity so must not be used during pregnancy or breastfeeding. Bitter melon should not be taken by people with glucose-6-phosphate dehydrogenase (G6PDH) deficiency (a genetic condition most common in people from the Mediterranean and Middle East) due to a risk of hemolytic anemia.*

Where to find *The fresh fruit is available in some supermarkets and Asian stores. Bitter melon supplements are available in health food stores or from a qualified herbalist.*

How to use

Traditionally bitter melon is taken as a fresh juice, decoction or tincture. Concentrated fruit, seed and whole herb extracts are also available as tablets, capsules or powders. Follow label instructions or take as professionally prescribed.

BLACK COHOSH *Cimicifuga racemosa*

use for ✓ ***Menopausal symptoms*** ✓ ***Natural fertility management***

FOR CENTURIES NATIVE AMERICANS took black cohosh to treat menstrual and other health problems, and New World colonists adopted the herb. In the late 1800s, it was one of five herbal ingredients in a highly successful and profitable medicine, launched by Lydia E. Pinkham (Lily the Pink). Pinkham's Vegetable Compound, which also contained a significant amount of alcohol, was marketed directly to women, offering relief from menstrual cramps and side effects of menopause such as depression and hot flashes.

Although evidence of its efficacy is not conclusive, the World Health Organization and the European Cooperative on Phytotherapy have listed black cohosh for menopausal symptoms. The German Commission E, which regulates herbs in Germany, has approved it for treating menstrual and menopausal problems.

How it works

The herb used to be described as a phytoestrogen, a plant whose compounds mimic the effects of estrogen, which may be helpful as falling estrogen levels are responsible for adverse effects of menopause. Researchers have now discovered that its estrogen-like action is limited to specific areas. These include the brain and bones, supporting its ability to relieve hot flashes and potentially to help prevent osteoporosis. It also appears to have some estrogen-like effects on the vagina but not on the breasts or uterus.

When taken alongside the fertility drug clomiphene, black cohosh was shown to more than double the pregnancy rate of women with unexplained infertility. In a 2005 German trial of 304 menopausal women, black cohosh extract relieved symptoms much better than a placebo; results were similar to those from earlier studies of hormone replacement therapy. A combination of black cohosh and St. John's wort (p. 274) proved effective for relieving hot flashes and menopausal depression in a 2007 Korean study.

Safety first *Black cohosh can cause occasional mild gastrointestinal problems and has been associated with liver damage in some women. Discontinue use and consult your doctor if you have a liver disorder or develop symptoms of liver trouble such as abdominal pain, dark urine, or jaundice while taking black cohosh.*

The safety of black cohosh during pregnancy and breastfeeding and for women who have breast cancer is uncertain and so it is best avoided or used only under medical supervision in these circumstances.

Where to find *Black cohosh products are available in health food stores and pharmacies or from a qualified herbalist.*

How to use

The herb is sold as capsules, tablets, tinctures, solutions and powders and is the main ingredient in many menopausal formulations. Follow label instructions or take as professionally prescribed. Black cohosh should not be taken continuously for more than six months.

BLACK RASPBERRY *Rubus occidentalis*

use for ✓ ***Gastroenteritis***

JUICY AND SWEET, WITH A REFRESHINGLY tart edge, black raspberries are a delicious summer treat when plucked and eaten straight from the garden. Not to be confused with the similar but less potent blackberry, this fruit is more than a tasty addition to a fruit salad or pie. Native American healers used the roots of this North American plant to treat stomach and bowel upsets and the berries were used to sweeten bitter remedies. Today, science supports these traditional uses while revealing some new potential health benefits.

How it works

The black raspberry's dark purple juice contains high levels of anthocyanins—compounds that boost the body's cell-protecting antioxidant defenses. Black raspberry is also a rich source of ellagic acid, a phenolic compound with antiviral, antibacterial and cancer-prevention properties. In a laboratory study, black raspberry juice has been shown to inhibit viral gastrointestinal tract infections.

Safety first *Black raspberry is safe when enjoyed as a food. There's no safety data available on the consequences of consuming larger and more concentrated quantities of the fruit or its active compounds, particularly for pregnant or breastfeeding women.*

Where to find *Black raspberries are widely available in supermarkets during the summer season. Look for black raspberry concentrates in capsules, liquid extracts and as a freeze-dried powder in health food stores.*

Evidence from animal studies suggests that compounds in black raspberries may protect against several types of cancer. In one Ohio State University study, a freeze-dried black raspberry extract flipped genetic switches on cells affected by cancer-causing toxins—restoring normal cell activity. In a 2010 animal study from the University of Illinois at Chicago, a daily dose of black raspberry powder reduced risk for colorectal cancer formation. Other research from Ohio State University points to the cell-guarding powers of anthocyanins in black raspberries to help explain this fruit's cancer-preventing potential.

How to use

Reaping the black raspberry's healthy rewards may be as simple as including this fruit in a healthy diet on a regular basis. In laboratory studies, researchers have tested extracts though there is scant evidence that these are any better than fresh or frozen fruit. When using capsules or other products, follow label instructions or take as professionally prescribed.

BORAGE *Borago officinalis*

use for ✓ ***Eczema***

WITH ITS TENDER LEAVES and star-shaped blue flowers, borage was a popular addition to kitchen gardens in western Europe long before the dawn of modern medicine. Borage's leaves and stems were used as remedies for fevers and lung problems. But today, alternative therapists and scientists alike focus more intently on the unique oil contained in this herb's tiny seeds.

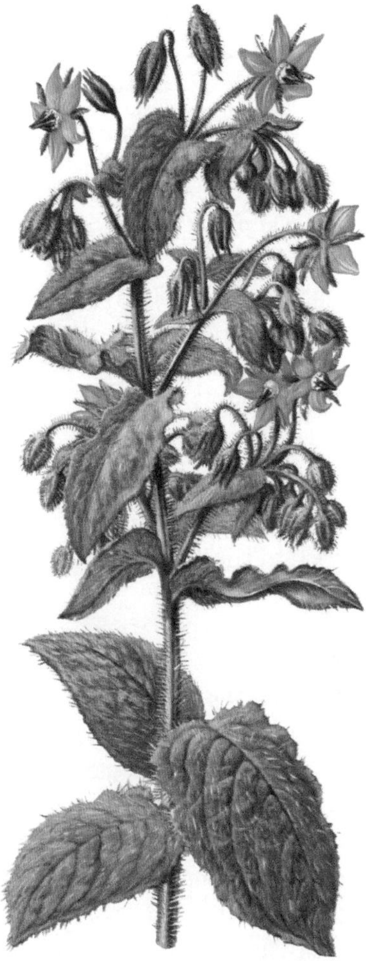

How it works

Borage seed oil is one of nature's top sources of gamma-linolenic acid (GLA)—a good fat in short supply in most people's diets. While evening primrose oil contains up to 10 percent GLA by weight and blackcurrant oil has up to 20 percent GLA, borage seed oil boasts an impressive 17–25 percent GLA.

GLA is an omega-6 fatty acid with anti-inflammatory effects that is used as a popular treatment for eczema in Europe. In one study, eczema symptoms improved in children who wore vests coated with borage seed oil. Some research also suggests that GLA-rich oils may help ease symptoms of rheumatoid arthritis. The reason? In the body, some GLA is converted into an anti-inflammatory compound called prostaglandin E1, which may help cool inflammation and ease joint pain.

How to use

Borage seed oil is usually taken in capsule form. Eating a healthy diet can help your body make best use of its treasure trove of GLA; getting enough magnesium, zinc and vitamins C and B_6 assist in the conversion of GLA into anti-inflammatory compounds. Take it with food and be patient. Herbalists say it can take several months to notice any benefits. Follow label instructions or take as professionally prescribed.

Safety first *Do not take borage seed oil or other GLA supplements if you have a seizure disorder; and consult your doctor about taking it before surgery, during pregnancy, while breastfeeding or if you are taking blood-thinning or other medications.*

Where to find *Borage seed oil is sold in bottles and in capsules. It is available in health food stores or from a qualified herbalist.*

BOSWELLIA *Boswellia serrata*

Also called: Indian frankincense

use for ✓ ***Asthma*** ✓ ***Bursitis and tendonitis*** ✓ ***Cancer support*** ✓ ***Chronic pain*** ✓ ***Osteoarthritis***

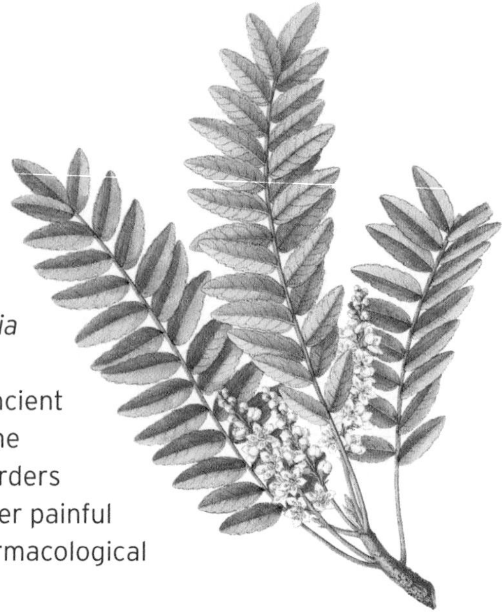

THE OILY GUM RESIN TAPPED from the Indian tree *Boswellia serrata*, also known as Indian frankincense, has been used ritually and medicinally for millennia. It is one of the most ancient and most highly valued of Ayurvedic herbs, cited in two of the earliest texts for its ability to treat rheumatic (arthritic) disorders and in later traditional texts as a remedy for a variety of other painful and inflammatory conditions. Modern science is finding pharmacological evidence to support many of these uses.

How it works

Studies suggest that the resin's anti-inflammatory effects are due to pentacyclic triterpenic acids, known as boswellic acids. Boswellic acids appear to block an enzyme that generates inflammatory molecules, called leukotrienes. Leukotrienes cause bronchoconstriction, the tightening of the airways during an asthma attack. They also trigger the pain and swelling associated with osteoarthritis.

In one German study of 40 asthmatic patients aged from 18 to 75 years, 70 percent had fewer attacks and significantly fewer symptoms such as breathlessness and wheezing after six weeks of treatment with a preparation of boswellia gum resin (compared to 27 percent of patients in the control group).

In a 2003 study, 15 patients with osteoarthritis of the knee received boswellia extract for eight weeks while a further 15 patients took a placebo. The first group then took the placebo and the second group the boswellia for a further eight weeks. After taking boswellia, all reported less knee pain, reduced swelling and greater flexibility of the knee joint. More recently osteoarthritis patients treated with boswellia resin in capsule and ointment form reported improved mobility and less pain. In another study, researchers found that patients with brain cancer who were given *Boswellia serrata* experienced significantly reduced brain swelling caused by radiation treatment. This suggests it may have potential as an alternative to steroids.

Safety first *While no serious side effects have been reported from clinical trials of standardized boswellia extract, it has not been widely tested during pregnancy or breast-feeding so it is best avoided or used only under medical supervision during these periods. Similarly avoid boswellia if you have kidney or liver disease.*

Where to find *Boswellia products are available in health food stores and pharmacies or from a qualified herbalist.*

How to use

Boswellia, sometimes marketed under its Sanskrit name *Shallaki*, is available as a standardized extract, in capsule or tablet form and as an ingredient in pain-relieving creams and ointments. Follow label instructions and consult your doctor first if you are taking other anti-inflammatory medications.

BOVINE COLOSTRUM

use for ✓ ***Diarrhea***

COLOSTRUM IS THE PREMILK FLUID PRODUCED by mammals a few days after giving birth. Bovine colostrum is obtained from cows. Sometimes referred to as a nutraceutical—a combination of nutritional supplement and pharmaceutical agent—colostrum contains large amounts of protein as well as growth and immune factors. It has been used for centuries in Ayurvedic medicine, especially for the care of newborns and has gained popularity in the West in recent years. In the 1950s Dr. Albert Sabin used bovine colostrum in the creation of the very successful oral antipolio vaccine.

How it works

Baby mammals are born without an active immune system. Colostrum contains high levels of antibodies that promote a healthy immune system in the infant mammal. The antibodies help the body to defend itself from certain bacteria, fungi and viruses including candida, *E. coli*, cryptosporidium and salmonella. A super boosted bovine colostrum known as hyperimmune bovine colostrum (HBC) has been used in several studies. This super colostrum is taken from cows that have previously been inoculated against diseases including the rotovirus (which causes diarrhea) and HIV-1 (AIDS virus). HBC has been found to contain antibodies for these conditions.

Studies have shown HBC may be helpful in the treatment of debilitating diarrhea. Certain substances in the colostrum are thought to inhibit the adhesion of the bacteria to the bowel wall, thus preventing infection. Other potential uses for bovine colostrum include improving athletic performance as there are growth factors within colostrum that may improve muscle growth and strength, increasing stamina and enhancing postexercise recovery in the training athlete.

Bovine colostrum contains lactoferrin, an iron-containing protein. Lactoferrin stimulates the growth of beneficial intestinal flora including bifidobacterium. Lactoferrin also increases iron absorption, reduces cholesterol levels and is thought to have some cancer-fighting potential.

How to use

Bovine colostrum and HBC are available in tablet, serum, capsule and powder form. Follow label instructions or take as professionally prescribed.

Safety first *Bovine colostrum is generally well tolerated by adults and children, with gastrointestinal upsets being the only infrequent side effect. Bovine colostrum should be avoided by those with a sensitivity to dairy foods. It has not been widely tested during pregnancy or breastfeeding so it is best avoided or used only under medical supervision during these periods.*

Where to find *Bovine colostrum is available in some health food stores, but it is best to obtain it and HBC from a qualified naturopath or other health practitioner, who will also be able to advise you on how to take it.*

BOWEN TECHNIQUE

use for ✓ ***Back and neck pain*** ✓ ***Bursitis and tendonitis*** ✓ ***Frozen shoulder***

DEVELOPED IN THE 1950S BY A REMARKABLE, largely self-taught Australian physical therapist named Tom Bowen, the Bowen Technique uses a light touch and gentle rolling motions to ease stiff, achy joints. Tom Bowen was working as a carpenter when he began treating people with muscle and joint complaints. Bowen died in 1982, but today trained practitioners offer the technique around the world.

How it works

No one's quite sure how the technique works, but practitioners theorize that the gentle movements send signals to the brain, via nerve pathways, that prompt the body to reset, repair and balance itself. The technique is not like a conventional muscle massage. It doesn't involve kneading tissues to "break up" tight spots. Instead, practitioners work gently on the fascia—the stretchy, thin, collagen-packed material that encases muscles, nerves, organs, bones and blood vessels.

Restoring fascia to flexibility and health can improve posture, loosen stiff joints and muscles and more. The therapy may offer relief for most musculoskeletal problems, including bursitis, back pain and muscle strains. In a UK study of 39 migraine sufferers who had three Bowen Technique sessions, 31 reported fewer and/or less severe headaches. Other studies organized by the European College of Bowen Studies have found that the therapy eased neck and shoulder pain and reduced knee and ankle stiffness in most people who came in for treatment.

A visit to the Bowen Technique practitioner

When visiting a practitioner, you may wear light clothing, though some therapists would rather work directly on the skin. Practitioners often begin by working on the lower and mid back and legs as the client lies facedown on a therapy table, then move to the upper back, shoulders and neck.

Safety first *Tell the practitioner if you are pregnant and mention any medical condition you have and other treatments or medicines you are taking. A program will be tailored to your specific needs.*

Where to find *To find a qualified practitioner, visit The American Bowen Academy at www.americanbowen.academy or ask your doctor for a recommendation.*

You may be surprised by how gentle the technique is—practitioners say clients feel relaxed afterward but may not notice an immediate improvement. Signs that the technique is working may include fatigue, thirst, a temporary increase in symptoms and even feeling as if you have the flu. Bowen Technique proponents say it's important to go back for the next session despite these sensations in order to see improvement. Practitioners also ask that clients do not schedule other bodywork within a week of a session, so that any healing triggered by the technique isn't disturbed.

A session generally lasts 45–60 minutes. In general, practitioners recommend three to four sessions, spaced a week apart.

BUTTERBUR *Petasites hybridus*

use for ✓ ***Allergies*** ✓ ***Chronic pain*** ✓ ***Hay fever*** ✓ ***Migraines***

THIS TRADITIONAL HERBAL REMEDY is nicknamed "bog rhubarb," because it grows in damp, marshy areas. It was once used in Europe to treat the plague; today, it is used for seasonal allergies (such as hay fever), colds and flu, and asthma, as well as providing effective relief for migraines.

How it works

Butterbur has natural antiallergenic, anti-inflammatory, antispasmodic and mildly analgesic (pain-relieving) effects. It works by decreasing the secretion of histamine and leukotrienes by the immune cells, which are the main chemicals that the body releases during an allergic reaction to what it perceives as an invader such as pollen, dust or animal dander. Butterbur is considered to be as effective as commonly available over-the-counter antihistamines for treating and controlling seasonal allergies such as hay fever. It acts to both mediate the allergic reaction and fight the inflammation in the upper respiratory tract, thereby alleviating symptoms such as stuffy nose, sore throat, runny eyes, blocked ears and sneezing, but without causing drowsiness. The active compounds it contains, called petasins, stop the inflammation associated with hay fever and may improve the efficacy of conventional inhalant preventive medications for asthma. Although evidence for the effectiveness of butterbur on allergies is small, many natural therapists and herbalists have found it useful for their patients.

Taken daily as a preventive, butterbur extract can bring relief to migraine sufferers, with clinical trials showing that it reduced the frequency, duration and intensity of migraine episodes. In one study published in *Neurology*, butterbur extract was found to be significantly more effective in reducing the frequency of migraines than placebo. It may also assist in relieving joint pain and menstrual cramps.

Safety first *Butterbur has not been widely tested during pregnancy or breastfeeding and so it is best avoided or used only under medical supervision during these periods. In rare instances, it may cause gastrointestinal upset, diarrhea, rashes, itchy eyes or skin, or drowsiness. Note that the wild plant contains compounds called pyrrolizidine alkaloids (PAs) that are toxic. However, standardized extracts used in herbal medicine are purified and often labelled "PA free."*

Where to find *Butterbur is available in health food stores or from a qualified herbalist.*

How to use

Butterbur is available in tablet or capsule form. Look for a product containing a standardized extract of petasins. Some manufacturers combine butterbur with other antiallergenic and anti-inflammatory ingredients, such as rosmarinic acid, nettle, quercetin or vitamin C, in formulas to prevent hay fever. Dosage depends on the potency of the product chosen. Follow label instructions or take as professionally prescribed. It is beneficial both as a treatment and a preventive for hay fever or seasonal allergies; if taking as a preventive, begin treatment around four to six weeks prior to the time when your symptoms usually first appear.

CALCIUM

use for ✓ ***Celiac disease*** ✓ ***Cramps, muscle*** ✓ ***Fall prevention*** ✓ ***Indigestion*** ✓ ***Menstrual problems*** ✓ ***Osteoporosis*** ✓ ***Tooth and gum disorders***

DIETARY CALCIUM IS FOUND IN DAIRY FOODS and bony fish such as canned salmon and sardines. It is also available from plant sources such as legumes, almonds and leafy green vegetables, although the presence of fiber and other compounds in plants means that calcium tends to be more difficult to absorb from these foods.

Many people don't obtain sufficient calcium from their diets, and consequently are at increased risk of developing osteoporosis, muscle spasms and pain, dental problems and other health issues. People most at risk of calcium deficiency include older people, people with malabsorption problems such as celiac disease, and those who have taken certain prescription medications (e.g., corticosteroids) for long periods of time.

How it works

Although best known for the important structural role it plays in the bones and teeth, calcium is also required for many other functions in the body, including muscle and nerve function, blood clotting, hormonal balance, the production of energy, and the maintenance of a regular heartbeat.

Safety first *Do not exceed the upper limit (UL) for calcium of 2,500 mg/day. If you suffer from kidney disease, hyperparathyroidism, sarcoidosis or related conditions, do not take calcium supplements unless advised to do so by your doctor.*

Where to find *Calcium supplements are available in health food stores, pharmacies and supermarkets. Look for a calcium supplement that also contains vitamin D_3.*

How to use

The US Recommended Dietary Allowance (RDA) of calcium for adult men (19+) is 1,000 mg/day, increasing to 1,200 mg/day from 70 years of age. The RDA for adult women is 1,000 mg/day (including those who are pregnant or breastfeeding), increasing to 1,200 mg/day from 50 years of age.

Calcium supplements are recommended for anyone who does not obtain the RDA from their diets—especially older people. When taken with vitamin D_3 (which enhances calcium absorption), calcium supplements may help slow declines in bone density, reduce the risk of bone fractures and aid in the prevention of falls in older people.

Taking calcium supplements daily for several months may also help relieve menstrual symptoms such as period pain, fluid retention and food cravings. If you suffer from indigestion, chewing on calcium carbonate tablets may help relieve your symptoms.

CALENDULA *Calendula officinalis.* Also called: Marigold

use for ✓ ***Cuts and scrapes*** ✓ ***Eczema and dermatitis*** ✓ ***Skin rashes***

NAMED FOR ITS ALMOST YEAR-ROUND FLOWERING from the Latin *calendae*, meaning the first day of the month, calendula has been used since ancient times to treat wounds and inflamed skin conditions. It is a member of the marigold family, but should not be confused with another popular genus, *Tagetes*, which is not medicinal. Herbal and cosmetic products are made from *Calendula officinalis*. The herb is easy to grow and the yellow edible flowers can add a colorful touch to salads.

How it works

Although calendula has been used traditionally to treat stomach upsets, ulcers and menstrual problems, scientific research has centerd on its wound-healing properties. The dried petals—the parts used—contain high levels of flavonoids, including lutein and betacarotene, which are antioxidants that help protect against infection and cell damage caused by free radicals.

Laboratory and animal research has shown that calendula flower components have a marked anti-inflammatory and antibacterial action, and heal wounds by helping new blood vessels and new tissue to form. In patients with leg ulcers treated with either a calendula ointment or saline solution dressings, calendula helped ulcers heal much faster.

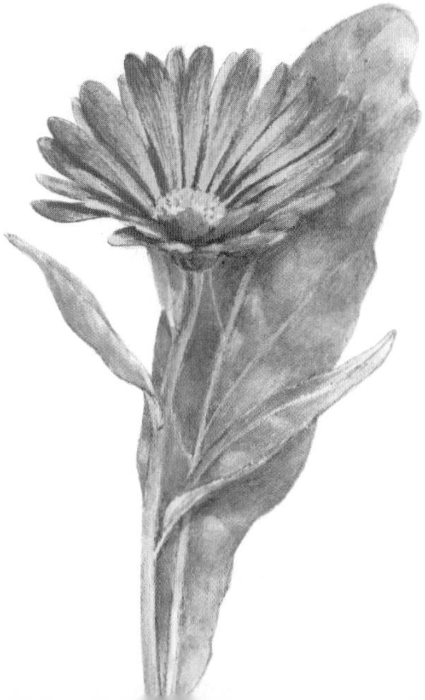

French researchers rated topical calendula "highly effective" for preventing dermatitis in women who had received radiation therapy for breast cancer.

How to use

There are many available creams, ointments, lotions, oils and more. Follow label instructions; or make your own soothing salve. Place dried flowers in a jar and fill with olive oil. Infuse for a few weeks, shaking the jar regularly. Strain the oil, then add beeswax—about 2 ounces (50 g) to a cup (250 ml) of oil—and then heat until the beeswax melts. Add a few drops of essential oil fragrance, if desired, plus a little vitamin E, then store in a bottle or jar.

You can also use an infusion of the flowers as a tea, a healing gargle or mouthwash, or in a compress to soothe wounds. Steep 1–2 teaspoons (5-10 ml) of petals in boiling water for 10–15 minutes and then strain.

Safety first *Calendula is considered very safe but be careful if you are taking sedatives, blood pressure or diabetes medications as it could enhance their effects.*

Where to find *Calendula products can be bought in health food stores, pharmacies or from a qualified herbalist.*

CARMINATIVE HERBS

Anise *(Pimpinella anisum)*, Caraway *(Carum carvi)*, Dill *(Anethum graveolens)*, Fennel *(Foeniculum vulgare)*

use for ✓ ***Bad breath and body odor*** ✓ ***Flatulence*** ✓ ***Indigestion***

ANISE, CARAWAY, DILL AND FENNEL are among the many "carminative" herbs, so-called for their time-honored ability to calm digestive problems. The Ancient Egyptians used caraway to ease the pain of intestinal gas. The digestive benefits of both fennel and dill were recorded in Anglo-Saxon times; the name "dill" comes from the Anglo-Saxon "dylle," meaning to lull or soothe. The Romans served aniseed cakes–*mustacae*–at the end of feasts as a digestive; anise is also mentioned for its capacity to sweeten the breath and relieve hiccups in John Gerard's *The Herball, or Generall Historie of Plantes* (1597). All four aromatic herbs are widely used in cooking, and as food and drink flavorings. Indian restaurants often provide patrons with a seed mix at the end of a meal to aid digestion.

How they work

It is the seeds of these plants that are used medicinally. Their constituents appear to have an antispasmodic effect and settle indigestion by dispelling gas and relaxing the smooth muscle in the gut. Russian research has shown that fennel seed oil is effective for soothing infant colic and reducing intestinal spasms. Fennel seeds also combat bad breath by increasing saliva flow and limiting the bacteria that cause the odor.

Dill, long known in Ayurveda for its carminative, stomachic and diuretic properties, is also used to treat colic. Extracts of both herbs are traditional ingredients in gripe water used to relieve infant colic and still found in modern brands. Anise, also used in Ayurveda, has muscle-relaxing effects and the potential to treat gastric ulcers and nausea among other disorders, according to a 2012 Iranian review of its properties. Caraway's capacity to ease the pain of intestinal gas has been shown in scientific studies where the oil was used in combination with peppermint and other carminative herbs.

How to use

To ease digestive problems, try chewing the seeds, or look for over-the-counter herbal products that contain them. One such remedy is **Iberogast** *(p. 213)*. You can make a soothing herbal tea by infusing 1–2 teaspoons (5–10 ml) of freshly crushed seeds in a cup of boiling water for up to 10 minutes. Take the essential oils in liquid or capsule form, as directed on the labels. Cooking with the aromatic herbs will counteract the gassy effects of beans and help prevent indigestion and flatulence.

Safety first *Carminative herbs are considered safe but always take essential oils and extracts as directed; excessive doses can be dangerous. Avoid fennel if taking the antibiotic ciprofloxacin as it may reduce its potency.*

Where to find *The herbs are available in supermarkets; health food stores stock the oils and supplements.*

Kitchen garden healers

Anise, caraway, dill and fennel all produce an abundance of tiny flowers held in large, compact flowerheads known as "umbels." It is the fruit of the flowers, the seeds, that are harvested for use medicinally to treat digestive complaints. In addition to their medicinal uses, all four herbs have culinary uses. Anise seeds are the source of the popular aniseed flavoring used in confectionery and liqueurs.

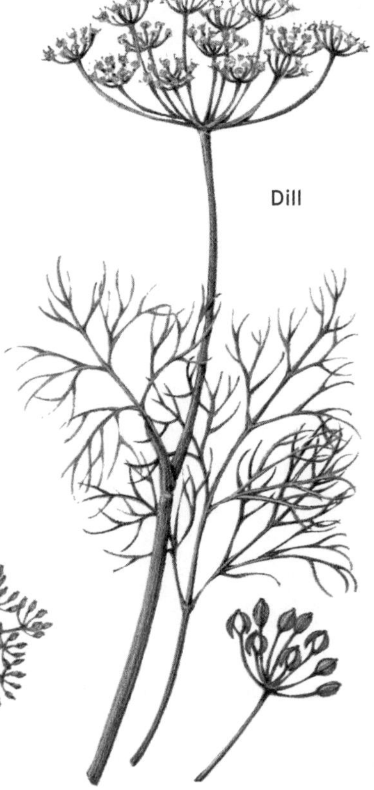

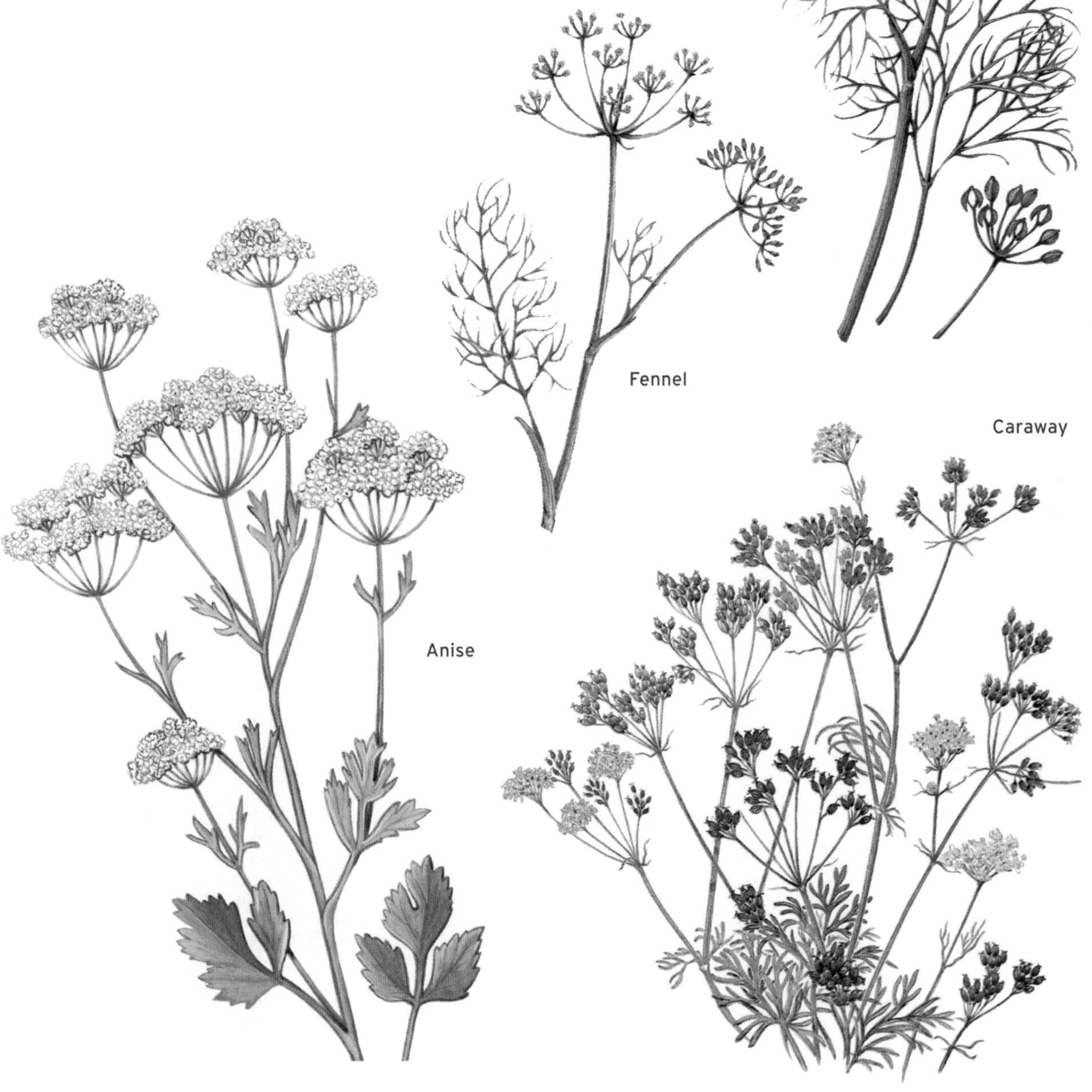

CAT'S CLAW *Uncaria tomentosa*

use for ✓ ***Warts***

WITH CURVED THORNS THAT RESEMBLE a cat's claws, this woody vine climbs tall trees in the uplands of the Peruvian rainforest. It is also native to other parts of Central and South America, where it has been used as a healing herb since the days of the Incas. Traditional applications for the inner bark and root include arthritis, stomach ulcers, inflammation, dysentery, fevers and even as a type of birth control.

Cat's claw reached a wider audience after an Australian botanical researcher learned about it from healer-priests of Peru's Ashinka people in the 1970s. Today, the herb is so popular that the Peruvian government allows harvesting only of the vine—sparing the plant's watermelon-sized roots to protect cat's claw from extinction in the wild. Today science is uncovering tantalizing clues to its possible uses.

How it works

Interest in cat's claw centers on suggestions from test tube studies that it may bolster immunity and scavenge free radicals—the rogue oxygen molecules that damage cells in ways that can raise the risk for cancer and heart disease. Cat's claw contains anti-inflammatory tannins and sterols as well as virus-fighting compounds.

Safety first *Do not take during pregnancy as cat's claw may cause miscarriage. Its safety in breastfeeding has not been studied, so avoid it while nursing, too. Skip cat's claw if you have low blood pressure, leukemia or an autoimmune disease like multiple sclerosis or lupus; it could make these conditions worse. Stop taking it two weeks before surgery; cat's claw may interfere with blood pressure control during a procedure.*

Where to find *Find cat's claw products in health food stores. Look for standardized bark extracts containing 3 percent alkaloids and 15 percent phenols.*

Though it is a traditional remedy for warts, cat's claw has not been clinically tested. However, its ability to strengthen the immune system could explain its use. Meanwhile, the herb is being investigated for use against a wide variety of other ailments including HIV, Crohn's disease, kidney trouble and Alzheimer's disease.

Cat's claw is also a popular rheumatoid arthritis (RA) remedy, though it can't prevent the progression of joint damage the way medication can.

How to use

Cat's claw can be taken as a liquid extract, capsules or as a tea made from crushed bark. Follow label instructions or take as professionally prescribed.

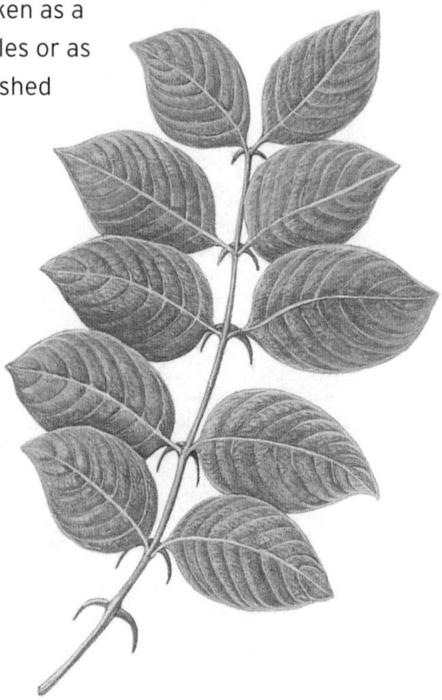

CAYENNE *Capsicum annuum*

use for ✓ ***Back and neck pain*** ✓ ***Neuralgia*** ✓ ***Osteoarthritis*** ✓ ***Shingles***

CAYENNE (A VARIETY OF CHILE PEPPER) is used as a culinary spice around the world, bringing heat and pungency to all manner of dishes. Herbalists of many different cultures have prized cayenne for its warming properties for centuries, and have used it to treat a wide variety of conditions traditionally associated with coldness, from chilblains and poor circulation to rheumatism and arthritis.

However, it has also long been known that cayenne is a remedy that needs to be used with great care. As far back as 1653, Culpeper wrote in his *Complete Herbal* that its effects on the skin could be "as if it had been burnt with fire, or scalded with hot water."

How it works

The heat of cayenne and other chile peppers is due to the presence of compounds called capsaicinoids, the most important of which is capsaicin. When capsaicin comes into contact with body tissues, it initially causes a burning or stinging sensation—the heat you experience on your tongue when you eat a chile is an example of this. With longer or more intensive exposure, capsaicin interferes with the way the nerves communicate pain signals to the brain leading to pain-relieving effects.

How to use

Adding cayenne powder or fresh chilies to your meals is an easy way to harness cayenne's warming properties and raise your body temperature or stimulate your circulation for a short time. Applied topically, capsaicin creams and gels can help relieve osteoarthritis and back pain. When using capsaicin products, follow label instructions.

Patches containing capsaicin can also be applied topically. The treatment needs to be administered by a doctor, however, often after giving you a local anaesthetic to numb the discomfort the capsaicin initially causes. This treatment can provide long-lasting pain relief for many different forms of neuralgia, including the neuralgia that sometimes persist after shingles (postherpetic neuralgia).

Safety first *Do not take medicinal quantities of cayenne if you are taking prescribed medicines (including blood-thinning medications), are suffering with digestive ulcers, or are allergic to plants in the Capsicum family.*

Do not allow cayenne or capsaicin products to come into contact with the eyes, mucous membranes or broken or irritated skin.

Cayenne has not been widely tested during pregnancy or breastfeeding so it is best avoided or used only under medical supervision during these periods.

Where to find *Cayenne powder can be found in health food stores and supermarkets. Capsaicin creams, gels and patches are available in pharmacies, and sometimes require a doctor's prescription.*

CELERY SEED *Apium graveolens*

use for ✓ ***Gout*** ✓ ***Osteoarthritis*** ✓ ***Rheumatoid arthritis*** ✓ ***Urinary tract infections***

CELERY IS A COMMON SALAD VEGETABLE, enjoyed for its slightly bitter and cleansing taste. Wine made from celery stalks, known as Selenites, was awarded to athletes in Ancient Greece. However, it is not the vegetable, but the ripe fruit of the celery, or celery seed, that is used in herbal medicine today.

How it works

The *British Herbal Pharmacopoeia* recommends celery seed as a remedy for rheumatoid arthritis. It is also found to be useful for gout and osteoarthritis. In a preclinical trial conducted in Australia, 15 patients with long-standing arthritic pain took regular doses of celery seed extract over a period of 12 weeks. After the third week there was a significant reduction of pain, and at the end of the trial many patients reported a reduction in the number of joints that had previously been painful.

One of the compounds present in celery seed extract, sedanolide, is believed to be responsible for the anti-inflammatory effect. The anti-inflammatory properties come without the gastric side effects that can be associated with medications such as the NSAIDs (nonsteroidal anti-inflammatory drugs).

Celery seed extract also has a diuretic effect, and works as a mild urinary antiseptic, making it a good remedy to choose in the treatment of cystitis. The same compounds that give celery its characteristic pungent aroma, phthalides, are responsible for the diuretic action.

Safety first *It is rare, but it is possible to be allergic to celery seed. Celery seed has not been widely tested during pregnancy or breast-feeding so it is best avoided or used only under medical supervision during these periods.*

Where to find *Celery seed preparations are available in health food stores or from a qualified herbalist.*

How to use

Celery seeds can be made into a tea using 1 teaspoon (5 ml) of seeds to a cup of boiling water. However, it is a bitter brew, and most people prefer to take it in a tincture, tablet or capsule form. Celery seed extract is often found in combination with other herbs that work in a supportive or synergistic way. Follow label instructions or take as professionally prescribed.

CHAMOMILE *Matricaria recutita, Chamaemelum nobile*

use for ✓ ***Eczema and dermatitis*** ✓ ***Indigestion*** ✓ ***Skin rashes***
✓ ***Sleeping problems***

THE DAISY-LIKE FLOWERS OF TWO different species—German chamomile *(Matricaria recutita)* and Roman chamomile *(Chamaemelum nobile)*—have similar active constituents and often interchangeable uses in herbal medicine. The herb was dubbed *kamai-melon* (ground apple) by the Ancient Greeks for its aromatic apple-like scent and throughout the centuries has been used traditionally to treat conditions ranging from chest colds and sore throats to anxiety, digestive problems and inflammatory skin conditions. Chamomile is also an ingredient in many skincare products and its essential oils are used in aromatherapy, while its calming tea is one of the world's most popular herbal brews.

How it works

The dried flowers are the parts used in teas and other preparations. Their constituents, including essential oils and flavonoids, have anti-inflammatory and antispasmodic properties. A topical preparation of *C. nobile* was as effective as a hydrocortisone cream for treating eczema in one German study. Recent laboratory and animal research suggests that *M. recutita* may heal wounds faster than two topical steroids. It appears that several of the active flavonoids in chamomile can penetrate the skin and be absorbed by the deeper layers.

Chamomile may help to induce sleep in several ways. It is thought to be mildly sedative, probably as a result of its flavonoid apigenin, which has a calming effect on the brain. US research has also shown that extract of German chamomile has a modest anxiolytic (antianxiety) action on patients with mild to moderate generalized anxiety disorder (GAD).

If an upset stomach is keeping you awake, chamomile may help. The herb eases indigestion by dispelling gas and relaxing the smooth muscle of the gut. Chamomile tea combined with other **carminative herbs** *(p. 143)* can also treat colic in children.

How to use

For skin complaints, look for a cream containing 3–10 percent chamomile. Follow label instructions. To relax, dispel anxiety and help digestion, make chamomile tea by pouring boiling water over 2–3 teaspoons (10-15 ml) of dried German chamomile flowers. Cooled chamomile tea can be used in a compress to soothe dry or inflamed skin.

Safety first *Chamomile is considered safe but in one documented case caused internal bleeding when used with the anticoagulant warfarin. Don't drink chamomile tea before driving, as it may make you drowsy.*

Where to find *Supermarkets often stock chamomile tea. Dried flowers and other preparations are available in health food stores, pharmacies or from a qualified herbalist.*

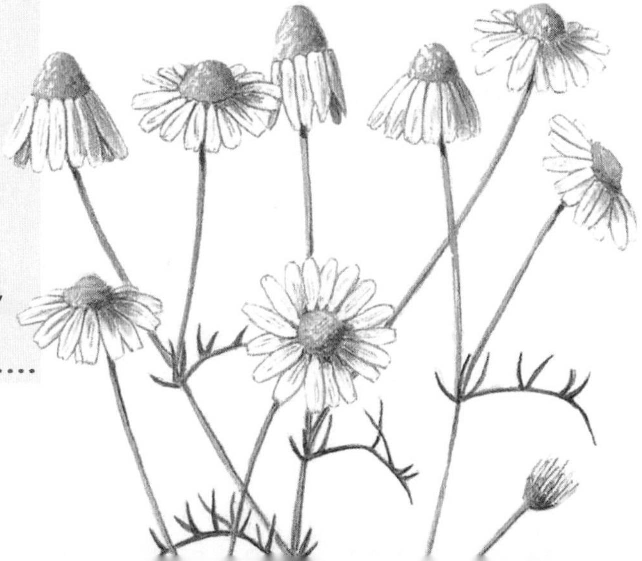

CHASTEBERRY *Vitex agnus-castus.* Also called: Chaste tree

use for ✓ ***Menstrual problems*** ✓ ***Natural fertility management***

THE ARCHETYPAL WOMEN'S HERB, chasteberry was recommended by Hippocrates in 450 BC and used extensively in Europe throughout the Middle Ages where the trees were commonly planted around monasteries and became known also as monks' pepper. One early prescription was for "sexual melancholia."

How it works

Chasteberry is commonly used as a hormonal normalizer in conditions where there is a hormonal imbalance, particularly in cases where there appears to be a relative estrogen dominance. Of the two main female hormones, estrogen and progesterone, a relative excess of estrogen is behind many female complaints including some cases of premenstrual syndrome (PMS), perimenopausal symptoms and female infertility. Although not proven to increase progesterone per se, chasteberry does appear to have a prolactin-lowering effect, which indirectly lowers progesterone levels. So paradoxically, by decreasing prolactin levels, progesterone levels are restored to normal, and this may relieve the relative excess of estrogen.

In a double-blind trial published in the *British Medical Journal* involving 170 women suffering from PMS, it was found that the women taking chasteberry experienced a significant reduction in symptoms including irritability, breast fullness, headache, anger and mood changes.

Several small trials have found that chasteberry improves fertility in women who were considered to be infertile. Other benefits of chasteberry include improving restless sleep, reducing the symptoms of polycystic ovarian syndrome, relieving tender and painful breasts and decreasing fluid retention.

How to use

Chasteberry is available in tincture or tablet form. Follow label instructions or take as professionally prescribed. Have patience—chasteberry is an effective herb, but it may take at least three menstrual cycles before improvement is noticed.

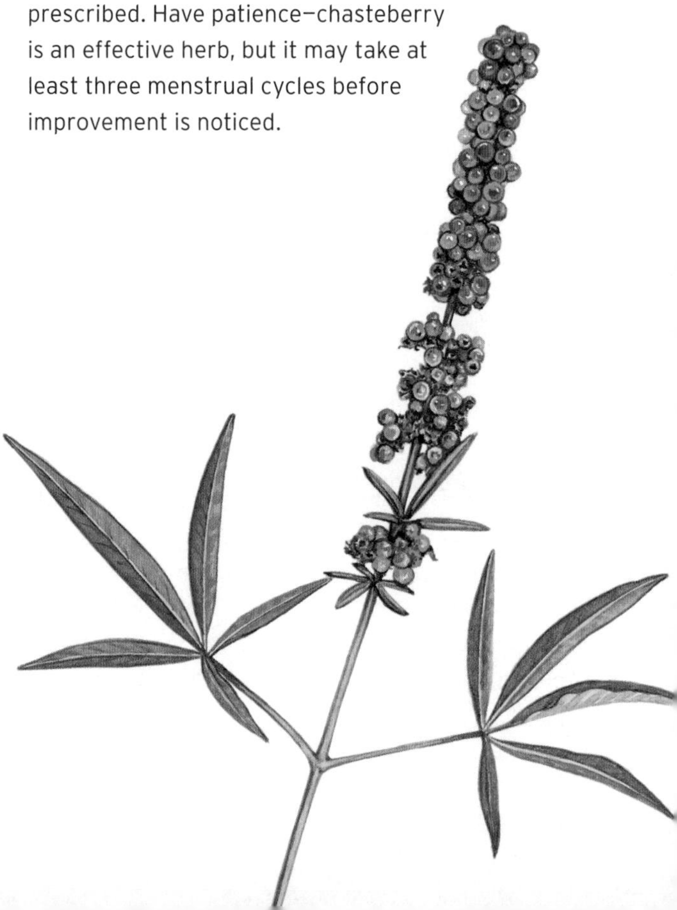

Safety first *Chasteberry is a generally safe and well-tolerated herb, but it is recommended to not take it in conjunction with hormone replacement therapy (HRT). However, it can be taken alongside the oral contraceptive pill (OCP) as clinical studies have found chasteberry reduces the symptoms of PMS, without affecting the efficacy of the OCP. Do not take chasteberry during pregnancy or while breastfeeding.*

Where to find *Chasteberry is available in health food stores or from a qualified herbalist.*

CHERRIES *Prunus* spp.

use for ✓ ***Gout***

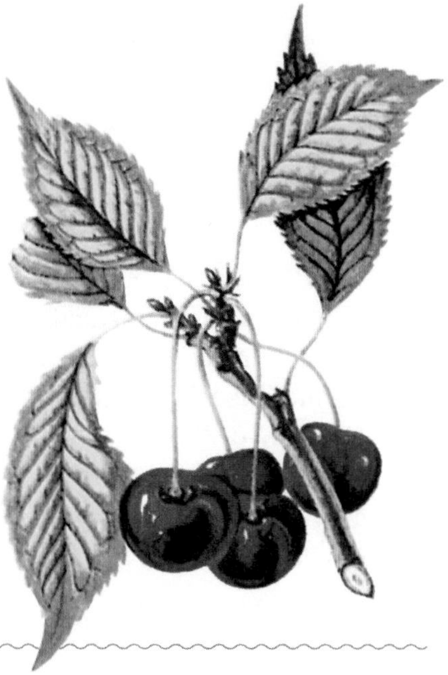

THE SMALL RED ORBS THAT SIGNAL the beginning of summer, cherries are delicious, nutritious and more than a little efficacious. Cherries belong to the *Prunus* genus, which includes plums, peaches, apricots and almonds. There are hundreds of varieties of cherries, although cherries are divided into two main groups: sweet *(P. avium)* and sour *(P. cerasus)*. Both types contain similar nutrients, but it was the sweet cherries that were chosen for the studies mentioned below.

How they work

Nutrient-dense yet low in kilojoules, cherries contain an assortment of beneficial nutrients including anthocyanins, quercetin and vitamin C. Anthocyanins are responsible for giving cherries their color, and cherries contain more of this compound than nearly all fruits. Anthocyanins are known to have antioxidant properties, protecting against free radicals (the rogue molecules that damage cells and increase the risk of cancer and heart disease). There is some evidence that anthocyanins may also help to reduce the risk of Alzheimer's disease. Anthocyanins are also helpful in reducing insulin resistance.

Safety first *If possible choose organically grown cherries as conventionally produced cherries are often heavily sprayed and may contain pesticide residues.*

Where to find *Fresh, frozen and canned cherries are available in supermarkets and greengrocers. Cherry juice is available in health food stores and some supermarkets.*

Combined with a low glycemic index (GI) of 22, cherries are a good choice of fruit to keep blood glucose stable, and help prevent diabetes. Cherries have a lower GI than other fruits, including peaches (GI 42), blueberries (GI 40) and apricots (GI 57).

Anthocyanins are also extremely anti-inflammatory and therefore counter inflammatory diseases such as arthritis and gout as well as heart disease, cancer and even obesity. Gout, caused by a buildup of uric acid in the body, is an excruciatingly painful condition that affects certain joints especially the big toe. In a study of 633 people suffering from gout, eating cherries was shown to decrease the risk of a gout attack by 35 percent. The study proposed two possible mechanisms for the improvement: through a reduction in inflammation, and by decreasing the amount of uric acid in the body.

How to use

Cherries, fresh or frozen, are a delicious addition to your daily fruit quota. Cherry juice is also available. There is no particular dosage recommendation; eat and drink liberally.

CHICKEN SOUP

use for ✓ ***Colds and flu***

THIS STAPLE OF JEWISH AND MANY other world cuisines could be much more than a comfort food. The great medieval rabbi, physician and philosopher Moses Maimonides recommended chicken soup for treating respiratory tract disorders in a 12th-century treatise and its healing potential was known centuries earlier. Today, science suggests that a warming bowl of chicken soup may be the ultimate nurturing food for convalescents, providing good nutrition and even hastening recovery. Modern research has confirmed that chicken-and-vegetable soup can help control cold symptoms, while a compound within the mix may also combat flu.

How it works

US researchers from the Nebraska Medical Center tested a traditional chicken soup recipe, which was cooked and liquidized for the laboratory experiment. It was also tested at different preparation stages to determine the individual actions of its ingredients and how they relieve cold symptoms.

The study, reported in *Chest* in 2000, showed that by inhibiting the movement of immune system cells called neutrophils, the soup helps suppress the body's natural inflammatory response to an infection, including the streaming flow of mucus that normally accompanies a cold. Each of the ingredients showed the same effect, suggesting that vegetarians could get similar effects from vegetable soup.

Later research, in 2012, pointed to the effects of chicken, which is rich in a compound called carnosine. According to researchers, carnosine influences the body's immune response and could further help fight off viruses. A variety of phytochemicals within the vegetables have medicinal properties, too. And, while simply drinking hot liquids is known to relieve congestion by loosening secretions, research shows that chicken soup does this much more effectively than mere hot water.

Safety first *No adverse effects of chicken soup are known, except when whole chicken bones or bone fragments have been swallowed.*

Where to find *All chicken soup ingredients can be found in supermarkets.*

How to use

Here are the basics of the traditional recipe used, though other versions can work just as well, according to the Nebraska researchers who tested commercial brands as a comparison.

INGREDIENTS

1 5 pound (2.5 kg) chicken
2 pounds (1 kg) chicken wings
3 large onions
1 large sweet potato
3 parsnips
2 turnips
2 large carrots
5 celery sticks
Parsley, salt and pepper to taste

Place the chicken in a large saucepan, cover with cold water and bring to a boil. Add all other vegetables except the celery and parsley and cook for 90 minutes. Add the celery and parsley, cook for another 45 minutes, then remove the chicken (which can be used in another dish). Purée the soup in a food processor; season to taste.

CHICKWEED *Stellaria media*

use for ✓ ***Eczema and dermatitis*** ✓ ***Skin rashes***

IN CENTURIES PAST, EUROPEAN FOLK HEALERS turned to this low-growing plant to relieve all manner of skin irritations—from eczema and acne to ulcers and rashes. The 1931 British botanical *A Modern Herbal* notes that: "The fresh leaves have been employed as a poultice for inflammation and indolent ulcers with most beneficial results." The stems and leaves of this mild herb still play a supporting role in skin-soothing remedies recommended by professional herbalists today.

How it works

Chickweed's age-old reputation as an anti-inflammatory herb for skin irritations is backed by science. This herb contains five types of apigenin according to a 2007 analysis from China's Shenyang Pharmaceutical University. Apigenin is an inflammation-cooling compound that works in ways similar to prescription anti-inflammatory COX-2 inhibitors. Saponins present in chickweed help. cleanse skin gently, too.

Safety first *Chickweed is safe to use as a food. Chickweed tea and supplements have not been widely tested during pregnancy or breast-feeding so are best avoided or used only under medical supervision during these periods.*

Where to find *Chickweed salves, ointments, teas and capsules are available in health food stores or from a qualified herbalist.*

How to use

Fresh chickweed leaves can be enjoyed in a salad or juiced; they can also be crushed and applied directly to the skin or mixed with coconut oil, petroleum jelly or lard to make an ointment for bruises, irritations and other skin problems. Chickweed can also be used as an extract, or in dried form in capsules, as a loose tea or in herbal ointments. Follow label instructions or take as professionally prescribed.

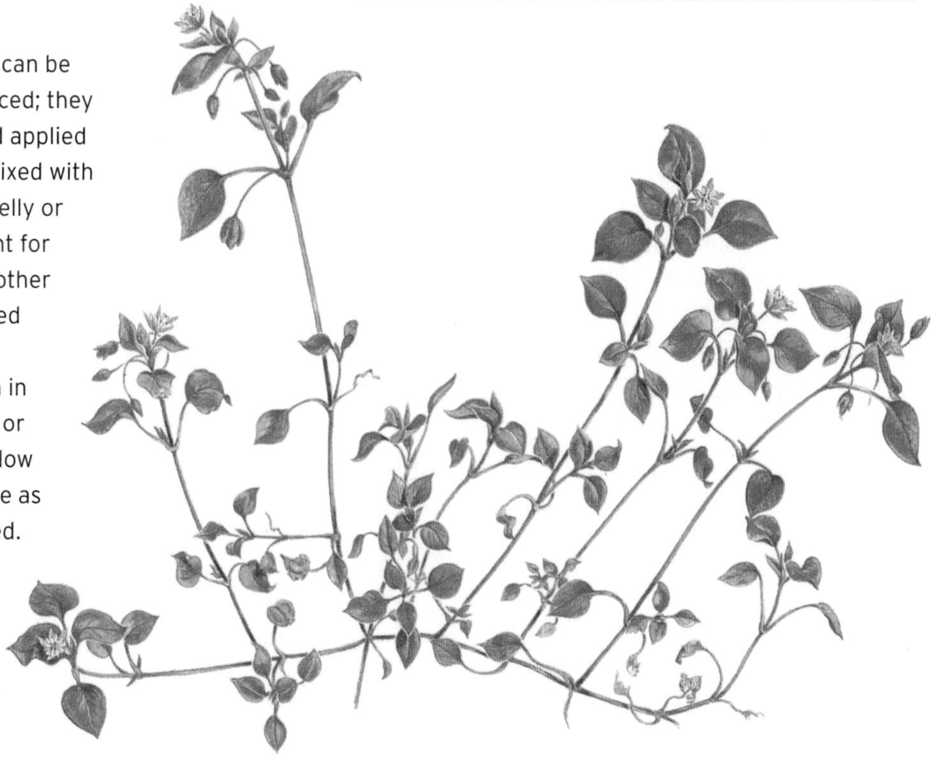

CHIROPRACTIC

use for ✓ ***Back and neck pain*** ✓ ***Headaches*** ✓ ***Jaw pain*** ✓ ***Migraines*** ✓ ***Neuralgia*** ✓ ***Strains and sprains***

IN THIS THERAPY, A PRACTITIONER manipulates the joints and the spine in order to rebalance the body's functions. A "magnetic healer" named Daniel David Palmer developed chiropractic in the late 19th century. He came up with the idea for the therapy when he found that some small bones in his deaf office cleaner's back had become dislocated and after he'd manipulated them back into position, the cleaner could hear again. Palmer went on to form the Palmer School of Chiropractic, coining the word from the Greek *cheiro*, meaning "hand," and *praktikis*, meaning "to do."

How it works

Palmer believed that all disease is associated with disorders of the spine and therefore chiropractors should be able to treat all sorts of illness, in addition to the more obvious examples of musculoskeletal injury. This philosophy has made chiropractic a controversial treatment in the past, though it is gaining recognition with doctors, especially for musculoskeletal problems.

Over 90 percent of patients who visit a chiropractor have musculoskeletal problems, such as lower back pain or postural pain due to sciatica, a pinched nerve or lumbago, as well as occipital and facial neuralgia or jaw or neck pain, strained muscles or sprained joints. The therapy can also benefit people who have suffered whiplash injuries, or those who experience migraines or tension headaches.

Safety first *Tell the chiropractor if you are pregnant and mention any medical condition you have and other treatments or medicines you are taking.*

Where to find *To find a qualified chiropractic practitioner, visit the American Chiropractic Association (www.acatoday.org) or ask your doctor for a recommendation.*

Some chiropractors, in keeping with Palmer's philosophy, consider treatment may benefit other complaints, given that back problems can cause pain or malfunction not only in the spine but in the shoulder, chest, arm, hips, knees or legs. Chiropractors may therefore use their skills to treat asthma, colitis, colic in babies, constipation and menstrual problems.

A visit to the chiropractor

A visit to a chiropractor will usually entail a detailed physical examination and medical history, plus an examination of any existing X-rays; further X-rays may be requested before the practitioner commences any manipulative work. You will then often be given gentle preparatory soft-tissue work, followed by any necessary adjustment or manipulation. This is rarely painful, though patients may report feeling a start or slight shock, particularly if the chiropractor makes a rapid thrust; this thrusting action is sometimes responsible for the "clicking" sound, but this does not always occur.

Often, if pain has been chronic, relief is immediate. In other cases, some stiffness may be experienced before the area loosens up and becomes more flexible. You may need several sessions, depending on the complaint and your body's response.

Nerve supply

Every vital organ in the body is connected to and controlled by nerves that link up with the spinal cord and brain. Nerves for the various organs connect with the spinal cord in different regions along the spine. Chiropractors believe that by manipulating the spine back into its correct alignment they can relieve pressure on nerves and so assist all manner of ailments, not just musculoskeletal problems.

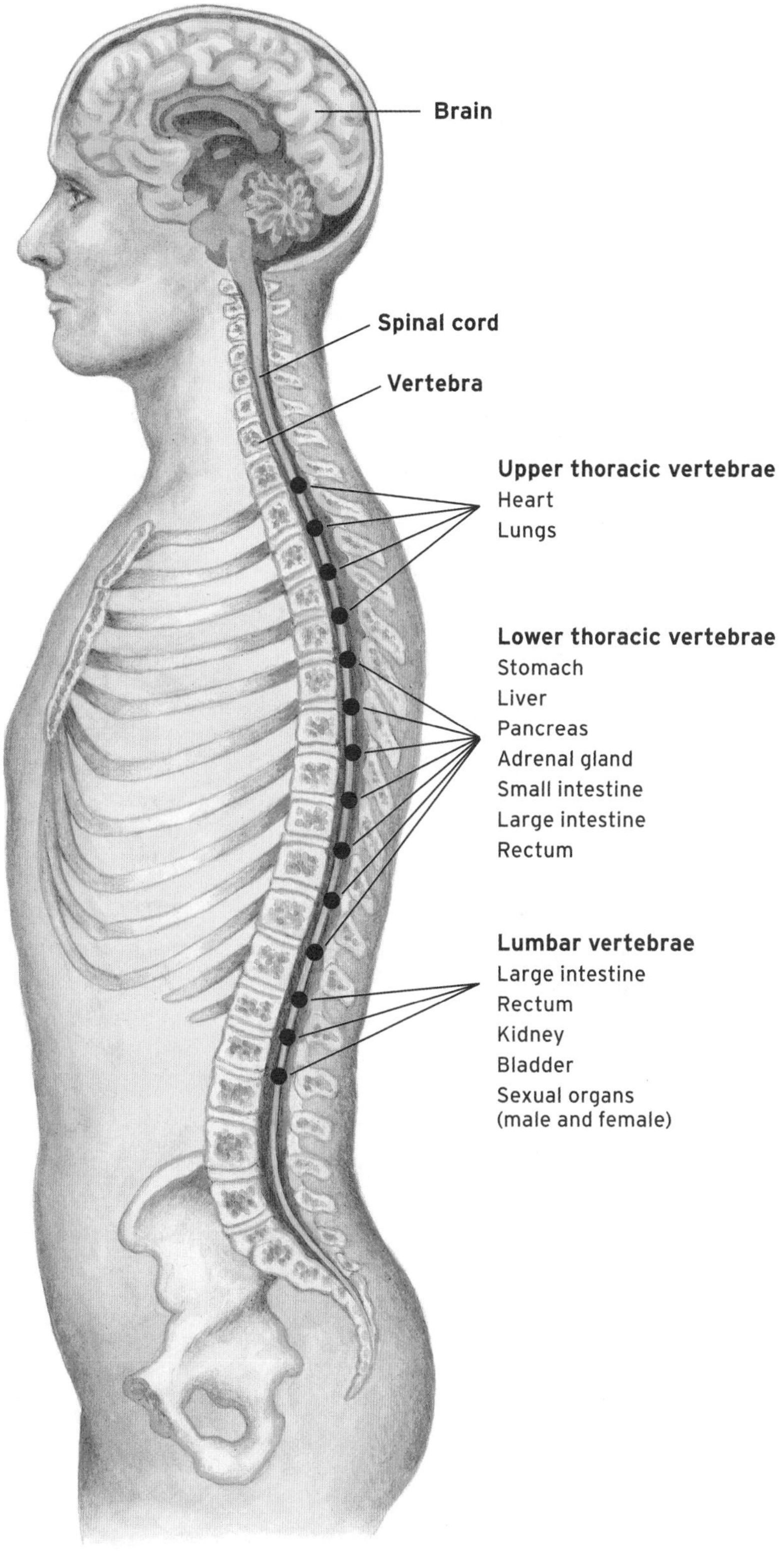

CHROMIUM

use for ✓ ***Diabetes and insulin resistance***

CHROMIUM IS A MINERAL FOUND in legumes, spices (especially black pepper), whole grains, cheese, eggs, bananas, spinach, broccoli, oysters and offal. Though needed in tiny amounts, diets high in refined sugar increase chromium excretion by more than 30-fold and chronic deficiency leads to an increased risk for heart disease, obesity and type 2 diabetes.

How it works

Chromium is the "go to" supplement for treating insulin resistance, a common precursor to type 2 diabetes. Insulin resistance occurs when cells fail to respond to the message from the hormone insulin, to allow glucose from the blood to be taken into the cell where it can be used for energy. This results in high circulating blood glucose levels—a red flag in blood results. Chromium does not increase insulin levels, but rather is believed to improve the action of insulin on the cell membrane, assisting the transfer of glucose from the blood into the cell.

Safety first *If you are taking diabetes medication, consult your doctor before taking chromium supplements as the mineral may alter the dosage needed for insulin or other diabetes medication. Chromium is safe to use during pregnancy and breastfeeding under the guidance of a health practitioner.*

Where to find *Chromium supplements can be found in health food stores and pharmacies. They can be prescribed by your doctor.*

Other conditions where chromium may be useful include cardiovascular disease. One study has shown that chromium supplementation decreased blood fats including triglycerides and LDL cholesterol while raising the protective HDL cholesterol. Obesity is another area where chromium may prove helpful. One study revealed a lowering of fat mass combined with an increase in lean body mass, a welcome outcome when treating obesity.

Other conditions where insulin resistance is a feature, and therefore chromium supplementation may be helpful, include polycystic ovarian syndrome, gestational diabetes and metabolic syndrome.

How to use

Health authorities in the US estimate an Adequate Intake (AI) of chromium for adult men (19+) is at least 35 mcg/day. Women need 25 mcg/day, increasing to 30 mcg/day during pregnancy and 45 mcg/day while breastfeeding. Different forms of chromium supplements are available, but the most bioavailable, and the ones used in studies, are chromium picolinate and chromium nicitinate (bound with niacin). Follow label instructions or take as professionally prescribed.

CINNAMON *Cinnamon verum, C. cassia*

use for ✓ ***Diabetes and insulin resistance*** ✓ ***Gastroenteritis*** ✓ ***Menstrual problems***

CINNAMON IS ONE OF THE OLDEST and most precious of spices. In the first century AD Pliny the Elder claimed that 1 pound of cinnamon (400 g) was equivalent to 10 months of a worker's wage. Widely used as a culinary spice, cinnamon is also prized for its medicinal value, particularly in Ayurvedic medicine, where it is used for chest infections as well as restoring the weak and debilitated. In traditional Chinese medicine (TCM), cinnamon is believed to invigorate and assist in the movement of blood in the abdominal area and cinnamon tea is routinely recommended for women who suffer from menstrual cramps. TCM also recommends cinnamon in cases where the person feels heat in the upper part of the body while simultaneously experiencing cold feet.

How it works

The European herbal tradition recommends cinnamon for its warming effect on the circulation in addition to its carminative properties, which are helpful for poor digestion. Hence, it is traditionally used in remedies for chilblains and venous insufficiency as well as bloating, flatulence and nausea.

A constituent of cinnamon, cinnamaldehyde, is thought to give cinnamon rather impressive antibacterial and antifungal properties. Cinnamon has been found to be effective against the bacteria *E. coli* and *Staphylococcus aureus*. Various studies have shown cinnamon to be helpful in the treatment and prevention of gum disease, chest infections and gastroenteritis.

In recent years there have been several studies looking at cinnamon's role in the treatment of type 2 diabetes. One study of 60 diabetics showed that as little as 1/4 teaspoon (1 g) of cinnamon taken daily over a period of 40 days reduced blood glucose levels and blood fats (triglycerides) in addition to lowering total cholesterol levels.

How to use

As a food, add cinnamon to your cooking, in fruit compotes, tagines, or stews, as well as simply adding a teaspoonful to smoothies. Cinnamon can be made into a tea, as it is in traditional Chai. Cinnamon is also available in tablet, capsule, essential oil and tincture form. Follow label instructions or take as professionally prescribed.

Safety first *Cinnamon in food is generally well tolerated. However, cinnamon has not been widely tested during pregnancy or breastfeeding so large amounts are best avoided or used only under medical supervision during these periods.*

Where to find *Supermarkets stock powdered cinnamon and cinnamon tea. Cinnamon supplements are available in health food stores or from a qualified herbalist.*

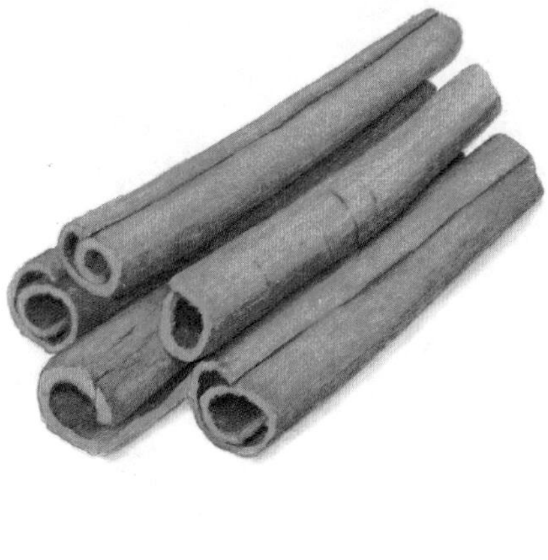

CLOVES *Syzygium aromaticum*

use for ✓ ***Tooth and gum disorders***

THE SWEET, PENETRATING AROMA and flavor of cloves have been valued for thousands of years. Cloves are the dried immature flower bud of the clove tree, indigenous to the Malaccas, today's Indonesia. Clove trees can live to over 150 years. In 17th-century Europe pomanders of oranges liberally studded with cloves were carried in an attempt to stave off the plague. It is the oil of clove that is most often used for medicinal purposes.

How they work

The old wives' tale of clove oil helping take away the pain of toothache is backed up by science. Eugenol, the main active component in clove oil, has profound anesthetic and analgesic (pain-relieving) properties. It appears to block certain pain receptors, the effect beginning after about five minutes and lasting up to 15 minutes. One study showed clove oil to be as effective as benzocaine, a dental local analgesic, when used before needle insertion. Due to its antiseptic properties, clove oil is useful in preventing gum disease.

Safety first **Clove oil can be toxic if ingested.** *There is also the potential for topical application to be a skin irritant. Clove oil has not been widely tested during pregnancy or breast-feeding so it is best avoided or used only under medical supervision during these periods.*

Where to find *Clove oil and enteric-coated capsules are available in health food stores or from a qualified herbalist.*

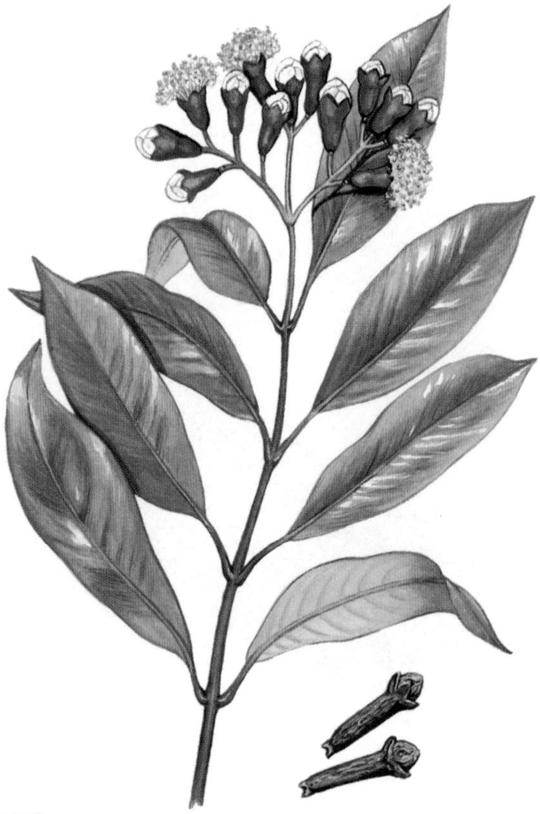

While the essential oil is most often used in remedies, clove powder has been found to be very effective as a deworming agent and in Ayurvedic medicine cloves are used to help treat nausea, flatulence and indigestion. Naturopaths often use clove oil or powder to reduce intestinal fungal, bacterial and/or parasitic overgrowth.

How to use

For headaches, dab a drop of clove oil onto each temple and massage with firm pressure in small circles. For toothache, chew on a clove or apply a single drop of clove oil to the affected area. For a mouthwash, add 2–3 drops of clove oil to 2 tablespoons (30 ml) of water, gargle, swill and spit out. For intestinal worms or bacterial overgrowth, capsules are available that contain dried cloves or clove oil. Follow label instructions or take as professionally prescribed.

COENZYME Q_{10}

use for ✓ ***Blood pressure, high*** ✓ ***Heart and circulatory health***

THE ALTERNATIVE NAME FOR COENZYME Q_{10} is ubiquinone, which reflects the fact that it is found ubiquitously throughout the body, but especially in the heart and muscle tissue. The body can synthesize its own coenzyme Q_{10} from the amino acid tyrosine; nevertheless levels of coenzyme Q_{10} decrease with age. In the diet coenzyme Q_{10} is found in meat and fish and in lesser amounts in broccoli, cauliflower, nuts, spinach and soy.

How it works

Coenzyme Q_{10} has two main roles in the body, first as an important player in the creation of energy within mitochondria, the energy powerhouse of cells. The second role of coenzyme Q_{10} is as an antioxidant, protecting all cell membranes, including those of the mitochondria, from being damaged by free radicals. Deficiency signs may include fatigue, muscle ache and pain, and gum disease.

Coenzyme Q_{10} has been thoroughly researched since the 1970s, particularly with respect to its role in protecting against heart disease. One study showed that patients taking coenzyme Q_{10} prior to heart surgery had a shorter hospital stay and faster recovery time. Other heart-related conditions where coenzyme Q_{10} has been shown to be useful include high blood pressure, ischemic heart disease, mitral valve prolapse and congestive heart failure.

If you are taking statins, ask your doctor if it might be worth taking coenzyme Q_{10}. Statins are often prescribed to lower cholesterol levels, because they inhibit an enzyme involved in the synthesis of cholesterol. Unfortunately, this same enzyme is involved in the synthesis of coenzyme Q_{10} in the body. This explains why muscle pain, muscle soreness and fatigue, which are commonly caused by statins, can be relieved by coenzyme Q_{10}.

Coenzyme Q_{10} is also recommended for gum disease, with improvement noticed in as short a time as one week. In one small study a supplement of coenzyme Q_{10} was found to alleviate symptoms of tinnitus in patients who initially had low levels of coenzyme Q_{10} in their blood.

Safety first *Coenzyme Q_{10} is relatively safe, although it may interact with certain medications such as warfarin, so check with your doctor if you are taking any kind of blood-thinning or anticoagulant medication. Coenzyme Q_{10} has not been widely tested during pregnancy or breastfeeding so it is best avoided or used only under medical supervision during these periods.*

Where to find *Coenzyme Q_{10} can be found in health food stores and pharmacies or may be available from your doctor.*

How to use

There is no official Recommended Dietary Allowance (RDA) for coenzyme Q_{10}. Follow label instructions or take as professionally prescribed. It is generally found in capsule form. For gum disease, take orally as well as applying topically to the gums.

COFFEE *Coffea arabica, C. canephora*

use for ✓ ***Asthma*** ✓ ***Concentration, improved*** ✓ ***Depression*** ✓ ***Fatigue*** ✓ ***Headaches*** ✓ ***Migraines*** ✓ ***Overweight and obesity*** ✓ ***Stroke prevention***

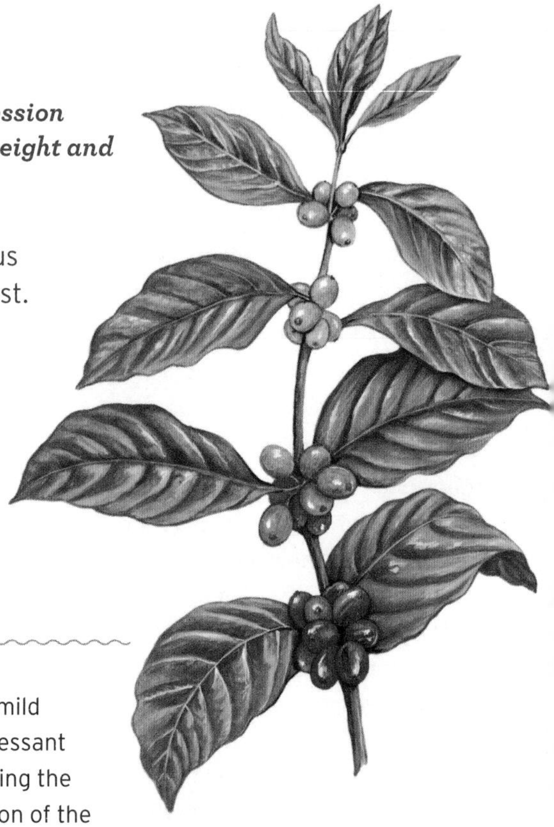

ITS RICH AROMA, ARRESTING TASTE and ability to wake us up has made coffee a global favorite, especially at breakfast. Since the opening of the first coffee house in Mecca in the 15th century, worldwide coffee production has risen astronomically; it reached over 8.8 billion tons in 2010. Is all this coffee good for us? Medical experts have been divided, but studies are now revealing physical and mental benefits of moderate consumption. An extract of raw green coffee beans that may speed weight loss is also attracting attention.

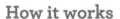

How it works

Caffeine, coffee's best-known constituent, has a stimulating effect on the central nervous system that combats fatigue and makes us feel alert—or jittery, anxious and sleepless if taken to excess. Lifelong coffee drinking appears to safeguard memory and cognitive function in older age; caffeine is thought to stimulate neurotransmitters that protect against the beta-amyloid damage that heralds diseases such as Alzheimer's and Parkinson's. Caffeine may also act as a mild antidepressant by boosting the production of the "feel-good" chemicals serotonin and dopamine.

Coffee's many antioxidants and other phytochemicals may protect against type 2 diabetes, heart disease and stroke by strengthening blood vessels, reducing blood pressure, regulating cholesterol and stabilizing blood glucose levels.

Chlorogenic acids from raw green coffee beans have been shown to reduce high blood pressure levels significantly. They also influence the way the body metabolizes glucose and fat; several studies have shown that taking green coffee bean extract can help to reduce weight.

How to use

Drinking coffee can boost concentration and protect against chronic diseases. Drink it filtered or instant to avoid the grounds, which contain two chemicals, cafestol and kahweol, that raise cholesterol levels and cardiovascular risk. In an asthma emergency, two strong cups of coffee can be used if an inhaler is unavailable. Caffeine has similar properties to theophylline, a medication used to treat asthma.

Safety first *To avoid the risk of miscarriage or low birth weight, pregnant women should drink no more than one cup of espresso-style coffee or three cups of instant a day. For other adults, up to four cups a day is considered safe. Regular coffee drinkers may experience caffeine withdrawal headaches if they are deprived of their "fix." For green coffee bean extract (GCBE) follow label instructions or take as professionally prescribed.*

Where to find *Supermarkets stock coffee while GCBE is available in health food stores.*

COGNITIVE BEHAVIORAL THERAPY

use for ✓ ***Anxiety*** ✓ ***Chronic pain*** ✓ ***Depression*** ✓ ***Phobias*** ✓ ***Sleeping problems***

COGNITIVE BEHAVIORAL THERAPY (CBT) focuses on discovering and changing the thoughts and feelings that trigger self-defeating actions. Unlike traditional "talking therapies," CBT is usually brief (about 12 sessions, on average) and focused on finding solutions to specific problems.

CBT began in the 1960s, when a University of Pennsylvania psychiatrist realized that his depressed patients experienced onslaughts of spontaneous, negative thoughts about themselves and the world around them. Identifying and challenging the thoughts helped many of them feel better. Today, this well-researched therapy is practiced around the world and has been proven in research studies to ease a wide variety of conditions.

How it works

The premise of CBT is that our perceptions influence our feelings and our behavior. Finding, challenging and changing negative, automatic thoughts (such as "I'm worthless" or "I'll never get to sleep") can actually change your reality.

Scientific research shows that it works—often better than medication alone. In a 2012 UK study of 469 people with treatment-resistant depression, those who received CBT plus medication were three times more likely to get at least a 50 percent improvement in their symptoms than those who received only antidepressants. In a Harvard University (US) study that compared the short- and long-term effects of CBT to a prescription sleeping pill for 63 people with insomnia, CBT helped participants fall asleep faster and sleep with fewer interruptions. And they were still sleeping better a year later. CBT can even ameliorate chronic pain (such as back pain, cancer pain and joint pain) by improving coping skills.

Brain scans reveal that CBT may subtly change the brain. In a 2006 University of Pittsburgh study, functional MRI images showed that activity in the brain's subgenual cingulate cortex (a region associated with mood regulation) was low in people with depression but increased after 12 weeks of CBT. Other research has uncovered beneficial increases in brain activity after CBT for people with post-traumatic stress disorder, obsessive-compulsive disorder and panic disorder, too.

> ***Where to find*** *For more information about CBT or to find a therapist, visit the Association for Behavioral and Cognitive Therapies (www.abct.org) or ask your doctor or local clinic for a referral.*

A visit to a cognitive behavioral therapist

A CBT session generally lasts 45 minutes to one hour. Your therapist will help you become aware of negative thoughts, emotions and beliefs and pay attention to how they affect your actions. You will also be asked to challenge negative, distorted perceptions—a step that can be difficult at first as you question long-held ways of thinking, but that will become a valuable new skill over time. You will also most likely have homework to do between sessions, as you apply what you've learned.

COGNITIVE CHALLENGE

use for ✓ ***Dementia*** ✓ ***Memory problems***

COULD "USE IT, OR LOSE IT" APPLY to your ability to balance your checkbook quickly, remember your neighbor's first name or prevent dementia? A growing body of evidence suggests that the answer is yes. Engaging your brain–by socializing with friends, taking up a new hobby, exposing yourself to new ideas through the arts or science, or participating in computerized "brain-training" programs–is a proven way to keep your mind sharp.

How it works

Cognitive challenges stimulate the growth of new brain cells and new connections between those cells. Some experts say it prompts brain cells to release neurotrophins–fertilizer-like compounds that fuel the growth of more and bigger connections between brain cells. This is important for the ageing brain because these connections can shrink with age.

A dramatic 2011 study from University College London found proof. Researchers used brain scans and found that London taxi drivers who memorized the city's maze of 25,000 streets and thousands of landmarks developed more gray matter in the hippocampus (the brain region that forms, organizes and stores memories). They outperformed other cabbies on memory tests, too.

It works in everyday people, too. In a 2013 University of California San Francisco study, older adults aged 60–85 who played a specially designed driving game for 12 hours over the course of a month developed multitasking skills superior to those of 20-year-olds. The working memory of participants also improved as well as the ability to focus for longer periods of time.

Other fun, leisure-time activities can help keep your mind active and sharp. In a ground-breaking 2003 study that tracked 469 older adults for more than five years, those who spent the most time reading, playing board games, playing a musical instrument or dancing had up to 63 percent lower risk for developing dementia compared to those who spent the least time enjoying challenging activities.

Where to find *AARP offers a selection of brain games (www.aarp.org/health/brain-health/brain_games.html) or visit Lumosity (www.lumosity.com) and other services that offer personalized brain training if you sign up.*

How to use

Seek out activities that challenge your little gray cells. Some experts say you'll get the best results by doing something new such as learning a new language, switching from crossword puzzles to maths games (or vice versa) or learning a new musical instrument. There's also growing evidence that well-designed brain-training computer games have benefits as well. Simple steps, like brushing your teeth or putting your fork in your nondominant hand, also serve to stimulate the brain.

COLD THERAPY

use for ✓ ***Acne*** ✓ ***Bruises*** ✓ ***Bursitis and tendonitis*** ✓ ***Cramps, muscle*** ✓ ***Frozen shoulder*** ✓ ***Gout*** ✓ ***Nausea and vomiting*** ✓ ***Rheumatoid arthritis*** ✓ ***Strains and sprains***

THE ACRONYM RICE (REST, ICE, COMPRESSION AND ELEVATION) is familiar to anyone who has attended a basic first aid course, or been inside a football locker room. Cold therapy includes the application of ice packs, cold water and cold compresses to an area to hasten the healing process after a soft tissue injury.

Cold therapy has been used throughout history. Barron de Larrey, an army surgeon in Napoleon's army, in the absence of anesthetics, used to pack limbs in ice prior to amputation. However, cold therapy is usually applied in less dramatic situations, often on the sports field, gym or after a fall.

How it works

After an injury the body's immediate reaction is to send blood hurtling to the affected area, marked by redness, heat and swelling. Cold therapy has the effect of slowing everything down and thereby avoiding tissue damage. The cold compress or ice pack draws out the heat and the lower temperature means that the cells' metabolic rate drops rapidly and so cell death is slowed or prevented.

The cold makes local blood vessels constrict, so there is less blood or fluids reaching the injury, reducing swelling. The cold may also have a numbing effect. As well as reducing inflammation, cold therapy can lessen bruising, pain and muscle spasm. Conditions that respond well to cold therapy include frozen shoulder, tendonitis, bursitis, sprains and muscle cramping.

Safety first *Never apply ice directly onto skin. Check the color of the skin after five minutes; if bright pink or red, remove the cold pack. Do not use an ice pack if the patient has an open wound, suffers from cold urticaria or has a history of frostbite.*

Where to find *Instant ice packs can be found in pharmacies and online.*

A cold compress, applied gently can relieve the pain of gout and rheumatoid arthritis. Additionally, a cold compress placed on the forehead may help relieve nausea. An ice cube pressed directly onto a pimple can reduce the redness of acne. Cold therapy can also be applied to rashes and inflamed areas of skin caused by minor burns, sunburn and insect bites.

How to use

Cold packs can be made by folding ice cubes into a damp cloth. A bag of frozen peas makes an excellent emergency cold pack. Instant cold packs can also be purchased. These are stored at room temperature and contain a chemical such as ammonium nitrate that undergoes an endothermic reaction when the packet is twisted or crushed, turning the pack cold. A cold compress is simply made from a clean cloth soaked in ice cold water and wrung out.

The key is to apply the cold pack swiftly. Within 10 minutes of an injury, apply the cold pack for 20–30 minutes; repeat every two to three hours. After 48 hours, it is likely that **heat therapy** (p. 204) will be more beneficial.

COMFREY

use for ✓ ***Back and neck pain*** ✓ ***Bruises*** ✓ ***Strains and sprains***

COMFREY HAS BEEN EMPLOYED for muscle, bone and joint problems for centuries, and has been known by a number of names that reflect these uses, including knitbone, boneset and bruisewort. Even its botanical name is derived from a Latin term meaning "grow together"—a reference to its long-held reputation for enhancing the repair of fractures.

Research has confirmed the validity of many of comfrey's traditional uses when applied topically, but has also revealed that the plant may be toxic when taken internally.

How it works

Although scientists have not yet fully determined how comfrey works, it is known to have pain-relieving and anti-inflammatory properties, as well as an ability to stimulate the regeneration of damaged tissue.

How to use

Both the leaves and the root of the comfrey plant can be used therapeutically, but most scientific research has utilized comfrey root preparations. For example, comfrey root cream has been shown to relieve muscular back pain.

Safety first **Comfrey can be toxic if taken internally.** *Short-term topical use is not believed to carry the same risks. Nevertheless, comfrey products should not be applied to broken or irritated skin, and should not be used by women who are pregnant or breastfeeding.*

Talk to your doctor before using comfrey if you have cancer, liver disease or an immune system disorder, or if you are using prescribed medicines (internally or topically).

Where to find Comfrey creams and ointments are available in health food stores or from a qualified herbalist.

Comfrey ointment also reduces the pain and swelling of sprained ankles, while simultaneously improving joint mobility. Its efficacy when applied to sprained ankles is similar to that seen with diclofenac gel (a topically applied nonsteroidal anti-inflammatory drug).

Comfrey root cream may also help relieve the symptoms and improve the healing of bruises in adults and children over three years.

When used three times daily for three weeks, comfrey root preparations have been shown to relieve the pain and other symptoms of osteoarthritis of the knee, and to improve quality of life. When using comfrey products, follow label instructions or use as professionally prescribed.

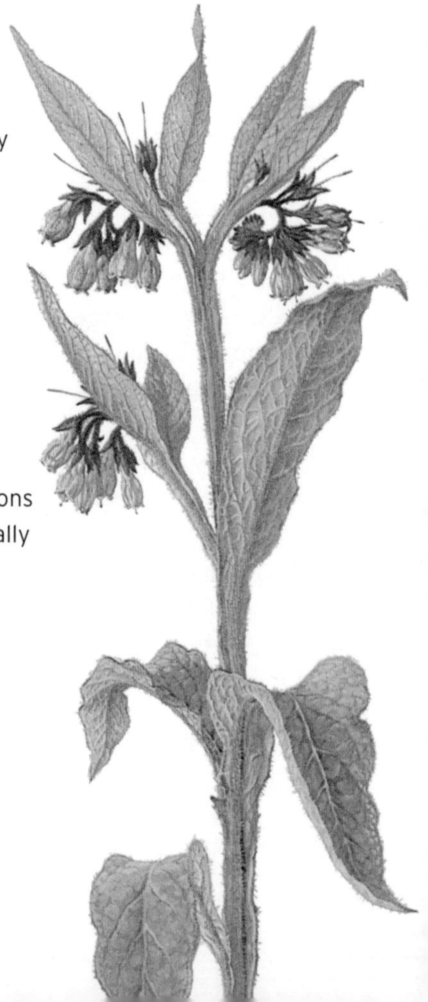

COMPRESSES AND POULTICES

use for ✓ ***Eczema*** ✓ ***Eye infections*** ✓ ***Fever*** ✓ ***Jaw pain***

SIMPLE AND SOOTHING, COMPRESSES AND POULTICES are natural ways to apply the healing properties of herbs (and healing foods and liquids) as well as heat and cold to the skin. While many people may think these two techniques are identical, there's actually a big difference: Compresses deliver warmth or cold as well as fluids (such as teas) while poultices act like a bandage to hold herbs or pastes in place and keep them covered.

These traditional techniques are worth learning and can help ease everything from eye ailments and headaches to fevers and muscle or joint pains.

How they work

Compresses help by cooling or warming the body. In one study of people with blepharitis—clogged, inflamed oil glands along the eye lids—a warm compress helped unblock blocked glands when the compress was sufficiently hot and used for a long enough period of time. In contrast, cool compresses soothed inflammation in a study of people with allergic conjunctivitis—red, swollen itchy eyes due to an allergic reaction. A warm compress can also relax stiff muscles and help ease jaw pain according to the Canadian Dental Association. Compresses can also be made with herbal tea. For example, some herbalists recommend a compress with cold lavender tea be applied to the forehead to ease a headache.

Poultices are not as well studied by scientists. But among traditional healers, they're a mainstay: a way to deliver herbs and other substances to the skin. Some poultices are intended to heal surface problems such as scratches, scrapes and rashes. Others are intended to do deeper work. One example of this is onion and garlic poultices, a popular, old-time home remedy for fever. The onion or garlic is usually chopped or sliced and applied to the feet either directly or wrapped in muslin, then covered with socks. Sometimes, poultices are topped with a warm or hot compress for bigger benefits.

How to use

To make a compress, soak a clean cloth or piece of flannel in hot or cold water or tea. Wring out and apply to the affected area. To make a poultice, apply your chosen healing material (such as chopped or crushed herbs or paste) directly to the skin or wrapped in muslin and cover with a clean cloth, secured to keep the material in place. Alternatively, wrap the material in a clean piece of flannel or muslin and apply to the area either continuously or intermittently in short bursts.

Safety first *If a compress feels too hot or too cold, remove it. Follow the same rule if a compress or poultice irritates your skin. Take particular care with poultices applied to babies and infants, who have much more sensitive skin than adults.*

CORN SILK *Zea mays*

use for ✓ ***Kidney stone prevention*** ✓ ***Urinary tract infections***

CORN SILK IS THE TERM USED TO describe the stigmas of the corn plant—the long silky strings of fibrous material found between a cob of corn and the leaves that encase it. Also known as maize, corn was first domesticated in Mexico over 9,000 years ago, and is now consumed as a food all over the world.

Corn silk has also been embraced for its medicinal effects in many different corners of the globe. Traditional therapeutic uses, predominantly for conditions affecting the urinary tract, have been documented in regions as far afield as North America, China, France, Turkey, Indonesia and Fiji.

How it works

Corn silk is attributed with diuretic actions, antioxidant and anti-inflammatory effects, and an ability to soothe inflamed and irritated urinary tissues. At least some of these actions are believed to be due to the presence of potassium and compounds called saponins that have soapy qualities in water.

Safety first *If you think you may have a kidney infection or kidney stone, or if you are experiencing cystitis symptoms, seek medical advice immediately. Although corn silk may help to ease the symptoms of these conditions, it does not treat the underlying condition.*

Corn silk has not been widely tested during pregnancy or breastfeeding so it is best avoided or used only under medical supervision during these periods.

Where to find *Corn silk supplements are available in health food stores or from a qualified herbalist. Corn silk can also be obtained from fresh corn cobs sold in farmers' markets and grocery stores.*

Although there is little scientific evidence to support the practice, corn silk is frequently taken to help ease the symptoms of cystitis and kidney infections, often being used alongside antibiotics or herbs that have antimicrobial properties.

Corn silk has also traditionally been regarded as having the ability to help address kidney stones. Research indicates that while it doesn't break the stones down, it may make them easier to pass, perhaps due to its anti-inflammatory effects on the urinary mucous membranes.

How to use

Corn silk is often included in herbal formulations that contain other urinary tract herbs. Follow label instructions or take as professionally prescribed. It can also be consumed as a tea, prepared by pouring boiling water over about 2 tablespoons (30 ml) of chopped fresh or dried corn silk and brewing it for 15 minutes prior to drinking.

DANCING

use for ✓ ***Dementia*** ✓ ***Depression***

DANCING MUST BE ONE OF THE MOST joyful forms of exercise—full of happy, exuberant and romantic associations. Its benefits stretch far beyond the physical—touching our emotions, forging friendships and, as researchers are beginning to discover, keeping our brains alert and active as we get older. Wherever and however you do it—from modern Zumba or salsa to ecstatic dance and five rhythms to the more sedate tea dances—dancing offers enormous benefits for every age group.

How it works

Important US research has shown that regular dancing can protect against dementia in older people. The 21-year study of several hundred older people compared the effects of various pastimes, including reading, doing crosswords, playing golf and walking. Frequent dancing offered the greatest protection for any cognitive or physical activity with a 76 percent reduction in the risk of dementia compared to a 35 percent reduction with reading and 47 percent reduction with regular crosswords.

Why? Scientists say that challenging our brains makes them more resilient to damage and disease, helping to establish new neural pathways that improve cognitive function. Dancing is mentally and physically demanding; you have to make split-second decisions, and remember steps and sequences, which also boosts memory skills. Like other physical activities, dancing also keeps you fit, helps to regulate blood pressure and boosts blood circulation, all of which benefit the brain. It improves posture and balance, too, which often deteriorate in old age. Studies show that various dances, especially the tango, can reduce the severity of Parkinson's disease symptoms, improving both balance and spatial awareness, and reducing falls.

Such health benefits as well as the social nature of dancing are likely to contribute to general well-being, happiness and confidence. Dance has been shown to reduce stress, depression and insomnia, and raise levels of the "feel-good" hormone serotonin. This may be true even for patients suffering from dementia. A Swedish study showed that social dancing alleviated symptoms, boosted positive feelings and helped patients communicate better.

Safety first *If you suffer any health problems, consult your doctor before starting a dance class to help determine how energetic your class should be.*

Where to find *Look for classes in your local newspaper or library, or check on community websites and listings.*

How to use

Join a local dance class and choose a style that suits you. If you, or a relative, live in a retirement or care home, ask if classes can be arranged. Physical limitation need not be a problem as dancing can be performed with any part of the body. To get you started, there are some popular easy dance steps on the next page.

continued on page 166

DANCING *continued*

Waltz

A favorite of the ballroom, this romantic dance is one of the easiest to learn. Waltz comes from the German word *walzen*, which means "to revolve," and the dance is made up of a series of graceful turns. It is set to a 3/4 time signature with six steps counted as "one-two-three, one-two-three."

THE STEPS The lead (traditionally the man) steps forward with his left foot (1), to the right with his right foot (2) then brings the left foot next to the right (3). Then he steps back with his right foot (4), back to the left with his left foot (5) and brings his right foot next to the left (6). These are the six moves that make up the basic "box step." The dance partner's steps are a mirror image of the lead's moves.

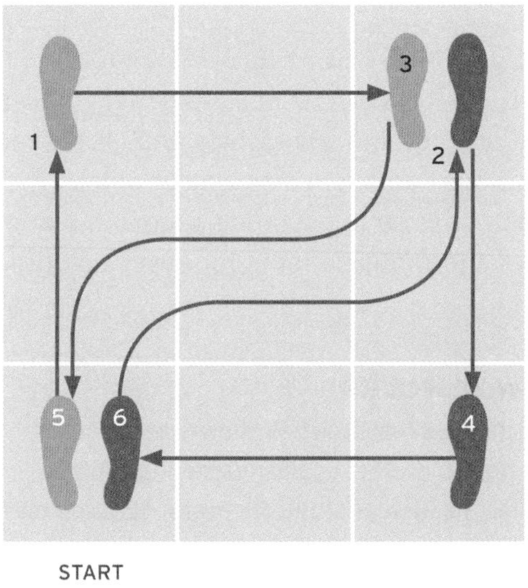

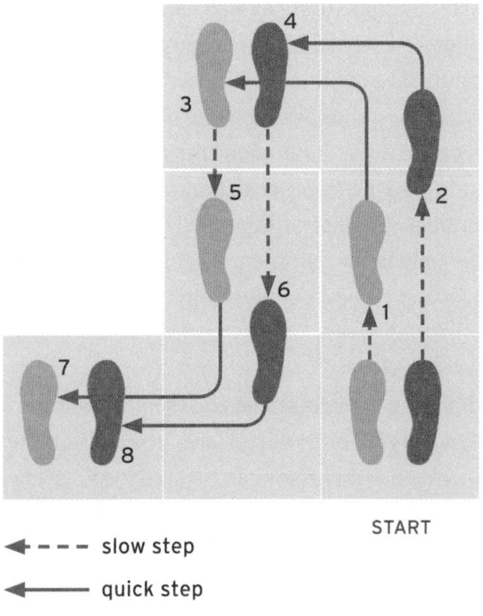

Foxtrot

Famously performed by Ginger Rogers and Fred Astaire, try this if you are feeling energetic. Moving to a slow-slow-quick-quick rhythm, follow the steps at left. You should soon cover much of the dance floor as you move forward, to the side, backward and to the side.

THE STEPS Once again the steps shown are for the lead dancer; the partner follows, with mirror-image footwork. *Slow-slow*: begin with two slow steps forward, left then right (1 and 2). *Quick-quick*: take a quick step to the side with the left foot (3) and then the right (4). *Slow-slow*: now take two slow steps backward, left (5) then right (6). *Quick-quick*: two steps to the left (7 and 8) complete the sequence.

DARK CHOCOLATE

use for ✓ ***Concentration, improved*** ✓ ***Depression*** ✓ ***Fatigue***

OVER THE YEARS, CHOCOLATE LOVERS have had a difficult time justifying their passion–until recently. News of high levels of antioxidants found in chocolate and the associated health benefits spread like wildfire among the chocoholics of the world. It seems that the occasional cube or two of the dark kind is good for you.

Chocolate is produced from the seeds of the cacao tree *(Theobroma cacao)*, which are fermented to provide cocoa powder and cocoa butter. These ingredients are then combined with sugar and milk to form chocolate. It is the cocoa powder that contains most of the beneficial phytonutrients. When buying chocolate, the higher the percentage of cocoa, the better the chocolate will be for your health.

How it works

Cocoa contains concentrated amounts of antioxidants including the highly prized catechins–more than either green tea or red wine. Dark chocolate contains 53.5 mg catechins per 3½ ounces (100 g), while milk chocolate contains 15.9 mg per 3½ ounces (100 g). (White chocolate contains none at all because it doesn't contain cocoa powder.) Cocoa also contains caffeine, theobromine, phenylethylamine and reasonable amounts of magnesium, calcium, iron, copper, potassium and zinc.

Dark chocolate has been shown to be helpful in depression, which could be due to chemicals in the cocoa such as phenylethylamine, caffeine and theobromine, which have the effect of boosting chemicals in the brain that improve cognitive function and mood. There are many studies showing chocolate's beneficial effect on the cardiovascular system, including lowering blood pressure, lipid levels and insulin resistance. One study on athletes showed that eating chocolate 15 minutes before exercising increases stamina, delays postexercise fatigue and enhances glycogen stores.

How to use

For the most benefit, choose good quality dark chocolate, with at least 70 percent cocoa. Studies have used up to 3½ ounces (100 g) per day with good effect, but you should balance your intake with your activity levels as chocolate is high in calories. Alternatively, have one to two cups of hot chocolate each day made with good quality cocoa powder.

Safety first *Although cited as a trigger for headaches, migraines and acne, there is little evidence backing these claims. Rarely, chocolate sensitivity may occur. Chocolate is considered safe during pregnancy.*

Where to find *Supermarkets, health food stores and department stores sell chocolate.*

DEVIL'S CLAW *Harpagophytum procumbens.*

Also called: Grapple plant

use for ✓ ***Back and neck pain*** ✓ ***Chronic pain*** ✓ ***Osteoarthritis***

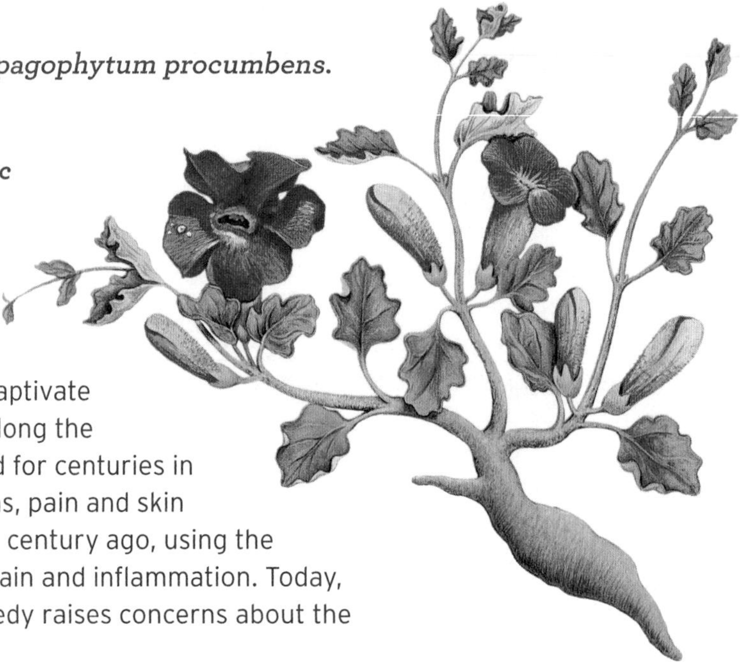

SEEDS WITH LONG, swooping hooks and fruit with a spiny outer rind inspired this African plant's English name. But it's the roots and potato-like tubers that captivate herbalists. This endangered plant grows along the edges of the Kalahari Desert and was used for centuries in traditional remedies for digestion problems, pain and skin sores. Europeans discovered devil's claw a century ago, using the dried root to ease heartburn and soothe pain and inflammation. Today, its widespread popularity as a herbal remedy raises concerns about the plant's survival in the wild.

How it works

Devil's claw contains bitter-tasting chemicals called iridoid glycosides, which may have anti-inflammatory effects. It is an especially rich source of one particular iridoid, called harpagoside, which may both soothe inflammation and ease pain. Research suggests this traditional remedy works: In one study, taking devil's claw for four months brought as much pain relief to people with osteoarthritis of the knee as a commercial painkiller, and a review of a dozen studies concluded that it eased pain caused by arthritis of the spine, back and knees. The bonus? Fewer side effects.

Other research suggests it can also be used to conquer back and neck pain. In one small study, it worked as well as a powerful, anti-inflammatory prescription painkiller.

This herb's extremely bitter taste also makes it excellent at enhancing digestion, say herbalists, since it stimulates secretion of stomach acids.

Safety first *About one in 12 people who take devil's claw develop diarrhea. Talk with your doctor before taking devil's claw if you have diabetes, gallstones, high or low blood pressure, a heart condition or a peptic ulcer; it may affect blood glucose, heart rate, bile production (which could make gallstones worse) and production of stomach acid. Devil's claw has not been widely tested during pregnancy or breastfeeding so it is best avoided or used only under medical supervision during these periods.*

Where to find *Devil's claw is available in health food stores or from a qualified herbalist.*

How to use

Devil's claw is available in liquid extracts, capsules and tablets. The dried root can also be used to make tea—though because devil's claw is among the most bitter-tasting of herbs, it may not be a pleasant cup. Follow label instructions or take as professionally prescribed.

ECHINACEA *Echinacea angustifolia, E. purpurea, E. pallida*

use for ✓ ***Colds and flu*** ✓ ***Cuts and scrapes*** ✓ ***Fever*** ✓ ***Frequent illness***

ECHINACEA'S DAISY-LIKE FLOWERS have crimson, mauve or white petals. The herb takes its name from the Greek word for sea urchin *(echino)* after the characteristic spiky raised cone at the center of its flowers.

Native Americans used echinacea for all manner of infections, wounds, bites and stings—even snakebites! Its use as a blood purifier and anti-infective agent became mainstream in the US during the 1800s, and by the turn of the 20th century it was the most popular herbal preparation in the country, only falling from favor as antibiotics emerged as the predominant means of treating infections.

How it works

A number of echinacea's constituents have pharmacological activity, the most important of which include alkylamides, polysaccharides and caffeic acid derivatives. The herb enhances immunity in a number of ways, including priming immune system cells for activity and stimulating the process by which immune system cells engulf and destroy invading organisms.

Safety first *Do not take echinacea if you are pregnant, breastfeeding, or have been diagnosed with an autoimmune disease or immunodeficiency disorder; safety under these circumstances has not been established. Do not take echinacea if you are allergic to plants from the Compositae (Asteraceae) family, which also contains daisies, sunflowers and feverfew.*

Where to find *Echinacea products are available in health food stores, pharmacies and supermarkets. Products prepared from E. purpurea have performed the most consistently in clinical studies.*

How to use

Many people take echinacea throughout winter to support immunity and build resistance to frequent illnesses such as colds and flu. Alternatively, when taken as soon as possible after symptoms develop, echinacea may relieve colds and hasten recovery.

On the whole, the scientific evidence supports echinacea's reputation as an immune system tonic and effective treatment for upper respiratory tract infections when taken by adults, but it appears to be less effective for children.

Herbalists have traditionally attributed echinacea with wound-healing properties, too, and there is some evidence to support topical applications of *E. purpurea* juice for skin conditions such as cuts, scrapes, abscesses and ulcers.

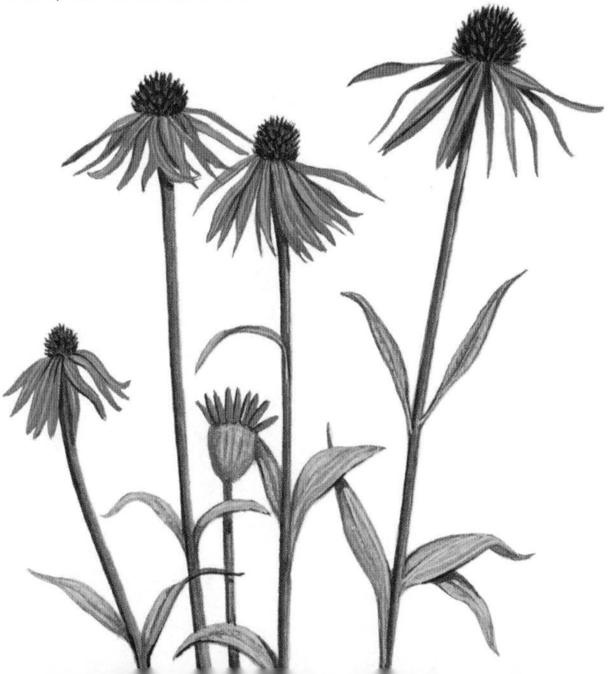

ELDER *Sambucus nigra*

use for ✓ ***Colds and flu*** ✓ ***Fever***

IN PAGAN MYTHOLOGY, THE ELDER tree was thought to have magical powers and the Druids used it to both bless and curse. Medieval herbalist John Evelyn described it as "a kind of Catholicon against all Infirmities whatever." Today elderflower tea and elderberry syrup are still popular herbal remedies for colds, flu and any accompanying fever—with some scientific backing. The berries and flowers are used to flavor cordials and wines.

How it works

Elderflower tea is used medicinally—especially in Germany, where it has been officially approved for treating feverish colds. It has a confirmed diaphoretic (sweat-inducing) effect and also increases bronchial secretions, making it helpful for treating fevers and respiratory infections. Its phenols and flavonoids, including the antioxidants quercetin and rutin, are thought responsible for these effects.

The berries, rich in vitamin C as well as protective flavonoids, have attracted more attention in recent years. The Israeli virologist Dr. Madeleine Mumcuoglu showed that elderberry constituents could deactivate spike-shaped proteins on the surface of flu viruses, preventing them from entering body cells and replicating. Elderberry also appears to boost the immune response, encouraging defensive white blood cells to fight off viral invaders.

Mumcuoglu turned her research into an antiviral flu treatment, an elderberry extract that small trials have shown is effective against both A and B strains of flu and, in a slightly different formulation, against swine flu, too. Another extract, in lozenge form, has shown promise against flu, while a combination of herbs, including elder, appears to treat bacterial sinusitis.

Safety first *Avoid unripe elderberries, which contain the mildly toxic substance sambunigrin. Ripe berries and flowers are considered safe, though they might interact with certain medications so check first with your doctor if taking prescription drugs.*

Where to find *Dried elderflowers and elder products are available in health food stores.*

How to use

To make an elderflower tea, steep a teaspoon of dried flowers in a cup of boiling water for 10–15 minutes. Commercial elder products are available as liquids, syrups, teas and tinctures or as capsules or lozenges. Follow label instructions or take as professionally prescribed.

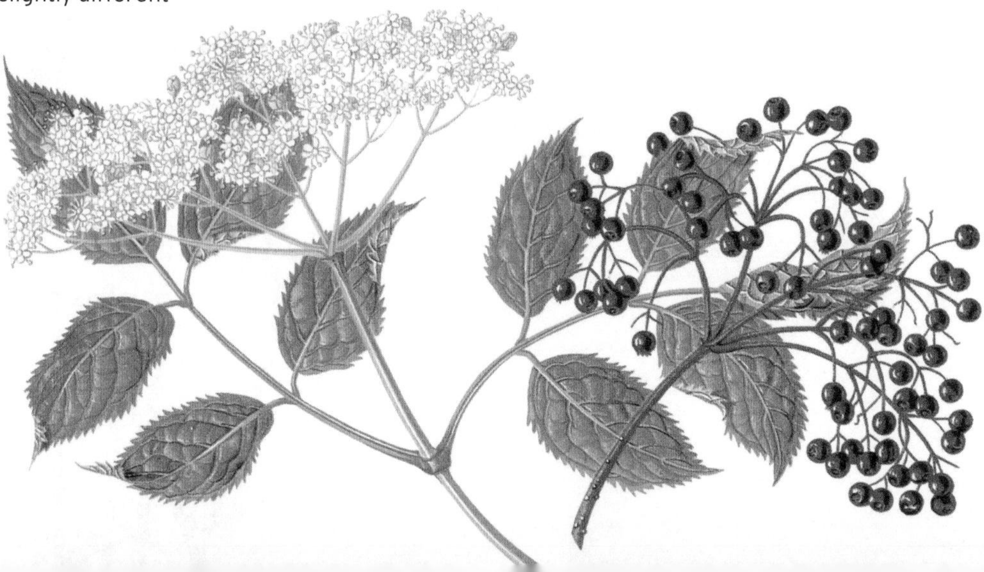

ELIMINATION DIET

use for ✓ ***Allergies*** ✓ ***Eczema and dermatitis*** ✓ ***Food intolerances*** ✓ ***Headaches*** ✓ ***Irritable bowel syndrome*** ✓ ***Migraines*** ✓ ***Rheumatoid arthritis***

THERE'S GROWING PROOF THAT FOODS can activate and worsen a wide variety of health conditions—from allergy symptoms to painful joints. Identifying and eliminating troublemakers can reduce symptoms or at least help prevent them from growing worse. Elimination diets are widely recommended for uncovering food culprits. The details of the diet vary for different conditions and you should ask your doctor about your particular situation. Here is a basic outline of how an elimination diet works.

How it works

By removing specific foods and ingredients that you suspect are causing a reaction, you can pinpoint triggers and keep them off your plate—and out of your body. This helps eliminate a wide variety of food reactions. Trigger foods can push your immune system into overdrive causing digestive upset, fatigue and a feeling of unease, as well as boosting inflammation, worsening eczema, rheumatoid arthritis and other inflammatory conditions.

How to use

An elimination diet is a four-step process. First, determine what could be causing problems. You may need to track your symptoms and diet for a week or more to find suspects. **(See Journaling, *p. 215.*)**

Common food allergy and intolerance triggers include wheat, gluten-containing products, milk, eggs, citrus, nuts and soy as well as certain chemical food additives such as monosodium glutamate. Headache triggers can include the compound tyramine (found in many cheeses, processed meats, red wine and other foods) as well as food additives such as nitrites and colorings. Foods that may worsen rheumatoid arthritis symptoms include red meat, sugar, fats, salt, caffeine, gluten, tomatoes and eggplant. Eczema flare-ups may commonly be fueled by dairy, eggs or nuts; but citrus, wheat, seafood and food additives have also been implicated.

Having decided on the potential triggers, the next step is to eliminate them all for one to two weeks. Be sure to replace key nutrients and keep your diet balanced. If your symptoms don't improve, go back to your regular diet and consult your doctor.

If your symptoms do improve, the next step is to reintroduce trigger foods one by one every three days to see which foods cause a reaction. If you don't have symptoms for a day or so after a food is reintroduced then the food is likely to be safe to eat.

Finally, create a new, healthy diet plan for yourself that does not include your trigger food(s).

Safety first *Long-term elimination diets can lead to malnutrition; don't follow one for longer than two or three weeks. And if you have a dangerous or life-threatening food allergy, do not try to reintroduce trigger foods.*

ENZYMES

Alpha-galactosidase, bromelain, lactase

use for ✓ ***Bruises*** ✓ ***Flatulence*** ✓ ***Food intolerances*** ✓ ***Gout*** ✓ ***Sinusitis*** ✓ ***Wound healing***

ENZYMES ARE MOLECULES THAT TRIGGER or speed up processes in the body. There are many different types of enzyme and our bodies need them for a multitude of purposes. Their many functions include digesting food, processing toxins, activating the immune system and stimulating muscle contraction. Most of us can make the enzymes we need in our bodies, but sometimes taking a supplemental enzyme can be helpful.

How they work

Enzyme supplements are sometimes used to supplement the body's enzyme production. For example, lactose-intolerant people often take the enzyme lactase to allow them to consume dairy foods more comfortably.

Bromelain is a combination of enzymes derived from pineapple plants that has well-documented anti-inflammatory and anti–blood clotting properties.

Safety first *The safety of some enzymes has not been determined for people with heart, kidney or liver disease and during childhood, pregnancy, breastfeeding or while taking some prescription medications.*

Bromelain has been associated with numerous drug interactions, side effects and allergic reactions. It is not suitable for use prior to surgery or by those with bleeding disorders, stomach ulcers or bleeding wounds. Talk to your doctor before use and seek medical advice if you experience side effects such as gastrointestinal discomfort, diarrhea or drowsiness.

Where to find *Enzyme supplements are available in health food stores. Lactose-free milk and milk with added lactase are available in health food stores and some supermarkets.*

How to use

Specific enzymes may aid the management of some (but not all) food intolerances. For example, taking lactase supplements or adding lactase drops to dairy foods enables some lactose-intolerant people to tolerate dairy products in greater quantities.

If you experience flatulence, bloating and digestive discomfort after eating legumes, taking the enzyme alpha-galactosidase just before you consume them may help relieve symptoms.

Bromelain supplements may reduce swelling, bruising and pain following surgical procedures and trauma, and may also accelerate wound healing. Bromelain may offer pain relief and have anti-inflammatory effects in other conditions, too. For example, it may relieve swelling, improve breathing and reduce recovery time in sinusitis. It is also sometimes recommended for gout, osteoarthritis and rheumatoid arthritis, although its efficacy in these conditions has not been verified by clinical research. When taking enzyme supplements follow label instructions or take as professionally prescribed.

EUCALYPTUS *Eucalyptus* spp. Also called: Blue gum

use for ✓ ***Asthma*** ✓ ***Bad breath and body odour*** ✓ ***Bronchitis*** ✓ ***Colds and flu*** ✓ ***Fungal infections*** ✓ ***Sinusitis***

AUSTRALIAN ABORIGINES TRADITIONALLY used infusions of eucalyptus leaves to relieve respiratory congestion, coughs and fevers, and as topical applications for sore muscles. Essential oil was distilled from eucalyptus trees not long after the first European settlers arrived in Australia. Commercial production commenced in the mid-1800s, and the oil soon came to be highly prized around the world for its antiseptic and antibacterial properties.

How it works

Eucalyptus oil contains several active constituents. The most important is 1,8-cineole (sometimes referred to as eucalyptol), which has an antimicrobial effect against a wide range of disease-causing bacteria, viruses and fungi.

How to use

For respiratory conditions such as asthma, sinusitis, bronchitis, colds and flu, eucalyptus oil is often used as an inhalation—commonly via a nebulizer or vaporizer in which the oil is diluted in steaming water. It is sometimes also used in a cream or ointment that is rubbed onto the chest, delivering the therapeutic actions through a combination of inhalation and the penetration of the oil through the skin. It is also sometimes included in throat lozenges or cough mixtures in minute quantities.

Topical applications of eucalyptus essential oil (usually in dilute concentrations) can also be used to treat infections of various kinds. For example, the essential oil and/or 1,8-cineole derived from it are often included in mouthwash products to help kill the bacteria that cause plaque, gingivitis and bad breath. Eucalyptus oil can also be added to laundry to kill dust mites in sheets, disinfect clothes and leave the washing smelling fresh.

Research also suggests that an ointment containing eucalyptus oil and other antimicrobial substances may be beneficial in the treatment of fungal toenail infections.

Safety first **Eucalyptus oil should not be taken internally.** *The topical use of the oil is not suitable for babies, children, pregnant or breastfeeding women, or people allergic to* Eucalyptus *spp. Caution is advised with eucalyptus inhalations as they can irritate the eyes, mucous membranes and skin.*

Where to find *Eucalyptus essential oil is available in health food stores and pharmacies or from a qualified aromatherapist.*

EVENING PRIMROSE *Oenothera biennis*

use for ✓ ***Eczema and dermatitis*** ✓ ***Rheumatoid arthritis***

HIDDEN WITHIN THIS EDIBLE PLANT'S TINY, spherical seeds is a beneficial fat called gamma-linolenic acid (GLA) that has benefits for a wide variety of health conditions. A native of North America, the evening primrose plant was used by Native Americans to make poultices to relieve bruises, heal sores and soothe hemorrhoids. English settlers took evening primrose back to the British Isles, where its roots were eaten as a food and its seeds used in place of poppy seeds. Today, herbalists and medical researchers focus their attention on evening primrose oil (EPO).

How it works

The human body converts GLA into a chemical that inhibits inflammation-boosting compounds. As a result, EPO may reduce the breast tenderness and swelling that happens in the second half of the menstrual cycle. In two studies, diabetes-related nerve pain was eased with a daily dose of EPO. Research also suggests that EPO can calm the swelling, itching, crusting and redness of eczema and help reduce the use of painkillers in people with rheumatoid arthritis. However, EPO research has not been unanimously positive; some studies have found little benefit, leading researchers to speculate that it may work better for some people than for others.

Safety first *Since EPO will not stop the progressive joint damage of rheumatoid arthritis, do not use it in place of medication. Skip EPO if you have or are at risk of prostate cancer (it is thought GLA may promote growth of prostate cancer cells). Avoid if you have seizures; there are reports that GLA may trigger seizures in people with seizure disorders. Avoid EPO in pregnancy due to concerns that GLA-rich oils could harm the fetus.*

Where to find *EPO is available in health food stores, supermarkets and, in some countries, by prescription from your doctor.*

How to use

EPO is usually taken in capsule form. Experts say you may have to take it for several weeks or months to see results. For rheumatoid arthritis pain relief, some experts recommend taking EPO along with fish oil capsules. Follow label instructions or take as professionally prescribed.

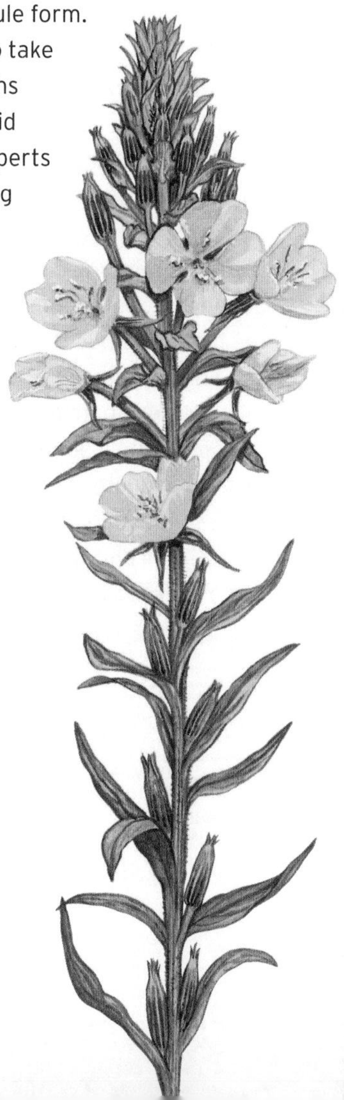

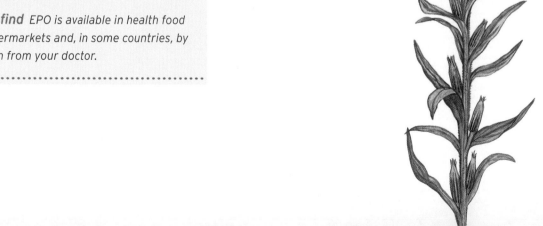

EXERCISE

use for ✓ ***Anxiety*** ✓ ***Constipation*** ✓ ***Dementia*** ✓ ***Depression*** ✓ ***Diabetes and insulin resistance*** ✓ ***Fall prevention*** ✓ ***Fatigue*** ✓ ***Frequent illness*** ✓ ***Heart and circulatory health*** ✓ ***Inflammatory bowel disease*** ✓ ***Osteoarthritis*** ✓ ***Overweight and obesity*** ✓ ***Phobias*** ✓ ***Sleeping problems*** ✓ ***Strains and sprains*** ✓ ***Stroke prevention*** ✓ ***Tooth and gum disorders***

GO AHEAD—GET MOVING! A growing stack of impressive research proves that physical activity is powerful medicine. By burning calories, activating muscles, getting the blood pumping, relieving stress and pampering brain cells, exercise (or "vitamin x") is a natural, drug-free strategy for better all-around health. And you don't have to work out like an Olympic athlete to get results. There's growing evidence that short exercise sessions are beneficial—as are routines where you set the pace and choose activities you enjoy most.

How it works

The health benefits of exercise reach into virtually every corner of your mind and body. Added to this is an overwhelming variety of physical activities to choose from. But the key to reaping the benefits of exercise is to find an activity that you'll happily do *regularly*. Exercise can be adapted to suit everyone's ability and lifestyle—you just need to find out what's right for you. Here's a roundup of how "vitamin x" could benefit you.

Safety first *Moderate activity is safe for most people. However, check with your doctor first if you have a chronic health condition such as heart disease, arthritis or diabetes. Always keep within your limits and if you feel faint or uncomfortably breathless, or experience any kind of pain: stop.*

Where to find *Local gyms and adult-education centers offer exercise classes for beginners. Your doctor should be able to give you more information about local resources.*

For weight loss

Physical activity helps you lose excess weight and keep it off by burning energy; as you move, your muscles use up blood glucose and fat. If you burn more than you consume, the weight comes off. But that's just the beginning of a positive spiral. Regular exercise helps control the appetite by reducing levels of the hunger hormone ghrelin, raising levels of an appetite-suppressing hormone called peptide YY and making brain cells more sensitive to leptin, the "satisfaction" hormone, so you feel full sooner.

Adding strength training to your routine has even more benefits. Starting in our midthirties, we lose 2 percent or more of our muscle mass each decade. Studies show that after just two and a half months of regular strength training two or three times per week you can build about 2 pounds (1 kg) of muscle and lose slightly more fat. Rebuilding muscle boosts your metabolism, because muscle burns more calories than fat "round the clock." It also looks sleeker than fat, giving your body a more toned appearance.

continued on page 176

EXERCISE *continued*

For a healthy heart, arteries and better blood glucose control

Aerobic exercise reduces levels of stress hormones and boosts levels of artery-relaxing nitric oxide in blood vessels, which helps lower blood pressure. It raises levels of heart-protecting HDL cholesterol, improves sensitivity to insulin (the hormone that tells cells to absorb blood glucose) and also prompts muscle cells to sip more glucose directly from your bloodstream for an immediate, blood glucose–lowering effect. Strength training improved insulin sensitivity by 30 percent and lowered blood pressure by as much as five points in studies done at Tufts University, and it reduced heart-threatening LDL cholesterol in a recent Greek study.

For strong bones

Weight-bearing exercise, such as walking, jogging, aerobics or strength training, prompts bone to grow more densely—helping reduce the risk of fractures. By building muscle, which acts as a shock absorber, and keeping joints flexible, gentle strength training can reduce the pain of osteoarthritis, too.

For your brain and mind

Exercise boosts mood, eases stress and anxiety, improves sleep and helps to lift depression, with regular exercise being as effective as some medications in relieving mild depression. Exercise also helps protect against dementia by boosting blood circulation in the brain, protecting brain cells from injury and by fueling the growth of new brain cells and new connections between those cells.

It's never too late to start. In one 2008 study of 2,263 men, aged 71–92, inactive volunteers who started an exercise program cut their risk of dementia in half. In another study published in the *New England Journal of Medicine* that examined risk of dementia and cognitive and physical activities in people over 75 years, **dancing** *(p. 165)* was found to be the most effective activity, reducing the risk of dementia by as much as 76 percent.

As well as remediating the conditions mentioned above, regular exercise may have far-reaching effects into all sorts of body systems. For example, by reducing inflammation and supporting a healthy immune system, regular exercise may even lower your risk for tooth and gum problems and inflammatory bowel disease flare-ups. So get into the habit—and start today.

How to use

Aim for 150 minutes of moderately paced exercise or 75 minutes of vigorous exercise each week. That could be a brisk, 30-minute stroll five days a week, three strenuous, 25-minute workouts or similar amounts of time spent in exercise classes, using fitness equipment or enjoying other activities such as cycling, swimming or playing an active sport. You're exercising at a moderate pace if you can still hold a conversation comfortably; you've reached a vigorous pace when exercise is intense enough that chatting is too difficult. If you don't have time for a 30-minute workout, two 15-minute or three 10-minute sessions a day can be just as beneficial.

The US Centers for Disease Control and Prevention recommends also making time for two strength-training sessions a week that target all major muscle groups (legs, hips, back, abdomen, chest, shoulders and arms). You can use weight machines, hand weights, resistance bands or moves that use your own body weight such as pushups. Always leave at least one day off between strength-training workouts for optimal muscle recovery. Start with light weights or resistance bands and easy moves so that you can work out with proper form. If you are new to strength training, consider taking a class to learn more.

Be creative and have fun. Any activity that gets you moving helps. Gardening, raking leaves, active fun like playing outdoor games or sports, dancing, even a morning of heavy housework burns energy and activates your muscles. Get moving and enjoy the benefits in your body and mind.

STRENGTHENING YOUR LOWER BODY

INNER THIGHS Lie on your right side with your left leg angled in front of you and the inside edge of your left foot resting on the floor. Place your left hand on the floor for balance. Keep your right leg straight without locking your knee, with the ankle, knee, hip and shoulder in a straight line. Raise your right leg as high as you comfortably can (lower picture). Hold for one second, then lower it slowly to within 1 inch (2.5 cm) of the floor. Hold, then repeat. For this and the exercise below, do two sets of 10–12 repetitions, switching sides between sets.

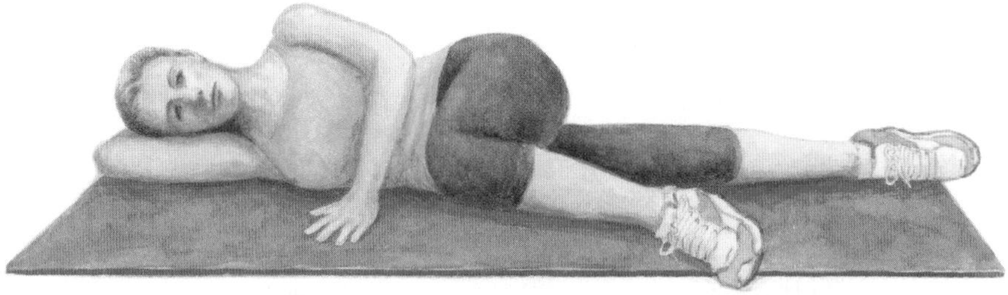

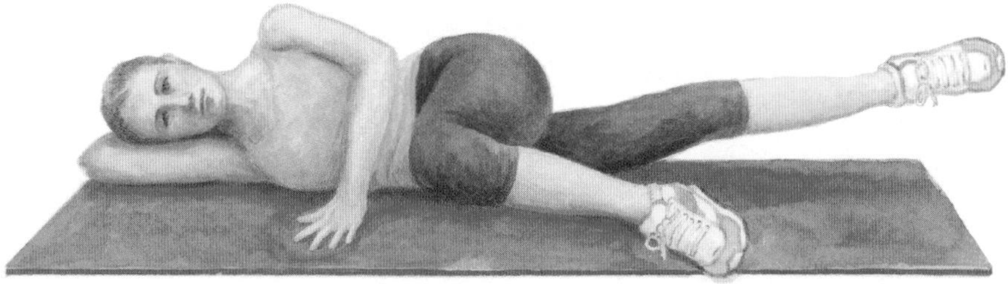

OUTER THIGHS Lie on your right side with your right knee and hip bent. Keep your upper leg and torso straight. Raise your upper leg as high as you comfortably can. Hold for one second, then slowly lower it until it is almost touching your lower leg. Repeat.

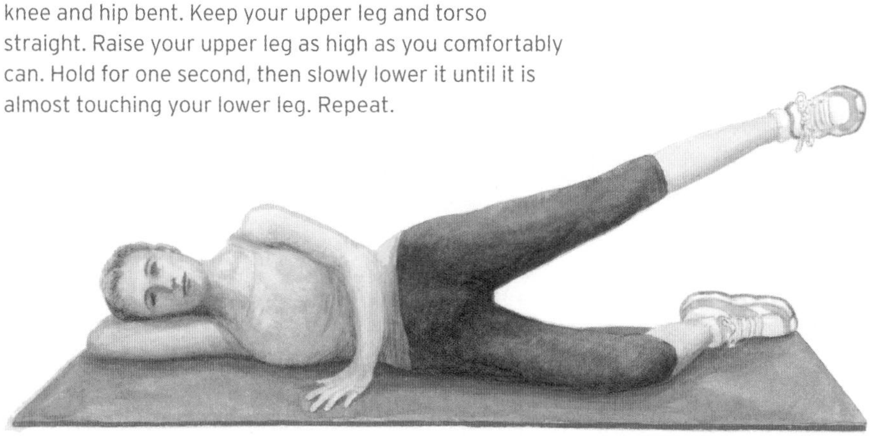

continued on page 178

KICKBACKS These exercises improve your arm strength. Rest your left knee and left hand on a bench or chair and extend your right leg behind you, your right foot flat on the floor. Grasp a small weight in your right hand, your arm bent at a 45-degree angle. Exhale as you straighten your right arm almost fully. Keep your elbow at your side and move only your forearm. Pause, then inhale as you lower your arm to its original position. After each set, switch to your other arm. Start with two to three sets of 10–12 repetitions, resting briefly between each set.

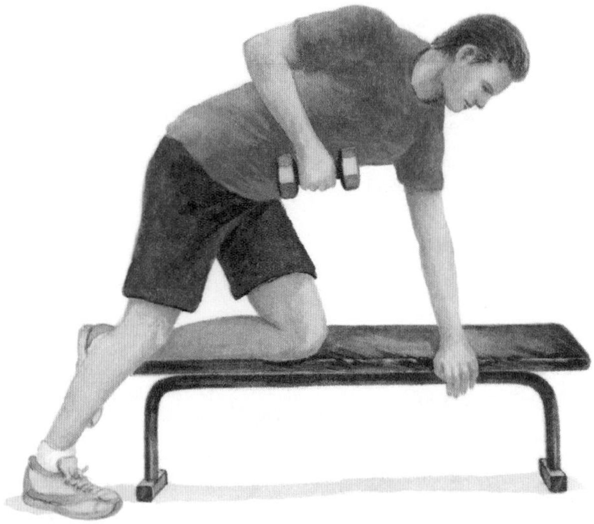

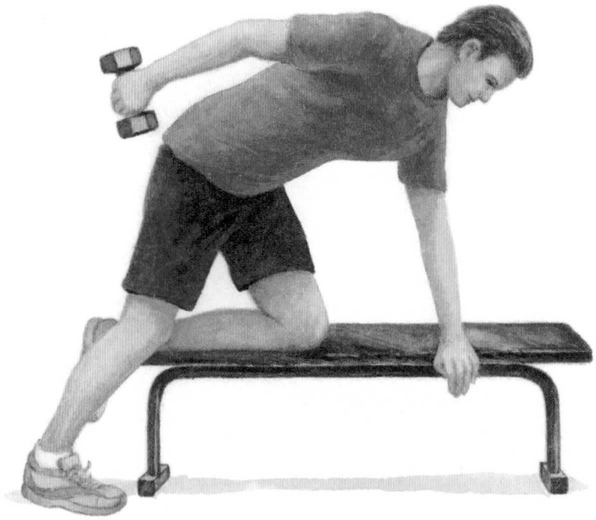

STRENGTHENING YOUR CORE

CRUNCHES Keeping your core or midsection strong is important for maintaining mobility and a healthy back. Crunches are a well-known favorite. Lie down with knees bent and heels on the floor with toes pointing up. Place hands gently behind your head and focus on your abdominal muscles, which should be doing all the work. Exhale as you slowly curl your upper body toward your thighs to about 30 degrees, keeping your lower back firmly on the mat. Pause and inhale as you lower yourself back down. Do two sets of 15 repetitions to begin with.

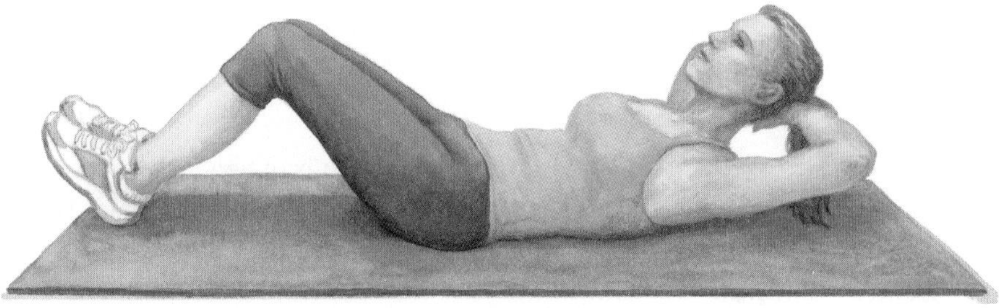

REVERSE CRUNCH This exercise focuses on your lower abdominal muscles. From a lying position, raise your legs (one at a time) so that the soles of your feet face the ceiling. Keep your lower back on the floor but raise your head slightly, placing your hands gently behind the head for support. Exhale and contract your abdominal muscles to pull your legs by about 30 degrees toward your head. Focus on your lower abs as you do this. Inhale as you relax back to the starting position. Do two sets of 15 repetitions to begin with.

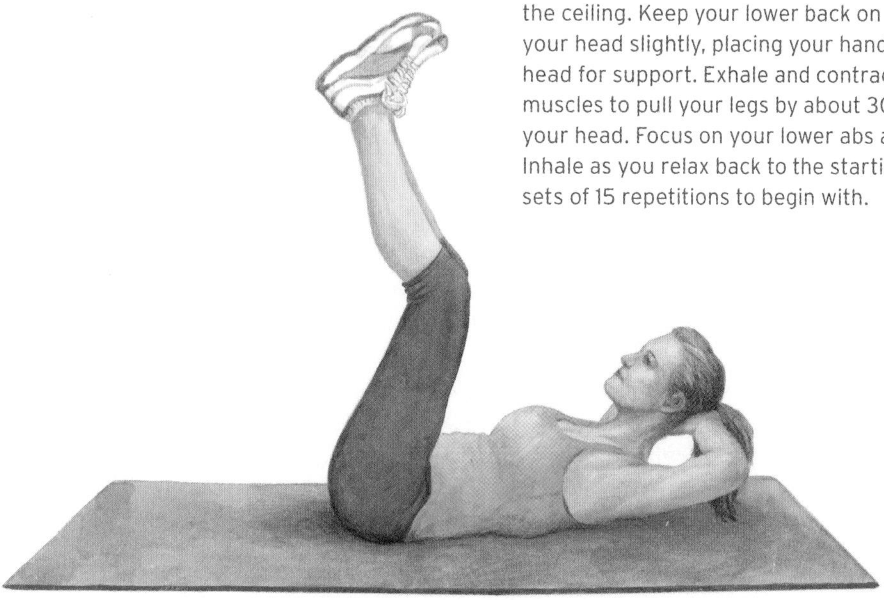

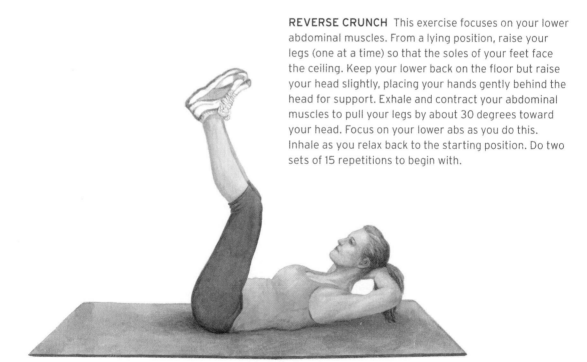

FELDENKRAIS METHOD

use for ✓ ***Back and neck pain*** ✓ ***Bursitis and tendonitis*** ✓ ***Fall prevention*** ✓ ***Osteoarthritis***

THE FELDENKRAIS METHOD (FELDENKRAIS) is an exercise-based therapy that was developed in the 1940s aimed at improving the way you move. It is often used as a supportive or rehabilitative measure for people affected by musculoskeletal conditions, and is popular among athletes, musicians and artists, who use it to enhance their physical performance.

Its founder, Dr. Moshe Feldenkrais, said that the aim of the technique is to create "...a body that is organized to move with minimum effort and maximum efficiency, not through muscular strength, but [through] increased consciousness of how it works."

How it works

Proponents claim that Feldenkrais improves physical, mental and emotional well-being by increasing sensory awareness, enhancing the integration between the body and mind, promoting dexterity, and fostering the development of new and improved motor skills. In a practical sense, retraining the body to move and hold itself more appropriately means that Feldenkrais may help prevent or address biomechanical issues caused by repeatedly performing specific movements or holding certain postures. In turn, it is of benefit for musculoskeletal conditions that arise from those issues such as bursitis and neck and back pain.

Safety first *Tell your practitioner if you are pregnant or affected by musculoskeletal injuries or chronic disease (such as cardiovascular disease) to ensure your program is tailored to your specific needs.*

Where to find *Seek out a qualified practitioner. The International Feldenkrais Federation (www.feldenkrais-method.org) provides contact details for the Feldenkrais Guilds and Associations responsible for practitioner accreditation in each country.*

A visit to a Feldenkrais practitioner

Feldenkrais utilizes a combination of group classes, and one-on-one private treatments called Functional Integration (FI) or manipulation sessions. During group classes, participants are guided through movement sequences designed to draw attention to different types of movements such as those involved in walking. Feldenkrais classes have been shown to improve older people's balance (which may in turn help prevent falls) and reduce some of the symptoms and disability associated with osteoarthritis.

During an FI session, the practitioner places his or her hands on your body to guide you through specific movements so that you become aware of the way you currently move and hold your body. The practitioner then shows you how you could move more efficiently in the future. Some massage techniques may also be employed. Group classes and FI sessions are performed fully clothed.

The pelvic clock

This exercise is used in Feldenkrais to explore the movements of the pelvis and how it relates to the spine and body. Movements are very subtle and slow. The person imagines a clock face on the pelvis with 12 at the top beneath the belly button and six at the bottom. When pressure is put on 12 o'clock, the back flattens; putting pressure on 6 o'clock makes the back arch slightly. The student rocks gently to and fro, noting the effect. Then the pelvis is tilted to 3 o'clock, with the right hip raised and 9 o'clock with the left hip raised and gently rocked between the two positions. Finally the student slowly circles through all four positions.

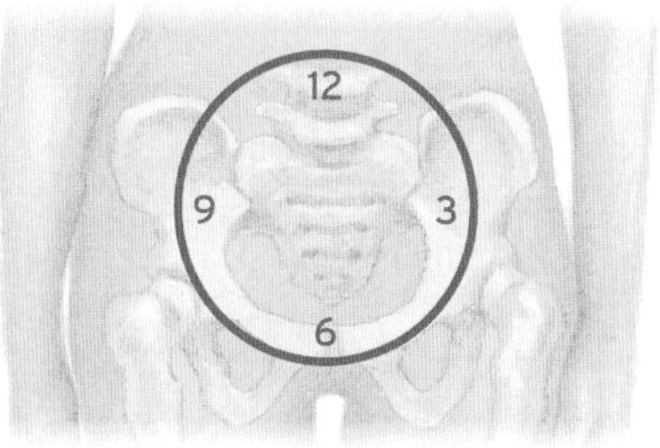

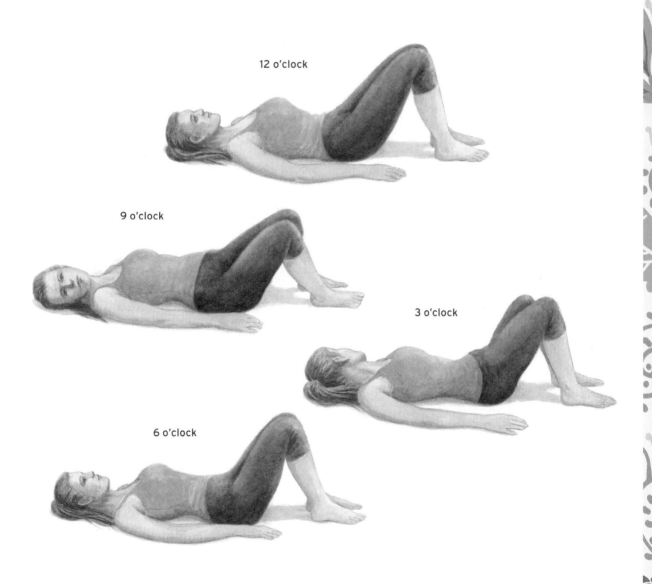

12 o'clock

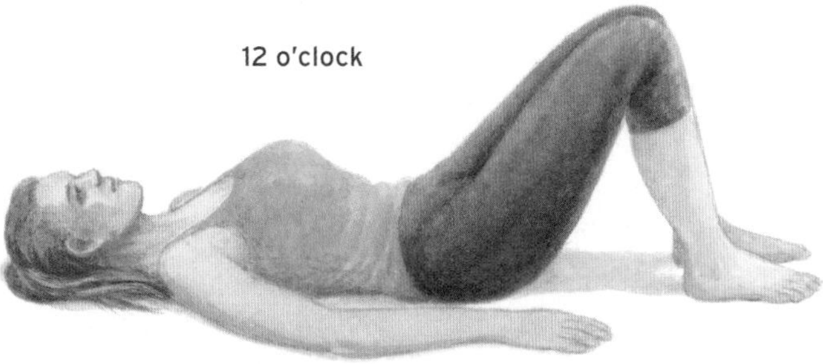

9 o'clock

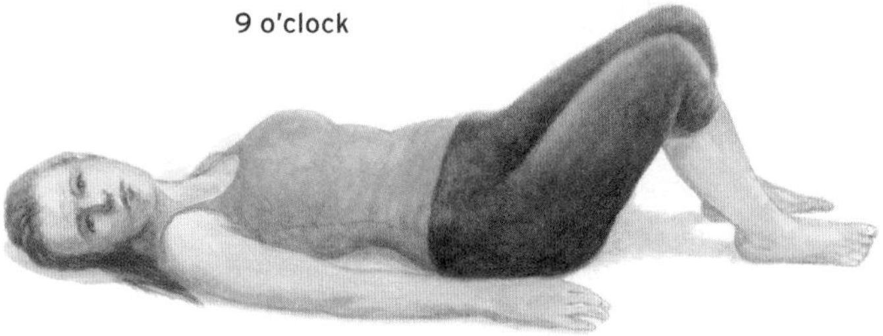

3 o'clock

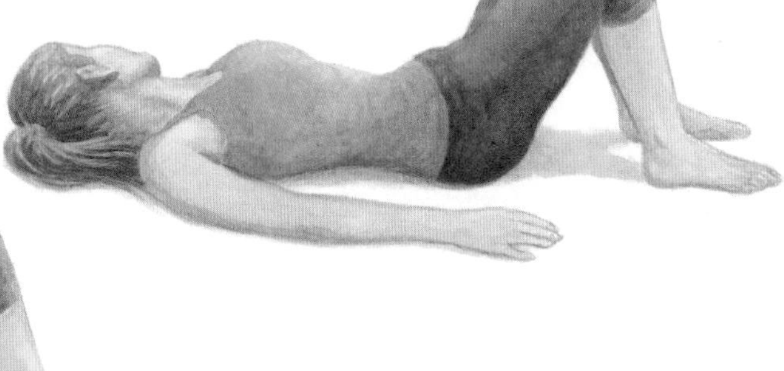

6 o'clock

FENUGREEK *Trigonella foenum-graecum*

use for ✓ ***Diabetes and insulin resistance***

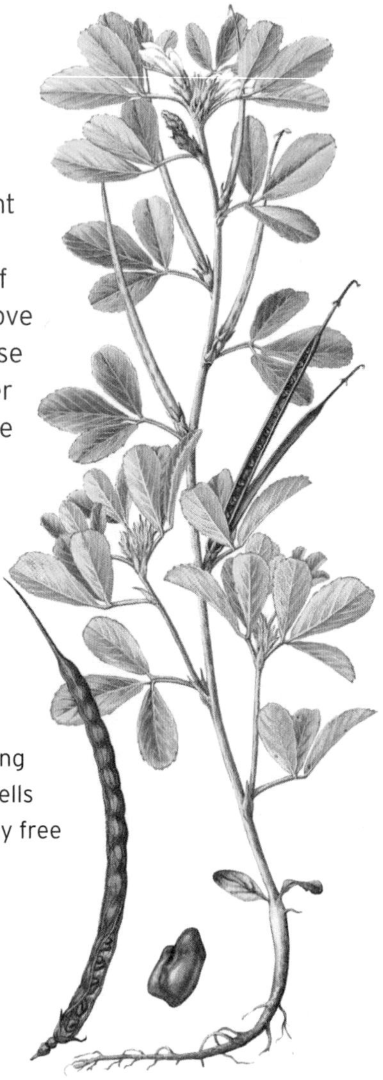

SEEDS OF THIS ANNUAL HERB, A MEMBER of the pea family, were found in Tutankhamun's tomb and reference to it first appears on ancient Egyptian papyrus dated to 1500 BC. Its aromatic properties make it a staple of Indian and Middle Eastern cookery and it has a long history of uses in traditional medicine. Clinical trials have shown that it can improve metabolic symptoms associated with diabetes by lowering blood glucose levels and improving glucose tolerance. It is alleged to offer many other health benefits (including the relief of digestive problems, gout, erectile dysfunction and eczema) and has been used for centuries by women who are breastfeeding to promote milk production.

How it works

In multiple trials fenugreek has been shown to decrease blood glucose and cholesterol. The powdered seed, available as capsules, is high in soluble fiber that slows the absorption of sugars in the stomach, while the presence of the amino acid 4-hydroxyisoleucine may help to stimulate insulin production. One small trial found that adding about 1-2 ounces per day (25-50 g) per day of powdered fenugreek seed to the diet reduced blood levels of triglycerides and LDL ("bad cholesterol") over a 20-day period.

Fenugreek seeds are also a good source of vitamins, minerals and antioxidants, helping to protect the body's cells from damage caused by free radicals.

How to use

Fenugreek leaves and seeds can be used to add a slightly sweet, nutty flavor to savory dishes. Fenugreek can also be taken as capsules, tablets or as a tea. (Some people soak seeds overnight to produce fenugreek water to consume in the morning.) With all products, follow label instructions or take as professionally prescribed.

Mild diarrhea, gas or bloating can occur during the first few days of use, but these side effects usually pass quickly.

Safety first *Fenugreek is safe when consumed in food but check with your doctor before using supplements if you are taking prescribed diabetes medications or anticoagulant medications such as warfarin or aspirin.*

Fenugreek is best avoided during pregnancy, when it could cause early contractions.

Where to find *Fenugreek capsules are available in health food stores and supermarkets. Fenugreek–or "Methi"–leaves can be found in Asian supermarkets or from a qualified herbalist.*

FEVERFEW *Tanacetum parthenium*

use for ✓ ***Migraines***

FEVERFEW HAS BEEN USED MEDICINALLY for thousands of years. Its common name is testament to its historical usage as a medicine to reduce fevers, while its botanical name, *Tanacetum parthenium,* is said to refer to it having saved a man's life when he fell from the Parthenon in Athens during its construction in the fifth century BC.

Historically, feverfew has been used to address headaches from a wide range of sources, as well as many other painful conditions. Today it is almost exclusively taken to reduce the frequency and intensity of migraines.

How it works

Feverfew appears to work in several ways to help prevent migraines, including decreasing blood vessel constriction and inhibiting the body's production of inflammatory chemicals called prostaglandins. A group of compounds called sesquiterpene lactones are believed to be the most medicinally active constituents of feverfew. Of those, a compound called parthenolide is present in the greatest quantity and is regarded as the most important; however, other compounds may also play significant roles in the herb's medicinal action.

How to use

Feverfew leaves can be consumed fresh or dried and in supplement form. Fresh feverfew leaves are bitter and may irritate the mucous membranes of the mouth so are best consumed with other food. Feverfew supplements won't stop a migraine once it has started, but when taken on an ongoing basis may help to reduce the frequency of migraine attacks and make them less severe. Follow label instructions or take as professionally prescribed.

Safety first *Do not take feverfew if you are allergic to plants from the Compositae (Asteraceae) family, which also contains daisies, sunflowers and echinacea.*

Feverfew has not been widely tested during pregnancy or breastfeeding so it is best avoided or used only under medical supervision during these periods.

Where to find *Feverfew supplements are available in health food stores or from a qualified herbalist.*

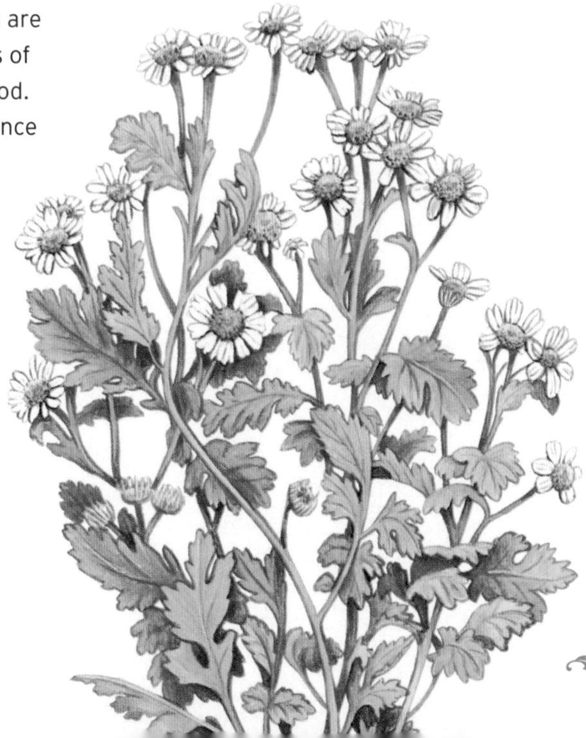

FIBER

use for ✓ ***Cancer support*** ✓ ***Cholesterol, high*** ✓ ***Constipation*** ✓ ***Diabetes and insulin resistance*** ✓ ***Hemorrhoids*** ✓ ***Stroke prevention***

THE TERM DIETARY FIBER REFERS to components in food that are indigestible. Fiber is a form of carbohydrate, and is exclusively found in foods derived from plants. It is described as either soluble or insoluble, depending on whether or not it dissolves in water. Fiber is a key element in a healthy diet and has several associated health benefits.

How it works

During digestion, fiber moves through the gastrointestinal tract relatively untouched until it reaches the intestines, where it undergoes partial or complete fermentation depending on its solubility. Insoluble fiber (such as wheat bran) provides bulk to the stool and promotes the easy passage of the feces through the gut for excretion.

Soluble forms of fiber (such as psyllium and oat bran) bind to bile acids (which are made from cholesterol), enabling them to be excreted via the feces, and ultimately helping to lower cholesterol levels. They also slow down the conversion of carbohydrates to glucose and help to maintain stable blood glucose levels.

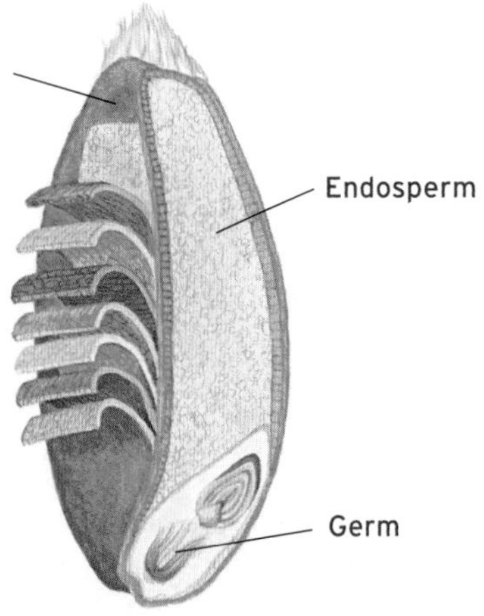

Whole grain is best for fiber

Foods that are "whole grain" are made from grain with its bran and vitamin-packed germ intact.

How to use

The US Institute of Medicine states that a daily adequate intake (AI) of fiber for adult men is 30 g, and that women should consume 25 g, increasing to 28 g during pregnancy and 30 g while breastfeeding. However, even greater levels may provide optimum health benefits.

Dietary surveys indicate that people whose diets contain large amounts of fiber enjoy a degree of protection against chronic conditions such as cardiovascular disease, diabetes and some forms of cancer (including colon and gastric cancer). In contrast, inadequate fiber often leads to constipation

Safety first *Introduce additional fiber into your diet slowly in order to avoid issues such as abdominal pain and flatulence. Note that increased fiber intake should always be accompanied by increased fluid intake.*

Some types of fiber can inhibit the absorption of certain nutrients and prescribed drugs, which may need to be taken several hours away from fiber supplements or high-fiber meals. Ask your doctor for more information.

Where to find *Fiber is naturally present in plant foods such as fruit and vegetables, grains, legumes, nuts and seeds. Fiber supplements are also available in supermarkets, pharmacies and health food stores, usually in powders that can be added to drinks.*

and associated conditions such as hemorrhoids. These problems are often simply addressed by eating more fruit and vegetables and choosing whole food options (such as whole grain bread) wherever possible, thus increasing your fiber intake. To help manage cholesterol levels and reduce your risk of other cardiovascular problems such as stroke, add oat bran, **psyllium** *(p. 264)* or other sources of soluble fiber to your diet on a regular basis.

Eating large amounts of soluble fiber also helps people with diabetes and insulin resistance to manage their blood glucose and insulin levels.

Fiber-rich foods

You can increase your fiber intake by eating more of the foods shown below. Seek out whole grain bread and brown rice and start the day with cereals containing seeds, nuts and oats, perhaps topped with fresh berries. Filling up on fiber also helps to make you feel full so you don't crave unhealthy sugary snacks.

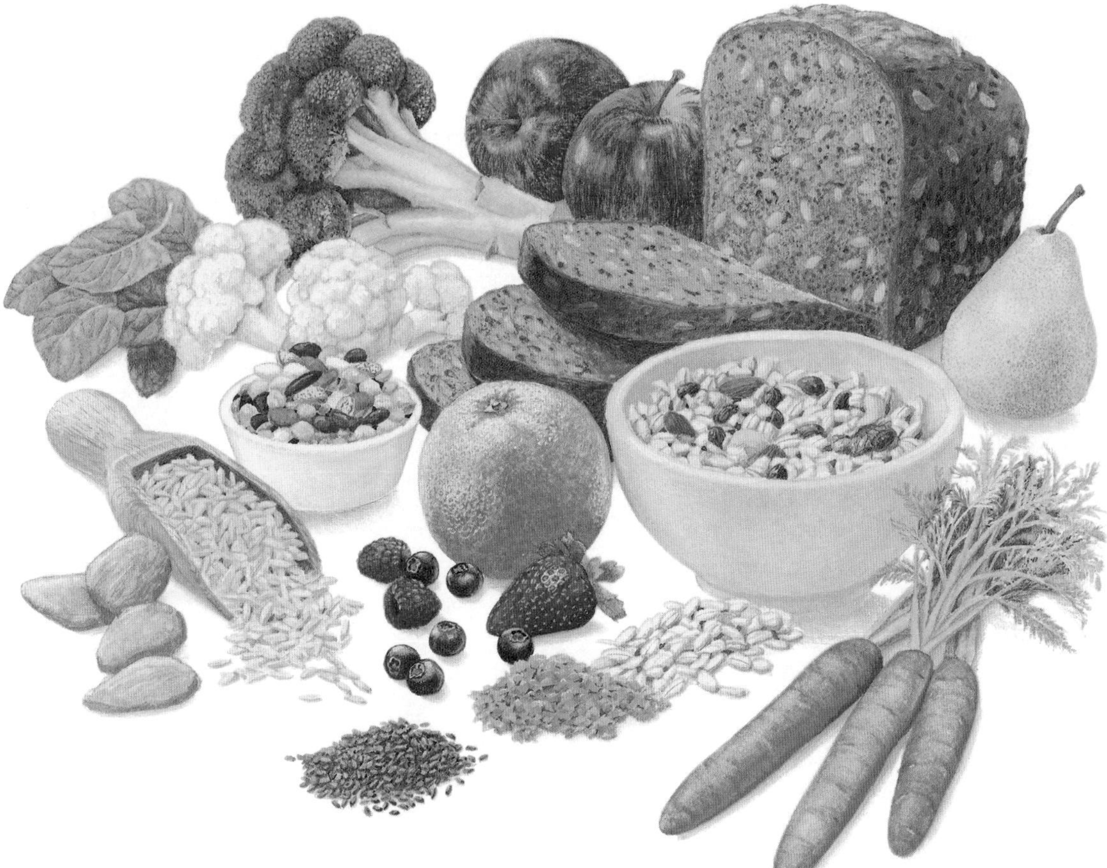

5-HTP (5-hydroxytryptophan)

use for ✓ ***Headaches***

THE COMPOUND KNOWN AS 5-HTP (5-hydroxytryptophan) is produced naturally in the body as an intermediate step in the conversion of the amino acid tryptophan to the neurotransmitter serotonin. Serotonin is sometimes referred to as one of the brain's "feel-good" chemicals, and is involved in regulating moods, appetite, pain and sleep (among other physiological functions). The 5-HTP used in supplements is usually derived from the seeds of a plant called *Griffonia simplicifolia*, which is native to Africa.

How it works

In order to produce serotonin, the body first needs to convert tryptophan into 5-HTP, a process that involves an enzyme called tryptophan hydrolase. If tryptophan hydrolase activity or the availability of tryptophan are inhibited (for example by stress, blood glucose problems or deficiencies of magnesium or vitamin B_6), the production of 5-HTP and subsequently serotonin may be compromised.

Taking 5-HTP as a supplement bypasses this issue, enabling serotonin production to occur regardless of tryptophan levels and tryptophan hydrolase activity, and ultimately resulting in increased levels of serotonin in the brain (as well as dopamine and melatonin). 5-HTP also has antioxidant properties.

Safety first *5-HTP has not been widely tested during pregnancy or breastfeeding so it is best avoided or used only under medical supervision during these periods.*

If you are taking prescribed medicines, do not take 5-HTP unless advised to do so by your doctor—numerous drug interactions are possible with this supplement.

Where to find *5-HTP is available in health food stores and from your doctor.*

How to use

Preliminary research suggests that 5-HTP may be beneficial for a wide range of health conditions influenced by serotonin levels, including headaches, mood problems, carbohydrate cravings, appetite problems, insomnia and fibromyalgia. However, more research will be required before 5-HTP's safety and efficacy are fully determined. The supplement should be used with caution and under the guidance of a health practitioner.

FLAVONOIDS

use for ✓ ***Allergies*** ✓ ***Bruises*** ✓ ***Hemorrhoids*** ✓ ***Skin rashes***

ABUNDANT IN ALL TYPES OF PLANTS, flavonoids (or bioflavonoids) comprise a large group of water-soluble compounds known for their antioxidant properties. Most are colorless but some are responsible for the yellow and red/blue hues seen in many fruits and vegetables. They are also found in chocolate and tea. Plants use these chemicals to attract pollinators, signal ripeness and to protect against attacks by microbes. For humans, the consumption of flavonoids, with their antioxidant, antimicrobial and anti-inflammatory characteristics, may help to boost the immune system and offer some protection against various ailments, including cancer and heart disease.

Of these more than 4,000 compounds, quercetin and the citrus flavonoids (including rutin, diosmin and hesperidin) are perhaps the best known.

How they work

Due to their low toxicity, humans can ingest significant quantities of flavonoids safely. In fact, nutritionists recommend at least seven daily servings of flavonoid-rich fruit and vegetables. The main health benefit of flavonoids is that they are antioxidants and neutralize free radicals—the unstable molecules that can cause cell damage. However, research is revealing other ways in which flavonoids help the body resist disease.

In test-tube experiments, quercetin was shown to prevent immune cells from releasing histamine, thereby offering relief from allergies, asthma, hay fever and hives. Experiments also suggest that it could reduce the risk of heart disease by lowering the levels of LDL (or "bad") cholesterol in the blood.

Citrus flavonoids are widely used to treat varicose veins, hemorrhoids, bruising, nosebleeds and cardiovascular diseases. Trials indicate that they work by strengthening the walls of blood vessels and reducing swelling.

How to use

A healthy, well-balanced diet should contain sufficient flavonoids from fruits and vegetables, although they are also available as supplements. They can be bought as tablets, capsules or lozenges; you can also buy a water-soluble form. Follow label instructions or take as professionally prescribed.

Safety first *Flavonoids are best consumed in fruits and vegetables. Supplements are generally considered safe for short-term use, but high doses may cause nausea, headaches or tingling of the extremities. If you take anticoagulant (blood-thinning) medications, check with your doctor before use.*

Flavonoid supplements have not been widely tested during pregnancy or breastfeeding and so are best avoided or used only under medical supervision during these periods.

Where to find *Supplements are available in health food stores.*

FLAXSEED *Linum usitatissimum.* Also called: Linseed

use for ✓ ***Constipation*** ✓ ***Menopausal symptoms***

THE FLAXSEED PLANT HAS BEEN DOMESTICATED since around 7000 BC but has been used by humans for much longer than that. Remnants of cords made from its fiber dating from the Palaeolithic era (approximately 30,000 years ago) indicate that prehistoric hunter-gatherers used the fiber to bind their stone tools together, weave baskets and make clothing. The medicinal and culinary use of the plant's seeds can be traced back to around 1000–500 BC, and continues today.

How it works

The seeds are a rich source of soluble fiber, and as such, can help manage constipation and blood glucose issues. They also contain estrogen-like compounds called lignans, which may have a number of health benefits for postmenopausal women.

In addition, flaxseed oil is the richest known plant source of omega-3 fatty acids, with a particularly high content of alpha-linolenic acid (ALA), from which the body can make the omega-3 fats eicosapentaenoic acid (EPA) and docosahexaenoic acid (DHA), albeit in smaller quantities than those obtained via the consumption of fish or fish oil supplements.

How to use

Eating whole seeds in bread or sprinkled over cereal is an easy way to increase your fiber intake, which may help manage constipation problems and improve the regularity and ease of bowel movements. However, whole seeds can pass through the digestive tract without being broken down, so you may not obtain the lignans and essential fatty acids they contain when you consume them in this way.

To gain the benefits of the lignans, which include helping to reduce cholesterol levels in post-menopausal women, grind whole seeds with a mortar and pestle before using them. Alternatively, choose flaxseed meal instead, sprinkling it over your cereal or adding it to smoothies.

Safety first *Choose flaxseed oil that has been cold-pressed and is stored in dark or opaque packaging. Store it in the refrigerator.*

Do not take high doses of flaxseed oil if you have prostate cancer or are considered at high risk of developing it.

Where to find *Whole seeds, as well as flaxseed meal, oil and capsules are available in health food stores and supermarkets.*

Flaxseed meal may also be beneficial for people with diabetes and other blood glucose problems, helping to lower blood glucose, glycated hemoglobin and cholesterol while also raising HDL cholesterol ("good" cholesterol).

Flaxseed oil is available in liquid and capsules for those seeking a concentrated vegetarian source of **omega-3 fatty acids** *(p. 250)*. Although it is often used as an alternative to fish oil supplements to support cardiovascular health and relieve inflammatory conditions, research suggests it is unlikely to be as effective due to inefficient conversion of ALA into EPA and DHA in the body.

FOLIC ACID

use for ✓ ***Anemia*** ✓ ***Celiac disease*** ✓ ***Dementia*** ✓ ***Natural fertility management***

FOLIC ACID IS A MEMBER OF THE B-COMPLEX group of vitamins, and along with related compounds, is commonly referred to as folate. Its name comes from the Latin word *folium*, which means leaf, and is a reference to the nutrient's widespread presence in green leafy vegetables. The body cannot store it for long so you need to replenish your supply daily.

How it works

Folic acid is essential for the production of DNA and the division of living cells, so is especially important at life stages in which rapid cell turnover occurs such as during fetal development. It is also required for the production of healthy blood cells, and anemia can occur if folic acid levels are low.

Along with vitamins B_6 and B_{12}, folic acid is required for the breakdown of a compound called homocysteine. Excessive levels of homocysteine in the body are associated with increased risk of some serious health problems including heart disease, stroke, peripheral vascular disease, age-related macular degeneration and dementia.

Safety first *If you are taking prescribed medicines, talk to your doctor before taking folic acid; it may interfere with your medication.*

The use of folic acid supplements can mask symptoms of vitamin B_{12} deficiency, so monitoring of your vitamin B_{12} levels may be required, especially if you are elderly or vegetarian. Ask your doctor.

Where to find *Folic acid supplements are available in health food stores and pharmacies. Foods such as bread and breakfast cereal are sometimes fortified with folic acid.*

How to use

The US Recommended Dietary Allowance (RDA) for adults (19+) is 400 mcg/day, increasing to 600 mcg for pregnant women and 500 mcg during breast-feeding. The upper limit is set at 1,000 mcg/day; however, higher doses may be prescribed by your doctor under some circumstances.

Folic acid is best obtained by eating a diet rich in green leafy vegetables such as spinach, broccoli and cabbage. However, folic acid supplements are recommended for pregnant women and those who may conceive. This ensures folic acid levels are adequate during the critical early stages of fetal development, and decreases your baby's risk of neural tube defects such as spina bifida.

Other people who may benefit from taking folic acid supplements include older people, those affected by diseases associated with compromised digestion (such as celiac disease and inflammatory bowel disease), and those who have taken certain prescribed medicines.

Your doctor may also advise you to take high-dose folic acid supplements (often with vitamins B_6 and B_{12}) in order to address or reduce your risk of problems such as anemia, dementia, age-related cognitive problems, depression, and heart and circulatory disease, especially if blood tests reveal that you have low levels of folic acid or high homocysteine levels.

GARCINIA *Garcinia gummi-gutta, G. cambogia.*

Also called: Malabar tamarind, Gambooge

use for ✓ ***Overweight and obesity***

IN KERALA, A COASTAL STATE IN southwest India, a small, pumpkin-shaped fruit called Malabar tamarind or gambooge lends a unique, sour flavor to traditional seafood curries. Gambooge also has a long history of use in Ayurveda, India's traditional healing system, to ease arthritis pain. Now, a compound found in the rind of this fruit is gaining attention as a weight-loss aid that might help control appetite and block fat production in the body. The effects sound sweet, but it is not yet clear whether this supplement lives up to the hype and research is ongoing.

How it works

The excitement–and controversy–over garcinia as a weight-loss aid focuses on the newly discovered compound in its rind, known as hydroxycitric acid (HCA). There is debate among experts as to how it works. Laboratory studies suggest that HCA may inhibit citrate lyase, an enzyme necessary for converting carbohydrates from the food we eat into fat. If it works the same way in humans, HCA might indeed be a "fat blocker" but so far, there's insufficient evidence to prove that this is happening.

However, HCA may help battle obesity in another way. In a 2002 animal study from Creighton University, in the US, HCA boosted levels of the feel-good brain chemical serotonin—leading HCA proponents to speculate that it is this mood-brightening lift that may act to discourage emotional eating in humans.

Meanwhile, there have been human studies that show promise. In one study, researchers tracked 60 extremely overweight people for eight weeks while they followed a low-calorie diet and received HCA or a placebo. The HCA group lost 5–6 percent of their body weight while the placebo group's benefits were "marginal or non-significant" according to the researchers. A 2012 review of garcinia's potential as an aid to weight loss concludes that the supplement has a modest effect in the short term, but more research and larger trials are needed.

Safety first *As a food, garcinia's fruit has been eaten safely for centuries. Less is known about the long-term safety of taking higher doses of HCA for longer periods of time. Garcinia has not been widely tested during pregnancy or breastfeeding so it is best avoided or used only under medical supervision during these periods.*

Talk with your doctor before using a garcinia or an HCA product if you take diabetes medications or a cholesterol-lowering statin drug. Avoid if you have Alzheimer's or dementia.

Where to find *Look for garcinia and HCA supplements in health food stores.*

How to use

Garcinia is sold as a supplement in tablet or capsule form. Some experts suggest looking for garcinia products that contain at least 50 percent HCA and that contain "HCA potassium salts," which may be the most effective. Follow label instructions or take as professionally prescribed.

GARLIC *Allium sativum*

use for ✓ ***Blood pressure, high*** ✓ ***Bronchitis*** ✓ ***Cancer support*** ✓ ***Cholesterol, high*** ✓ ***Colds and flu*** ✓ ***Fungal infections*** ✓ ***Heart and circulatory health*** ✓ ***Warts***

THE HEALTH BENEFITS OF GARLIC have been recorded for millennia. It has been used as a medicine in the world's oldest healing traditions, including Western herbalism, traditional Chinese medicine (TCM) and Ayurveda, India's medical system. The physician Charak, the "father of Ayurveda," wrote in 3000 BC that garlic "strengthens the heart and keeps the blood fluid," while the 16th-century British herbalist Nicholas Culpeper believed garlic to be a cure for many disorders, including coughs, colds and poor circulation.

How it works

Modern research continues to support garlic as being a potent natural medicine. Garlic contains a number of powerful antioxidants that may help prevent both cardiovascular disease and cancer, as well as the active compound allicin—responsible for garlic's sulfurous aroma—that helps to minimize the cellular oxidation and inflammation associated with these ailments. Garlic's specific heart-healthy benefits include reducing cholesterol, thinning the blood and reducing the development of plaque buildup on arterial walls. Both fresh garlic and garlic supplements have also been associated with lowering elevated blood pressure, a known major risk factor for heart disease and stroke. A review of clinical research, published in *BMC Cardiovascular Disorders*, suggested that garlic supplements have a significant effect, reducing systolic pressure and diastolic pressure by 8.4 mm Hg and 7.3 mm Hg, respectively.

Garlic has been shown to have antifungal, antibacterial and antiparasitic properties and so may help to boost the immune system. It also acts as a stimulant and expectorant, so may be of use in bronchitis or chest colds. It may be of assistance in supporting the body to fight fungal infections such as athlete's foot or candida.

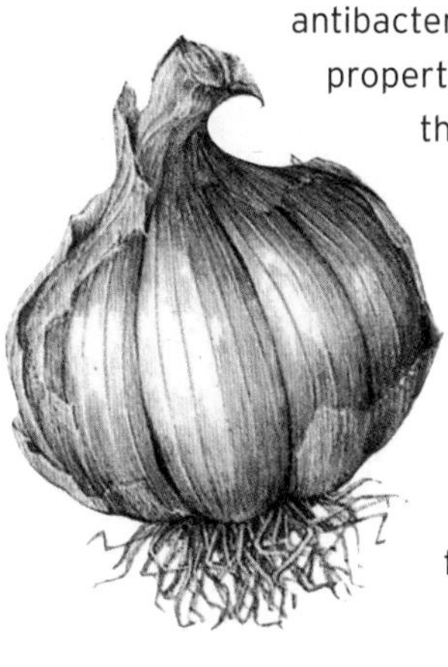

How to use

Garlic may be used liberally in cooking and also taken as a supplement in tablet, capsule or tincture form. When using supplements follow label instructions, or take as professionally prescribed.

Crushed garlic, applied as a poultice, is a time-honored treatment for an infection such as a boil or wart; a commercial preparation of garlic oil or gel may also be applied topically. Crushed garlic placed on a baby's feet between two pairs of socks (so that it is not in direct contact with the baby's skin) can help relieve a cold or stuffy nose.

When preparing fresh garlic it is important to let it sit for 10 minutes after slicing, chopping or mincing. This allows the enzyme allinase to form the sulfur-based compound allicin, which adds to garlic's medicinal properties as well as its pungent aroma and taste. If garlic is heated without letting it sit, the allinase is deactivated and no allicin will be formed.

Safety first *Check with your doctor before using garlic supplements if you are taking anticoagulant (blood-thinning) medications or medicine to reduce high blood pressure (antihypertensives).*

Where to find *Find fresh garlic in supermarkets. Garlic supplements are available in health food stores and supermarkets.*

GINGER *Zingiber officinale*

use for ✓ ***Bronchitis*** ✓ ***Cancer support*** ✓ ***Colds and flu***
✓ ***Heart and circulatory health*** ✓ ***Indigestion***
✓ ***Menstrual problems*** ✓ ***Nausea and vomiting***
✓ ***Osteoarthritis*** ✓ ***Rheumatoid arthritis***

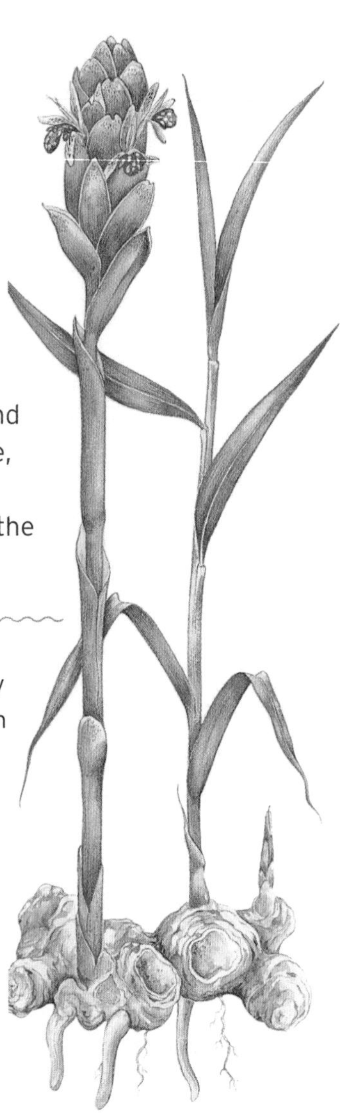

THIS TASTY SPICE HAS BEEN USED as both a condiment and a medicine for centuries. It was a staple at Roman banquets, to counter symptoms of overindulgence, and was much favored in ancient China and in India's Ayurvedic medicine as a remedy for indigestion, stomach-ache, respiratory congestion, constipation and diarrhea. It was also used as a tonic for women's gynecological conditions, being thought to stimulate the flow of *qi*, or energy, to the reproductive organs.

How it works

Ginger contains antioxidant substances called gingerols, which are thought to be responsible for its ability to alleviate nausea and indigestion. Unlike many conventional antinausea medications, ginger has the important benefit of not causing undesirable side effects such as a dry mouth or sleepiness. Research has shown that ginger can address nausea caused by a variety of causes, including food poisoning, motion sickness, pregnancy, postsurgical procedures, or the side effects of conventional drug treatment, notably chemotherapy. Similarly, ginger has been shown to alleviate symptoms of indigestion, including flatulence, bloating and griping pain.

The gingerols in ginger are also thought to account for its ability to alleviate some of the symptoms of rheumatoid arthritis, osteoarthritis and muscular discomfort such as pain, inflammation and swelling, possibly by inhibiting the production of inflammatory substances called prostaglandins and leukotrienes. This may also account for its ability to relieve menstrual cramping.

Ginger is often given as a tonic to fight colds and chills and improve circulation, with Taiwanese research confirming its benefits for circulatory health, as it does have mild blood-thinning properties. Ginger also has antimicrobial, carminative and diaphoretic (increases sweating) properties and may help to boost the immune system. These qualities make it of some benefit in treating coughs, colds, laryngitis or a sore throat where it is often combined with honey and lemon.

Safety first *Consult your doctor if using high doses of ginger while taking anticoagulant (blood-thinning) medications.*

Where to find *Ginger supplements and tinctures are available in health food stores. Fresh ginger is sold in supermarkets.*

How to use

Ginger can be eaten fresh or dried, or in pickled, jellied (candied), crystallized or syrup form, as a tea, or taken as a supplement, either as a tablet or capsule. When using supplements, follow label instructions or take as professionally prescribed.

GINKGO *Ginkgo biloba*. Also called: Maidenhair tree

use for ✓ ***Concentration, improved*** ✓ ***Memory problems*** ✓ ***Raynaud's disease*** ✓ ***Tinnitus*** ✓ ***Varicose veins***

FEW LIVING THINGS SURVIVED THE atomic attack on Hiroshima in 1945-among those that did were six *Ginkgo biloba* trees. Large and tenacious, the ginkgo is unique among trees, a "living fossil" that dates back to the days of the dinosaurs. Pyramidal in appearance with fan-shaped leaves, trees can grow to 115 feet (35 m) tall. Also known as the maidenhair tree, ginkgo is native to China where, as well as being eaten, ginkgo extract has various applications in traditional medicine.

Today, it is believed to enhance memory and concentration and is being investigated as a possible treatment for Alzheimer's disease. Ginkgo is also thought to aid circulation and improve oxygen use throughout the body.

How it works

Ginkgo leaf extract contains flavonoids—antioxidant compounds that may protect the body against free radicals—and terpenoids, which have an important function in all cellular membranes. The extract's most significant use, however, is as a memory and concentration enhancer, which it achieves by improving the oxygen supply to the brain and by stimulating nerve growth. For these reasons, it is also thought to help with depression, dizziness, tinnitus and headaches.

Ginkgo biloba has been shown to increase circulation to the fingertips and thus may offer relief to people with Raynaud's disease. The plant's alleged ability to improve circulation and strengthen blood vessels has also resulted in it being used to treat varicose veins and similar circulatory disorders.

Safety first *Ginkgo leaf extract is generally safe if the therapeutic dose is not exceeded. If it is, side effects including mild gastrointestinal disorders, restlessness, headaches, dizziness and allergic skin reactions have been reported.*

To avoid possible over-thinning of the blood, it is recommended that ginkgo be avoided a week before and up to two weeks after surgery.

Ginkgo should be avoided during pregnancy and lactation due to possible adverse effects.

Where to find *Ginkgo leaf extract is available in supermarkets and health food stores or from a qualified herbalist.*

How to use

The active ingredients of *Ginkgo biloba* are present in the leaves, and these are processed to extract the active phytochemicals for medicinal use. It is estimated that 50 fresh leaves yield one standard dose of the extract: 40 mg three times daily.

Ginkgo extracts are taken in tablet and capsule form or the dried leaves are steeped in freshly boiled water to make a "memory" tea. Follow label instructions or take as professionally prescribed.

GINSENG *Panax ginseng, P. quinquefolius, Eleutherococcus senticosus*

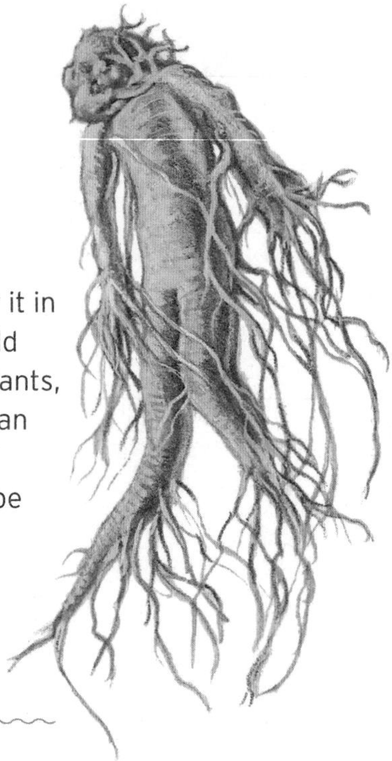

use for ✓ ***Colds and flu*** ✓ ***Concentration, improved*** ✓ ***Fatigue*** ✓ ***Natural fertility management***

FEW HERBS ARE AS HIGHLY PRIZED as ginseng. Wars were fought over it in China, where it has been used for 8,000 years. Today, a single root of wild *Panax ginseng* can command as much as $50,000. Of many ginseng variants, three are in common use. Asian/Korean ginseng *(P. ginseng)* and American ginseng *(P. quinquefolius)* are considered "true" ginseng, while Siberian/Russian ginseng is a more distant relative. The two Panax varieties may be white (the dried, unprocessed root) or red (the steamed, heat-dried root, thought to be pharmacologically more active). The uses of all three are primarily based on ginseng's reputation as an "adaptogen" that boosts immunity and enhances physical and mental performance.

How it works

Now widely cultivated, ginseng has been the subject of thousands of studies. The active constituents in the two Panax types are called ginsenosides, which act on the central nervous system. Research suggests that American and Asian ginseng boost the production of protective antibodies that help the body resist infections such as flu, the common cold and other respiratory illnesses; Asian ginseng may also offer some protection against cancer and speed recovery after treatment. Siberian ginseng, which can help combat flu and herpes viral infections, contains substances known as eleuthorosides that stimulate the immune system, encouraging the body to produce protective T-cells.

Various studies show that ginseng boosts memory and concentration, and combats fatigue. Two specific ginsenosides—Rb1 and Rg1—are thought to be responsible for improving cognitive function. Ginsenosides may also combat male impotence by reducing blood levels of the protein prolactin, which can cause erectile dysfunction. Asian ginseng appears to increase sperm levels and motility, as well as boosting sex drive; Korean red ginseng may also boost sexual arousal in women.

Safety first *Though considered generally safe,* Panax ginseng *may interact with diabetes medications, antidepressants and the blood thinner warfarin, and may enhance the effects of flu vaccines. Ginseng has not been widely tested during pregnancy or breastfeeding so it is best avoided or used only under medical supervision during these periods.*

Where to find *Varieties of ginseng are available in health food stores, some pharmacies or from a qualified herbalist.*

How to use

Many different types of ginseng are available in whole root, extract, powder, tablet and capsule form. You can also buy ginseng tea. Check to ensure you have the desired herb and follow label instructions or take as professionally prescribed.

GLOBE ARTICHOKE *Cynara scolymus*

use for ✓ ***Flatulence*** ✓ ***Indigestion*** ✓ ***Irritable bowel syndrome***

ONE OF THE WORLD'S OLDEST CULTIVATED plants, the artichoke is both a gourmet treat and a botanical remedy. With origins in Africa, this plant made its way to southern Europe, where the ancient Greeks and Romans regarded it as an important digestion soother. While artichoke's oversized flower buds are eaten as a vegetable, its leaves have long been used by European herbalists to jump-start the secretion of bile—a digestive fluid that helps the body break down fat from the food we eat. Herbalists still recommend artichoke leaf extract for a variety of gastrointestinal complaints.

How it works

Compounds in artichoke leaves called caffeoylquinic acids (such as cynarin) have been shown to stimulate the release of bile from the gall bladder. German researchers found that a single dose of an artichoke leaf extract more than doubled bile secretion in a small study of 20 people. Increased levels of this digestive fluid may explain why artichoke leaf extract eased indigestion in one study of 247 people.

Better digestion may also be the reason the extract reduced flatulence by 70 percent and abdominal pain by 78 percent in another German study of 203 people with gastrointestinal complaints. And in a 2004 UK study, people with irritable bowel syndrome who took artichoke leaf extract for two months said that their symptoms improved by 41 percent; many study volunteers reported that their bowel movements shifted from alternating constipation and diarrhea to a more normal pattern.

How to use

Artichoke leaf extract is taken orally as capsules or a fluid extract. Follow label instructions or take as professionally prescribed.

Safety first *Skip this herb if you have gallstones; it may trigger gall bladder contractions. Artichoke leaf extract has not been widely tested during pregnancy or breastfeeding and so it is best avoided or used only under medical supervision during these periods. Similarly it is best avoided by people with kidney or liver problems.*

Where to find *Artichoke leaf supplements are available in health food stores.*

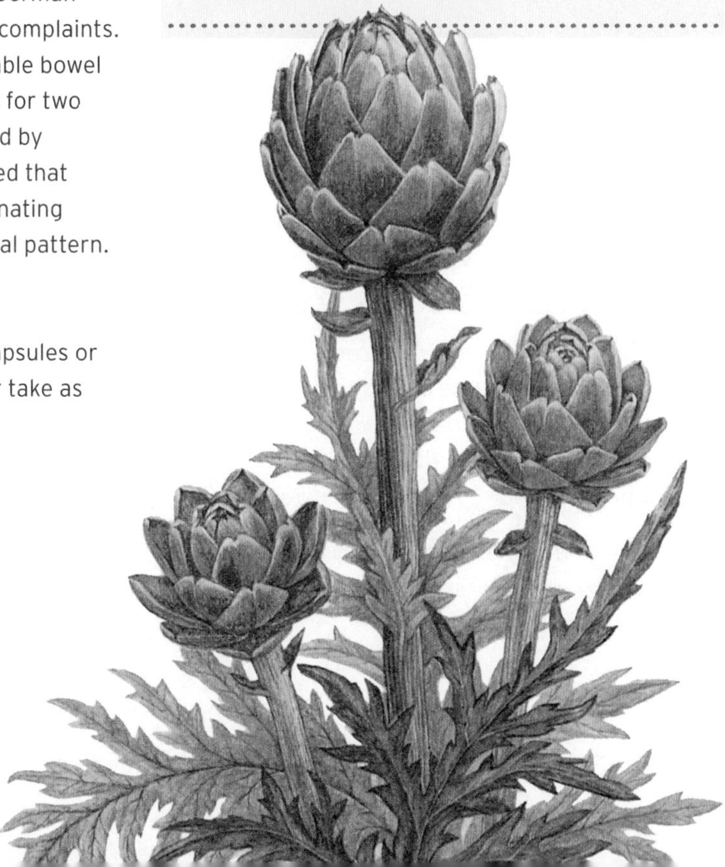

GLUCOSAMINE

use for ✓ ***Osteoarthritis*** ✓ ***Wound healing***

GLUCOSAMINE IS A SIMPLE MOLECULE that is used by the body to form connective tissue, tendons and ligaments. It helps to build cartilage—the cushioning at the tips of the bones—and protects and strengthens the joints. Although the body makes its own glucosamine, supplements can be helpful in some situations, especially since the natural sources of the substance are inedible. They include the shells of oysters, crabs and shrimp.

How it works

Glucosamine is found naturally in high concentrations in joint structures throughout the body. It has several complementary actions: it stimulates new joint cartilage; it helps to slow cartilage deterioration associated with ageing or injury; and it is involved in producing the synovial fluid that cushions joints. Glucosamine is available as a supplement, usually as glucosamine hydrochloride or glucosamine sulfate.

Glucosamine is often taken in conjunction with chondroitin sulfate, which is also thought to reduce joint pain and rebuild cartilage, and methylsulphonylmethane (MSM), an anti-inflammatory sulfur compound that has been shown to reduce joint pain significantly and improve mobility in patients with osteoarthritis (OA) of the knee. Formulations often contain all three substances.

Glucosamine, chondroitin and MSM help to combat both the causes and symptoms of osteoarthritis and rheumatoid arthritis; they may also be helpful for bursitis, osteoporosis and other degenerative bone diseases, as well as stimulating general wound healing. A large number of studies have been carried out on glucosamine, chondroitin and MSM; some have been inconclusive, but many have demonstrated worthwhile results. For example, a long-term study published in the *Lancet* of patients with knee OA who were given 1,500 mg/day of glucosamine sulfate, compared to a control group given a placebo, showed that the glucosamine resulted in a cessation of loss of cartilage. In addition there was no loss of space in the joint during that period, which in turn resulted in marked improvements in pain management, mobility and quality of life.

In a related study, published in *Osteoarthritis and Cartilage*, patients who had previously taken glucosamine supplements were less likely to go on to have knee replacements and were less reliant on anti-inflammatory medications. It is thought that glucosamine is most likely to be of benefit when some cartilage is still available, rather than when significant loss has already occurred. A review of glucosamine research suggests that the glucosamine sulfate is more effective than the hydrochloride form in treating osteoarthritis.

Safety first *Glucosamine may be sourced from the shells of crustaceans (shrimp, crab, lobster), so should not be taken by anyone with a seafood allergy. Check the label as some brands are synthesised from other materials.*

Where to find *Glucosamine supplements are available in pharmacies and health food stores or from a qualified naturopath.*

How to use

Glucosamine supplements come as tablets or capsules. A usual dose is 1,500 mg/day of glucosamine with 1,200 mg of chondroitin and 4,000–8,000 mg of MSM; however, dosages in over-the-counter products may vary depending on the potency of source material. Follow label instructions or take as professionally prescribed.

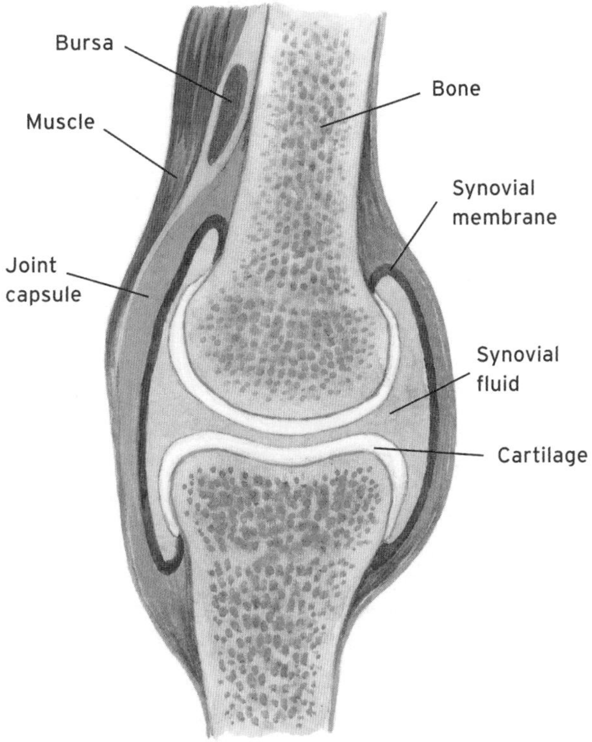

Normal joint

In a healthy joint, the ends of the bones are covered in a layer of cartilage that provides a smooth surface on which the two bones can move against each other. The synovial capsule that encloses the joint is filled with synovial fluid, which acts as a lubricant and provides nutrients for the structures within the joint.

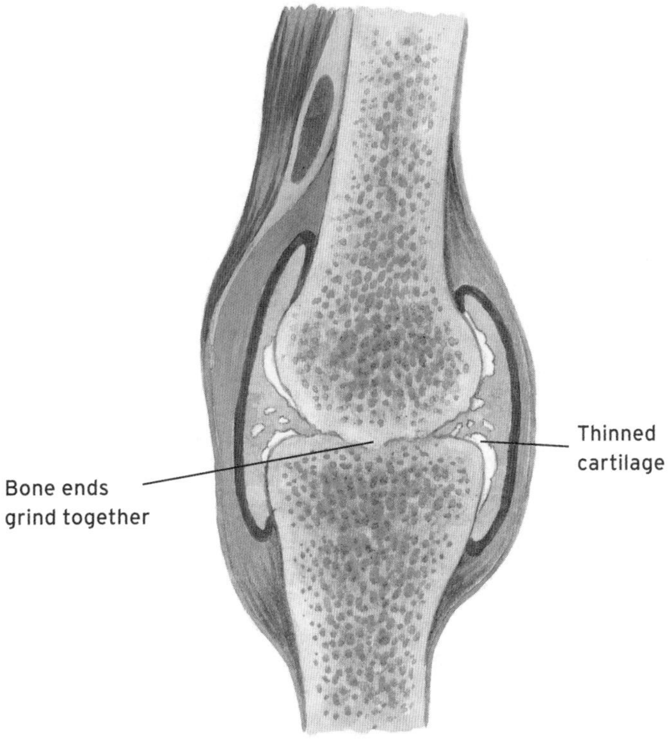

Arthritic joint

As a result of ageing or disease the cartilage at the ends of the bones can be worn down, leading to pain as the bones grind against each other. Glucosamine helps the body maintain healthy cartilage and is best taken as a preventive measure before significant loss has occurred.

GLUTEN-FREE DIET

use for ✓ ***Celiac disease*** ✓ ***Food intolerances*** ✓ ***Irritable bowel syndrome*** ✓ ***Psoriasis***

GLUTEN IS A TYPE OF PROTEIN IN GRAINS that gives dough its stretchy and elastic properties and holds baked goods together. It is found in products made from wheat (including specialist varieties of wheat, such as spelt and kamut), barley, rye and triticale. Gluten can also contaminate oat products during growing or processing, although gluten-free oats are available. Following a gluten-free diet can help relieve certain conditions.

How it works

For people with celiac disease, eating foods containing gluten damages the lining of the small intestine and interferes with digestion, compromising absorption and often causing symptoms such as diarrhea, bloating and abdominal cramps. Strictly following a gluten-free diet allows the intestine to heal and usually restores normal, healthy digestion.

As well as being essential for celiacs, gluten-free diets are often required by people who are allergic to or intolerant of wheat and other gluten-containing grains. Research suggests that people who experience frequent diarrhea due to irritable bowel syndrome may also find a gluten-free diet helpful.

In some circumstances, gluten-free diets may also be beneficial for people with psoriasis.

Safety first *Following a gluten-free diet means you need to take extra care to obtain all the nutrients your body requires. Ask your doctor whether you would benefit from vitamin, mineral or essential fatty acid supplements.*

Where to find *Gluten-free foods are available in health food stores and supermarkets and are increasingly available in cafés and restaurants.*

Following the diet

If you have celiac disease, you need to exclude gluten from your diet completely, as even tiny quantities can trigger digestive problems. On the other hand, people who have a nonceliac gluten or wheat intolerance can sometimes tolerate occasional small quantities of gluten-containing foods. Becoming gluten-free involves replacing many of your usual foods (such as bread, cookies, cakes, breakfast cereals and pasta) with versions made from grains that don't contain gluten such as gluten-free oats, rice, millet, quinoa and buckwheat.

You'll also need to become vigilant about reading the labels of packaged foods to find "hidden" sources of gluten. Gluten-containing ingredients are found in an extensive variety of food and drinks, from sausages to confectionery.

Luckily, you'll still be able to enjoy a balanced diet based on fresh fruit and vegetables, and containing meat, seafood, legumes, nuts and seeds, none of which contains gluten. Dairy products are also suitable for most people on gluten-free diets.

GOTU KOLA *Centella asiatica*

use for ✓ ***Burns*** ✓ ***Wound healing***

GOTU KOLA, ALSO KNOWN AS BRAHMI (not to be confused with *Bacopa monnieri*, which is also known as brahmi), is used in many herbal traditions. The original Tai Chi master, Li Ching-Yun, purportedly lived to be 256 by eating gotu kola leaves. And an old Sri Lankan saying is that by eating just two leaves of gotu kola a day you will keep old age away.

How it works

Western herbalists regard gotu kola as an excellent adaptogen. Adaptogens help the body deal with stress, whether it be physical—such as infection, injury or insufficient sleep—or psychological, including anxiety. One trial used gotu kola to treat 33 people with generalized anxiety for 60 days. At the end of the trial the majority of participants reported feeling less anxious and stressed. Its beneficial effect on the mind means that it can help improve memory, cognitive function and mood.

Many studies have shown that gotu kola improves the rate of healing by reducing inflammation and promoting the production of collagen. Collagen is the major protein in the body that forms skin, ligaments, blood vessels and bone. It is this collagen-enhancing attribute that makes gotu kola a favorite ingredient in top-quality cosmetics and face creams as it will improve the look and feel of the skin. Gotu kola has been found to be most beneficial in assisting the skin recover from burns and in the prevention and treatment of keloid scarring, a condition where there is an overgrowth of scar tissue.

Safety first *Gotu kola is considered an extremely safe herb.*

Where to find *Gotu kola is easy to grow, it can also be found in tablet or tincture form, and in creams and lotions, in health food stores or from a qualified herbalist.*

Gotu kola is no relation to the kola nut, a caffeine-containing ingredient of cola drinks. Gotu kola is caffeine-free.

How to use

Eat the small young leaves in salads, the older leaves can be stir-fried or stewed. Gotu kola is also available in tincture or tablet form. For skin conditions there are creams or lotions containing gotu kola. In all its forms, follow label instructions or take as professionally prescribed.

GRAPE SEED EXTRACT *Vitis vinifera*

use for ✓ ***Varicose veins***

BOTH THE ANCIENT EGYPTIANS AND GREEK philosophers praised the medicinal and nutritional value of grapes, often imbibed as wine, while European folk healers made an ointment from vine sap to treat skin and eye diseases. Modern grape seed extract is derived industrially from the seeds of red grapes. You can't gain the benefits simply by chewing on the pips, although the grapes themselves are nutritious.

Grape seed extract is a powerful antioxidant that may help to alleviate health problems associated with free radical damage. It also exerts a beneficial influence on blood vessels and is useful for conditions such as varicose veins. It may also be beneficial in the treatment of certain cardiovascular conditions and eye disease related to diabetes.

How it works

In a number of studies, antioxidants known as oligomeric proanthocyanidin complexes (OPCs) found in grape seed extract have been shown to reduce the symptoms associated with varicose veins and chronic venous insufficiency such as pain and swelling. Grape seed extract may also help to reduce swelling following surgery or caused by an injury—making it popular with some athletes—and it might lower cholesterol. Research conducted in test tubes suggests it could prevent the growth of certain types of cancer; however, this has yet to be tested successfully on humans. It has also been shown to reduce high blood pressure in animals.

How to use

Grape seed extract is derived from grapes and can be bought as capsules—often in combination with citrus **flavonoids** *(p. 187)*—as a powder for athletes to use during training or as a liquid and used as drops. No recommended dose has been established, though manufacturers suggest one 100 mg tablet a day or, in liquid form, 3 drops twice daily in water before a meal. Follow label instructions or take as professionally prescribed.

Safety first *Talk to your doctor before taking grape seed extract as it could affect the way certain medications are broken down in the liver. Common side effects include headache, sore throat, dizziness, itchy scalp, stomach-ache and nausea. It may also act as a blood thinner, so should not be used if you are taking anticoagulants or other blood-thinning medications. Nor should it be used by anyone with an allergy to grapes.*

Grape seed extract has not been widely tested during pregnancy or breastfeeding so is best avoided or used only under medical supervision during these periods.

Where to find *Buy tablets, drops or powder in health food stores or from a qualified herbalist.*

GREEN-LIPPED MUSSELS *Perna canalicula*

use for ✓ ***Asthma*** ✓ ***Osteoarthritis***

CHARACTERIZED BY THEIR DARK BROWN-GREEN shells with distinctive green edges, New Zealand green-lipped mussels are one of the largest mussel species, reaching up to about 10 inches (24 cm) in length. They attracted the interest of researchers who noticed that coastal Maori people whose diet included them in large numbers were fitter and had a lower incidence of arthritis than those who lived inland. A number of laboratory and human studies now suggest that green-lipped mussels may be helpful for controling symptoms of both asthma and osteoarthritis, though more research is necessary to confirm this.

How they work

Green-lipped mussel extract appears to have an anti-inflammatory effect, which may partly be due to its omega-3 fatty acids and antioxidants such as carotenoids. In population studies including the Japanese and Inuit, a high intake of fish oils (another type of omega-3 fat) has been associated with a lower risk of arthritis and other disorders associated with inflammation.

Conventional arthritis medications are usually aimed at blocking the action of an enzyme that causes pain and inflammation-known as Cox-2. Australian research has shown that green-lipped mussel extract blocks Cox-1 and Cox-2 enzymes and does so more effectively than fish oils.

Green-lipped mussel extract may also help reduce inflammation by influencing microorganisms in the gut. A 2013 study showed that green-lipped mussel extract inhibits inflammation-inducing clostridium bacteria in the gut, while encouraging more beneficial bacteria such as Lactobacillus species. These changes were associated with a decrease in osteoarthritis symptoms.

Safety first *Avoid green-lipped mussel products if you have a shellfish allergy.*

Where to find *Green-lipped mussel supplements are available in health food stores and pharmacies.*

Extracts of green-lipped mussels appear to treat asthma symptoms by blocking the activity of inflammatory molecules called leukotrienes. Overproduction of leukotrienes promotes inflammation and prompts the airways to tighten and secrete mucus during an asthma attack.

How to use

If you can obtain fresh green-lipped mussels, prepare and cook them as you would other mussels, taking care to discard any that are already open or any that remain closed when cooked. As a supplement, look for pure New Zealand green-lipped mussel oil or powder in capsule form. Follow label instructions or take as professionally prescribed.

GYMNEMA SYLVESTRE

use for ✓ ***Diabetes and insulin resistance***

ONE STRIKING FEATURE OF THIS TROPICAL climbing plant is its effect on the taste buds. Chewing its leaves temporarily blocks the sensation of sweetness, hence its Hindi name *gurmar*, meaning "destroyer of sugar." The leaves have been used principally to treat diabetes but Ayurveda, homeopathy and folk medicine prescribe gymnema for various conditions including asthma, inflammation and even snakebites.

How it works

Plant chemicals called gymnemic acids are responsible for the taste-bud phenomenon and the herb's apparent antidiabetic activity. Some researchers suggest that, because the acids and glucose molecules have a similar structure, gymnemic acids block receptors in the external layers of the intestine where glucose is absorbed, obstructing glucose uptake.

When people have diabetes, pancreatic beta cells that trigger the release of insulin may be destroyed or damaged making it difficult to maintain normal blood glucose levels. Studies have shown that gymnema leaf extract can regenerate or repair these cells, stimulate the pancreas to produce more insulin and consequently reduce blood glucose levels. The herb may also increase enzyme activity enabling the body to use glucose more efficiently. In two studies of patients with type 1 and type 2 diabetes, those who received the herb plus conventional treatment had better blood glucose control than those on conventional treatment alone.

Scientists have also been considering how *G. sylvestre* might help treat obesity. Obesity is strongly associated with type 2 diabetes—almost 80 percent of people with type 2 diabetes are obese—and fat cells have been shown to encourage production of the hormone resistin, which contributes to insulin resistance. Studies show that several *G. sylvestre* constituents may prevent the accumulation of fat in muscles and the liver, and help to reduce blood levels of fatty triglycerides.

Safety first *Consult your doctor before taking* G. sylvestre *as it could reduce blood glucose levels too far and cause hypoglycemia. The herb has not been widely tested during pregnancy or breastfeeding so it is best avoided or used only under medical supervision during these periods.*

Where to find G. sylvestre *supplements are available in health food stores and pharmacies.*

How to use

The water-soluble leaf extract is taken to support conventional treatment, rather than as a substitute, and is available in tablet, powder, liquid or capsule form. Follow label instructions or take as professionally prescribed.

HAWTHORN *Crataegus monogyna, C. oxyacantha.* Also called: May tree

use for ✓ ***Heart and circulatory health***

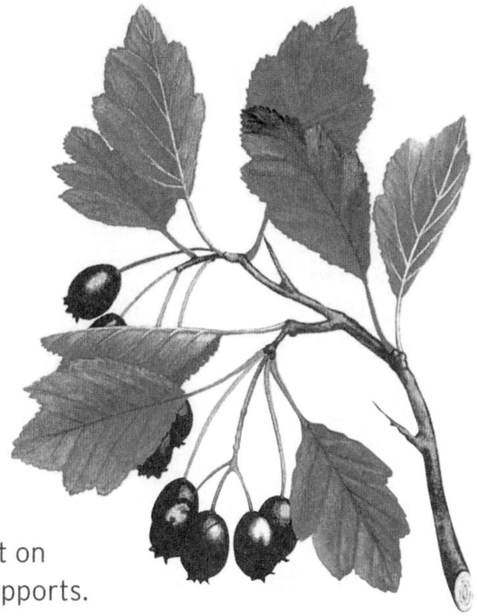

A PRICKLY HEDGE PLANT WITH bright red fruits, hawthorn is widespread in Europe. Traditionally, its flowers symbolized good luck and were used to decorate maypoles, hence its other name: May. However, hawthorn flowers brought indoors signaled death as their scent resembled that of the plague—"May in, coffin out," is one old adage. Yet, as early as the first century AD, the Greek herbalist Dioscorides recorded hawthorn's beneficial effect on certain heart conditions—findings that modern research supports.

How it works

The best evidence is for hawthorn leaf and flower extracts in combating both high blood pressure and heart disorders. Human studies have shown that hawthorn extract can improve heart function and boost blood circulation in people with congestive heart failure. Decreases in blood pressure, a drop in heart rate and significantly reduced arrhythmias (irregular heartbeats) have also been noted In heart patients suffering from borderline hypertension. A 2008 *Cochrane Review* of existing research indicated that hawthorn extract increased maximum heart rate and exercise tolerance, reduced oxygen consumption by the heart and reduced shortness of breath and fatigue.

Early evidence further suggests that hawthorn may combat angina (heart pain), and animal studies have demonstrated a cholesterol-lowering effect. With little or no clinical evidence to support it, hawthorn is also traditionally used to treat intestinal infections and minor sleep problems or applied topically to treat boils, sores, ulcers or even frostbite.

Safety first *Side effects are rare but may include mild nausea, dizziness and stomach complaints. Consult your doctor before using hawthorn if you are taking heart or blood pressure medication, as it can enhance the effects of such drugs. Hawthorn has not been widely tested during pregnancy or breastfeeding so it is best avoided or used only under medical supervision during these periods.*

Where to find *Hawthorn products are available in health food stores. Buy leaves, flowers and berries from a qualified herbalist.*

How to use

Hawthorn is available as extracts, capsules and tinctures. Follow label instructions or take as professionally prescribed. The leaves, flowers and berries may also be made into a tea. Put 1–2 teaspoons (5-10 ml) of dried flowerheads, or a teaspoon (5 ml) of the dried berries, in a cup of boiling water, infuse for 10 minutes, then strain before drinking.

HEAT THERAPY

use for ✓ ***Bursitis and tendonitis*** ✓ ***Cramps, muscle*** ✓ ***Frozen shoulder*** ✓ ***Menstrual problems*** ✓ ***Raynaud's disease*** ✓ ***Rheumatoid arthritis***

THE EGYPTIANS BELIEVED IN THE CURATIVE effects of heat as early as the fifth century BC, and used hot water, steam, sand and mud baths. The Greek physician Hippocrates prescribed heat for "spasticity," and pains in the extremities and torso, while the Chinese and Japanese were among the first to use natural hot springs to treat arthritic problems and many other disorders. Scientific research confirms the benefits of applied heat or "thermotherapy," which now comes in many forms from heating pads to ultrasound.

How it works

Studies show that heat therapy increases blood flow, raises the temperature of deep tissue and makes muscles more flexible. When blood flow is increased, more nutrients and oxygen can reach the injured area, helping it to heal. The application of heat also eases pain. In one study of 371 people suffering acute lower back pain, a heat wrap relieved pain and muscle stiffness, and improved flexibility significantly better than either ibuprofen or paracetamol. Functional brain-imaging research has shown that applied heat activates certain parts of the brain, which may mitigate the sensation of pain.

Safety first *People with diabetes, multiple sclerosis, poor circulation, spinal cord injuries or rheumatoid arthritis should take care as high-temperature therapies could exacerbate their condition, increase inflammation or cause burns and ulceration. Ultrasound therapy cannot be used on certain vulnerable parts of the body, or by people with joint replacements.*

Where to find *Seek a qualified physiotherapist for specialized heat treatments such as fluidotherapy, ultrasound or diathermy. Some heat treatments, such as paraffin wax baths, are provided by beauty clinics and health spas. Hot packs, wheat bags and heating pads are sold in pharmacies and health food stores.*

How to use

Take advice from a doctor or physiotherapist. Specialists divide heat treatments into three types: conduction, convection and conversion. Conducted heat therapies range from hot paraffin wax baths for arthritic disorders, to wheat bags, heating pads or wraps for acute muscular pain, to a simple hot-water bottle for menstrual pain.

Convection methods, such as moist or hot air baths, or fluidotherapy (a stream of dry heat), also work well for arthritic conditions, muscle spasms and muscle or joint injuries. Therapies using heat converted from another energy source, such as ultrasound or diathermy (high-frequency electromagnetic currents), can treat tendonitis, joint problems, muscle spasms and osteoarthritis; these are usually administered by a health professional and you should ask your doctor for a referral.

For certain injuries or conditions, such as bursitis and Raynaud's disease, alternating **cold therapy** *(p. 161)* and heat treatments may work best. When using home devices follow the instructions carefully so as to avoid burns.

HOLY BASIL *Ocimum tenuiflorum, O. sanctum.*

Also called: Tulsi, Tulasi, Sacred basil

use for ✓ ***Anxiety*** ✓ ***Bad breath*** ✓ ***Bronchitis*** ✓ ***Colds and flu*** ✓ ***Diabetes and insulin resistance*** ✓ ***Fatigue*** ✓ ***Fever*** ✓ ***Frequent illness*** ✓ ***Mouth ulcers*** ✓ ***Stroke prevention*** ✓ ***Tooth and gum disorders***

IN ADDITION TO ITS WIDESPREAD MEDICINAL and culinary use throughout Asia, southern Europe, northern Africa and the Middle East, holy basil is considered one of the most important plants within Ayurveda. It is one of the most sacred plants of Hinduism, where it is extensively used in purification ceremonies and religious rituals, and is regarded as the embodiment of the goddess Lakshmi (who represents prosperity and beauty). It is said that bowing in front of a holy basil plant is the same as bowing before the goddess herself.

How it works

Holy basil is an adaptogen—one of a class of herbal medicines that enhance the ability to cope with physical and mental stress. Among others, constituents of the plant that are believed to contribute to its medicinal properties include ocimumosides A and B, which have been shown to have beneficial effects on blood glucose, stress hormones and the adrenal glands.

As an adaptogen, holy basil has traditionally been used to address fatigue and stress-related issues, increase physical stamina and boost mental clarity. In patients with generalized anxiety disorder, taking holy basil may reduce anxiety, stress and depression.

Safety first *Holy basil is not advised for women who are pregnant or breastfeeding or men or women who are planning to conceive.*

Do not use holy basil if you are allergic to the Lamiaciae family of plants, which also includes other basils, mint, lavender and sage.

Where to find *Specialty markets such as Whole Foods may sell fresh holy basil and it can easily be grown in your garden. Holy basil tea, capsules and herbal liquids are available in health food stores or from a qualified herbalist.*

Research indicates that holy basil has antimicrobial activity and stimulates the activity of infection-fighting immune cells, making it useful against frequent illnesses such as colds, flu and bronchitis. Studies have also shown holy basil improves glucose control and other aspects of diabetes and metabolic syndrome, and that its antioxidant properties may protect the blood vessels of the brain, helping reduce the risk of stroke.

How to use

Fresh holy basil is a popular ingredient in many Thai stir-fries, but for medicinal purposes the herb is often taken as a tea. Steep a holy basil tea bag or one teaspoon (5 ml) of the dried leaves in boiling water for three to five minutes before drinking.

The same infusion can be left to cool and used as an iced tea that doubles as a mouthwash. It can help relieve mouth ulcers, bad breath and to reduce oral bacteria, including *Streptococcus mutans*, which is responsible for tooth decay.

Capsules and herbal liquids containing holy basil are also available. In all forms, follow label instructions or take as professionally prescribed.

HOPS *Humulus lupulus*

use for ✓ ***Anxiety*** ✓ ***Sleeping problems***

BEST KNOWN FOR THE BITTER FLAVOR they give to beer, hops have been used in food and therapeutically since ancient times. The aromatic, cone-like flowers feature in Ayurveda and traditional Chinese medicine as well as Western herbal medicine and have been prescribed for ailments including insomnia, nervous tension, indigestion and even leprosy. Hop compresses or poultices were also applied to bruises and boils, or to ease arthritic pain. Hops are still widely used to induce sleep and a sense of calm.

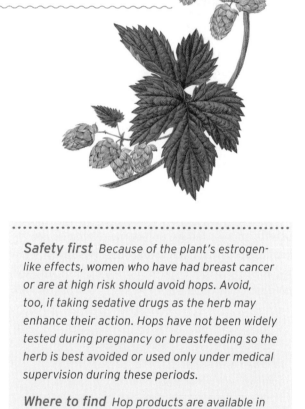

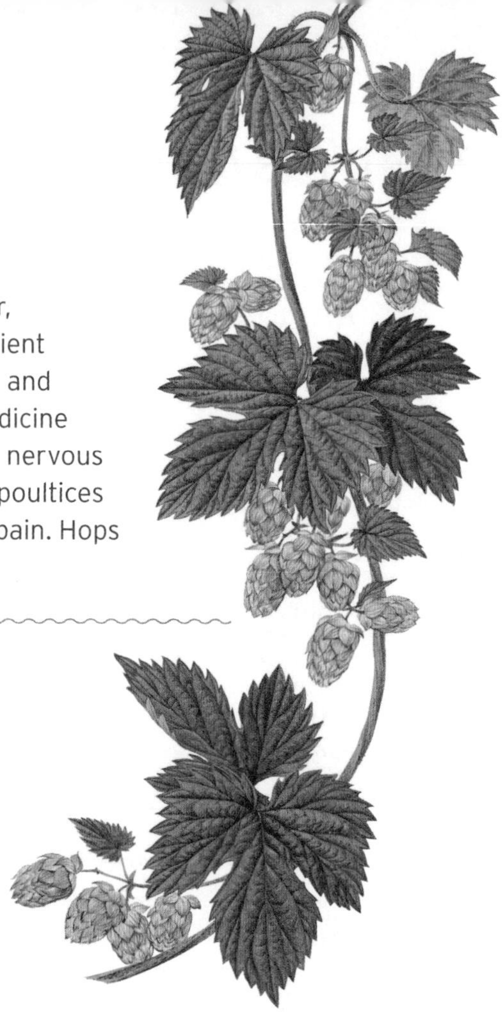

How they work

The herb is officially approved in Germany for treating anxiety and sleep disturbances with some scientific evidence of its efficacy. Hop plant constituents, such as its bitter acids, the flavonoid xanthohumol and the terpene myrcenol, appear to increase the activity of gamma-aminobutyric acid (GABA), a brain chemical that regulates anxiety.

In a recent Spanish study, nurses slept better after drinking about 12 ounces (350 ml) of nonalcoholic hop-flavored beer with supper each day for two weeks. In other human studies, hops combined with valerian have been shown to combat sleep disorders.

In Japanese research, a water extract of hops has been shown to reduce allergic reactions, while a special extract of hop bract polyphenols appears to combat dental plaque. Because the plant's constituents have a fairly strong estrogenic effect, certain hop formulations are said to help ease menopausal symptoms and enhance breast size, although there is no direct evidence for these effects.

How to use

Hop products are widely available as tablets, capsules and teas. Follow label instructions or take as professionally prescribed. You can also buy "sleep pillows" stuffed with dried hops.

Safety first *Because of the plant's estrogen-like effects, women who have had breast cancer or are at high risk should avoid hops. Avoid, too, if taking sedative drugs as the herb may enhance their action. Hops have not been widely tested during pregnancy or breastfeeding so the herb is best avoided or used only under medical supervision during these periods.*

Where to find *Hop products are available in health food stores and some pharmacies.*

HORSE CHESTNUT

Aesculus hippocastanum. Also called: Conker tree

use for ✓ ***Bruises*** ✓ ***Hemorrhoids*** ✓ ***Strains and sprains*** ✓ ***Varicose veins*** ✓ ***Wound healing***

THE HORSE CHESTNUT IS SO NAMED because it was once used to treat chest complaints in horses. The bark, leaves and seeds—better known as the conkers that children collect in autumn—have been used in traditional herbal medicine for coughs, fever, arthritis and rheumatism. Today, extracts from the seeds are a well-regarded and clinically validated treatment for varicose veins and other ailments pertaining to the circulatory system.

How it works

Horse chestnut has anti-inflammatory, antioxidant, astringent (tightening) and tonic properties. It contains a saponin known as aescin, which constricts blood vessels. Taken orally, or applied topically, horse chestnut helps to tighten tiny blood vessels and reduce cell wall permeability, preventing fluid leakage into surrounding tissue and helping to heal wounds.

Horse chestnut tones and strengthens vein walls, helping to prevent them from becoming slack or swollen and turning into varicose veins or hemorrhoids, as well as reducing the pain and swelling of existing varicose veins. In a study published in the *Lancet*, researchers found that taking horse chestnut extract might be as effective as using compression stockings.

Venous ulcers, spider veins and hemorrhoids may be improved with horse chestnut; it may also help to prevent nosebleeds. Horse chestnut may be of possible assistance in countering fluid retention in the legs and therefore help prevent deep vein thrombosis, as well as controlling the swelling associated with sprains and strains.

How to use

Horse chestnut is available as tablets, capsules and tinctures. Look for products containing standardized extracts of aescin. Follow label instructions or take as professionally prescribed. Horse chestnut may also be applied topically, via a lotion or a cream made by a herbalist.

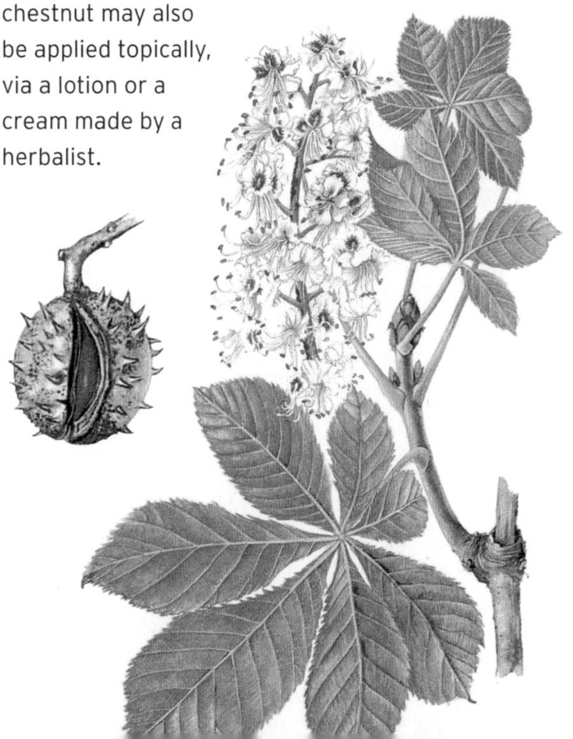

Safety first **The unprocessed seeds, bark, leaves and particularly flowers are poisonous.** *Don't take horse chestnut if you are taking anticoagulant or other blood-thinning medications, or if you have kidney or liver disorders, or are pregnant or breastfeeding. Side effects from taking horse chestnut are rare, but may include an itchy rash, upset stomach or nausea. Do not apply topically to broken skin.*

Where to find *Horse chestnut products can be found in health food stores and pharmacies, and from a qualified herbalist, who may supply it as a tincture combined with synergistic herbs.*

HORSERADISH *Armoracia rusticana*

use for ✓ ***Hay fever*** ✓ ***Sinusitis*** ✓ ***Urinary tract infections***

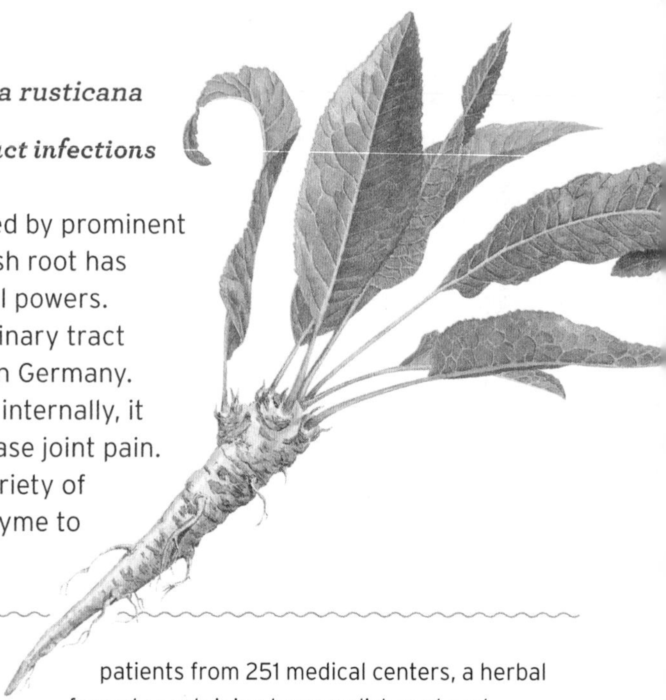

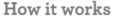

CULTIVATED SINCE ANCIENT TIMES and recorded by prominent herbalists including Nicholas Culpeper, horseradish root has long been popular for its fiery taste and medicinal powers. It is a traditional treatment for respiratory and urinary tract infections and officially approved for these uses in Germany. Applied topically in poultices or sometimes taken internally, it has also been used to reduce inflammation and ease joint pain. Scientists are currently studying the root for a variety of uses, including the potential of its peroxidase enzyme to help detect and target certain cancers.

How it works

Horseradish root's active chemicals include mustard oil and glucosinolates, bitter compounds also found in cruciferous vegetables that appear to have protective antimicrobial and antioxidant powers. Because the mustard-like constituents also help liquefy thickened mucus, horseradish can help relieve nasal congestion triggered by allergies, colds or sinusitis and may combat an underlying infection.

To date, however, there is relatively little human research to support these uses. In one German prospective cohort study involving hundreds of patients from 251 medical centers, a herbal formula containing horseradish root and nasturtium proved as effective as antibiotics for treating acute sinusitis, bronchitis and urinary tract infections. Another German study suggested that the same herbal combination could prevent new infections in people with recurrent bladder infections.

Safety first *While horseradish is relatively safe, it can burn the mouth or cause indigestion and, when applied to the skin, may cause irritation. Avoid contact with the eyes. Horseradish supplements have not been widely tested during pregnancy or breastfeeding so are best avoided or used only under medical supervision during these periods.*

Where to find *Fresh or dried horseradish root is sometimes available in supermarkets. Health food stores stock horseradish supplements.*

How to use

Fresh or dried horseradish root, often used as a condiment or in sauces, traditionally with beef, is safe for home remedies, too. To clear congestion, drink a little grated root about 1/2 teaspoon (2 ml) mixed with water or vegetable juice three times a day. If using externally to ease muscle or joint pain, wrap freshly grated root in a thin gauze and apply to the affected area. In supplement form, horseradish is often combined with other herbs such as garlic and with vitamin C. Follow label instructions or take as professionally prescribed.

HYDRATION

use for ✓ ***Colds and flu*** ✓ ***Diarrhea*** ✓ ***Fatigue*** ✓ ***Fever*** ✓ ***Gastroenteritis*** ✓ ***Gout*** ✓ ***Headaches*** ✓ ***Nausea and vomiting*** ✓ ***Snoring*** ✓ ***Urinary tract infections*** ✓ ***Vertigo*** ✓ ***Wound healing***

WATER IS THE MOST ABUNDANT MOLECULE in the body and ranges from over 75 percent of body mass in infants to around 60 percent in healthy adults. As we lose water from our bodies every day in sweat, urine, feces and water vapor—more in hot climates or during physical exertion—we must eat and drink enough to replenish that loss. Water plays a crucial role in numerous biological processes and during illness liquids help the body combat infection and promote healing, but water alone may not be enough. If a patient with a fever, streaming cold or diarrhea is losing excessive fluids, a rehydration drink that supplies additional nutrients may be necessary.

How it works

Our bodies use water to transport nutrients and waste products, regulate temperature, blood pressure and blood volume, lubricate joints and protect other organs. Good hydration keeps us functioning well, flushing out toxins, for instance, or preventing kidney stones.

While experts generally recommend 2 pints (1.2 L) of water a day, individual requirements are dictated by climate, activity levels and diet. A simple way to check whether you're drinking enough is to look at your urine. It should be a pale, straw color; if it's dark with a strong odor and you urinate infrequently, you may be dehydrated. Dehydration can also cause dizziness, headaches and fatigue.

Colds, fever and especially illnesses involving diarrhea or vomiting not only cause dehydration but also upset the body's delicate fluid-salt (electrolyte) balance by depleting levels of minerals such as calcium, sodium and potassium. So-called oral rehydration salts (ORS), which you can buy or make at home, will restore that balance.

Safety first *Water is rarely dangerous. Very occasionally athletes who drink too much water during an endurance event may overly dilute their body's sodium concentration, causing exercise-associated hyponatremia, a life-threatening condition.*

Where to find *Most pharmacies and health food stores stock rehydration drinks suitable for adults and children.*

How to use

A nutritious mineral-rich rehydration drink can be made by blending a fresh vegetable juice drink such as carrot or celery. Alternatively, try rice or barley water. Liquids should be sipped throughout the day. Follow label instructions on commercial rehydration drinks or take as professionally prescribed.

HYDROTHERAPY

use for ✓ ***Hemorrhoids*** ✓ ***Rheumatoid arthritis*** ✓ ***Varicose veins***

WATER THERAPY, OR HYDROTHERAPY, has long been used to treat disease and pain. There are many references to the healing uses of water, especially hot mineral springs and sea water, in ancient Hindu, Chinese and Native American teachings. Some springs, such as Lourdes, have been considered miraculous. At the basis of the hydrotherapy philosophy is the idea that water is the essence of life and a major part of the human body.

How it works

Modern hydrotherapy treatments stem from the 19th century and the work of Father Sebastian Kneipp, a Dominican monk. He founded one of the first health farms in Europe. The spa was located near a water source that was rich in sulfur, which helped with skin problems, arthritis and rheumatism. Kneipp's definitive "water contrast therapy," is still used today and involves alternating between hot and cold baths. Hot water draws blood to the surface, activating sweat glands and eliminating toxins. Cold water drives blood away from the surface and has an invigorating effect. Alternating hot and cold water baths can reduce inflammation and stimulate blood flow and lymphatic drainage.

Hydrotherapy can involve bathing in natural springs, which may have water with special qualities, doing exercises in a hydrotherapy pool, or simply taking a shower, bath or sitz bath (a small basin that you sit in with legs dangling outside so that the water covers only your lower abdomen, groin and upper thighs). Water for hydrotherapy can be supplemented by the addition of oils, salts, mud, volcanic rocks or seaweed (known as thalassotherapy from the Greek *thalassa*, meaning "sea") as well as pressure provided by jets or a therapist.

Naturopaths and physiotherapists have taken up many of Kneipp's ideas to treat all manner of ailments. For example, hot-and-cold water treatments may be used to improve circulation in the digestive area; sitz baths are useful for problems in the pelvic region or hemorrhoids; sprays of hot water and whirlpool spa baths may have a beneficial effect on back, joint or period pain.

A visit to the hydrotherapist

A naturopath or physiotherapist may refer you for specific hydrotherapy treatments, depending on the disorder. Treatments are readily available at natural hot springs and in health retreats and spas.

You can also practice hydrotherapy simply at home, for example with an Epsom salts bath, which induces perspiration and is useful for rheumatic conditions, colds and flu.

Safety first *Tell your practitioner if you are pregnant and mention any medical condition you have and other treatments or medicines you are taking.*

Where to find *Many health retreats offer hydrotherapy treatments. Physiotherapists may recommend treatments that are carried out in rehabilitation clinics or swimming pools.*

HYPNOTHERAPY

use for ✓ ***Cancer support*** ✓ ***Chronic pain*** ✓ ***Inflammatory bowel disease*** ✓ ***Neuralgia*** ✓ ***Phobias*** ✓ ***Warts***

FOR THOUSANDS OF YEARS, altered states of awareness—such as hypnogogic trance—have been employed for their psychological benefits. Using an individual's subconscious mind, a hypnotherapist will attempt to bring about change through the power of suggestion. Dealing with emotional issues, health problems, insomnia, phobias and weight loss are just some of the therapy's applications.

Forms of hypnosis were practiced by many ancient civilizations, including the Romans and the Druids of ancient Britain. As scholars gained a deeper understanding of human psychology the concept of hypnosis was refined from the 15th and 16th centuries onward.

It was the work of Austrian physician Dr. Franz Anton Mesmer in the 18th century that popularized hypnosis, though his methods were somewhat dubious. Indeed, the word "mesmerize" is derived from his name. Dr. James Braid, Dr. Emile Coue and Sigmund Freud did much to authenticate the practice and advanced our understanding of its applications.

William J. Bryan Jr. became the first full-time practitioner of hypnotherapy and created the American Institute of Hypnosis in 1955. Today, hypnotherapy is readily available and has been shown to offer a considerable range of health benefits.

How it works

The term "hypnosis" comes from the Greek word *hypnos*, which means "sleep"; however, people have described the hypnotized state as feeling more like daydreaming. A hypnotherapist will help a patient to enter a trancelike state by inducing deep relaxation. Then the therapist will direct beneficial suggestions (previously agreed with the patient) directly to the patient's subconscious mind. The patient remains in control while hypnotized and can bring themselves out of the hypnotic state at any time.

It is thought that hypnosis works by altering a patient's state of consciousness in such a way that the analytical left side of the brain is turned off and the nonanalytical right side becomes more alert. As the subconscious mind is deeper-rooted and more instinctive, this is the part that has to change for a person's behavior or physical state to alter. A person who is terrified of flying, for example, might consciously try everything they can to overcome this. However, the phobia will remain while the subconscious mind retains this terror.

Hypnotherapy is used to help with or alleviate a wide range of conditions. There is some evidence that it helps people suffering with cancer and other serious illnesses deal with the pain, stress and anxiety of their disease. The therapy can be used alone or alongside prescribed pain medication for pain management. Among the problems it has been used to manage are irritable bowel syndrome, sciatica, burns, joint pain, neck pain and other injuries and illnesses. Studies suggest that using hypnosis to treat chronic pain resulted in a significant reduction in perceived pain, which was often maintained for several months.

There is even evidence that hypnosis can be used to treat warts. One report cites a seven-year-old girl with 82 warts that disappeared after hypnotherapy, despite having failed to respond to other treatments for 18 months.

continued on page 212

HYPNOTHERAPY *continued*

A visit to the hypnotherapist

For hypnotherapy to be effective, a good rapport between client and therapist must be established. It is essential to feel at ease. Wear comfortable clothes and visit the bathroom before your appointment. And don't be afraid to ask questions before you start.

A hypnotherapist will begin by taking a detailed case history to establish your mindset, personality type, the problem you wish to address and the desired outcome. Next comes the hypnosis itself. The hypnotherapist's gently guiding voice will lead you into a state where body and mind are relaxed and almost asleep. At this stage, the therapist will introduce the things you wish to change or work on, as previously discussed and agreed on with you.

Finally, following the hypnosis, the therapist will encourage you to discuss your experiences during the session and any insights gained.

Safety first *Hypnotherapy should not be used on anyone suffering from psychosis or with a personality disorder, as it could make these conditions worse. If you do use a hypnotherapist, check that they are accredited and ensure they are trained specifically to work with your particular condition. Children should only be hypnotized by therapists trained to work with their age group.*

Where to find *It is important to find a therapist with extensive training and experience. No formal licensing exists in the US to govern hypnotherapists but your doctor should be able to refer you to a health professional experienced in hypnotherapy.*

How to use

In addition to attending sessions with a qualified hypnotherapist, self-hypnosis can be used to modify behavior, emotions and attitudes. Many people use self-hypnosis to help deal with everyday problems, to boost confidence and develop new skills. It can be used to relieve stress and anxiety, overcome problems such as overeating or smoking, or to boost the immune system. It is popular among athletes to improve performance. Self-hypnosis techniques include eye fixation and guided imagery.

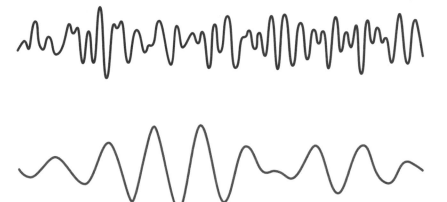

Beta waves

13–30 cycles/sec.

This is the normal, conscious state of mind. In highly alert states it can oscillate as much as 38 cycles/sec.

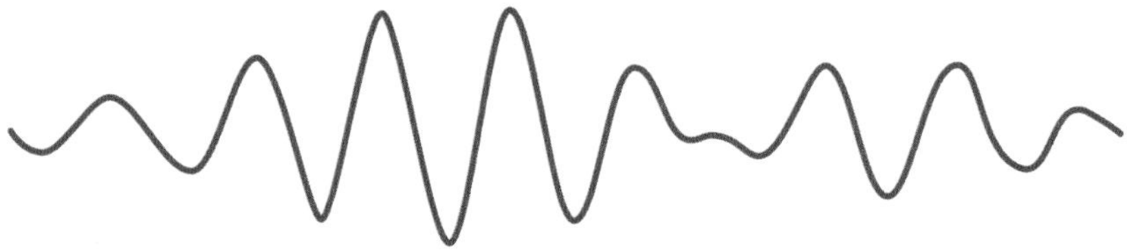

Alpha waves

8–12 cycles/sec.

Hypnosis slows the mind down to the alpha state, where it is relaxed, dreamy and open to suggestions.

IBEROGAST

use for ✓ ***Indigestion*** ✓ ***Irritable bowel syndrome***

IBEROGAST IS A PROPRIETARY HERBAL MEDICINE that has been on the market for more than 50 years, during which time it is estimated that more than 25 million people have taken it to relieve symptoms of indigestion, dyspepsia and irritable bowel syndrome. It is one of the most thoroughly researched complementary medicines in the world, having been the subject of numerous clinical trials involving more than 45,000 people.

How it works

Iberogast contains nine herbal medicines with a long history of traditional use for digestive complaints: **milk thistle** *(p. 238)*, **chamomile** *(p. 147)*, caraway, **lemon balm** *(p. 221)*, **peppermint** *(p. 255)*, **licorice** *(p. 222)*, greater celandine *(Chelidonium majus)*, angelica root *(Angelica archangelica)* and bitter candytuft (*Iberis amara*, from which the formulation takes its name).

Studies indicate that these herbs work together to relieve symptoms of gastrointestinal distress via a number of different mechanisms, including regulating the production of stomach acid, protecting the stomach lining, promoting normal gastrointestinal muscle tone and reducing intestinal spasms and gas production.

Safety first *Iberogast is considered very safe. However, if you are pregnant or breastfeeding, talk to your doctor before taking it, as its safety under these circumstances has not been determined.*

Where to find *Iberogast is available in health food stores, pharmacies and from natural health professionals.*

How to use

Iberogast can be used to relieve a wide range of gastrointestinal symptoms, including many of those that commonly characterize indigestion and irritable bowel syndrome such as heartburn, acid reflux, nausea and vomiting, flatulence, bloating, feelings of fullness, abdominal pain, constipation and diarrhea.

Iberogast comes in the form of a herbal liquid, which should be mixed with water and taken three times a day before or with meals at the dosage recommended on the label.

IRON

use for ✓ ***Anemia*** ✓ ***Celiac disease*** ✓ ***Fatigue*** ✓ ***Nail problems***

THE MINERAL IRON PLAYS A VITAL ROLE in transporting oxygen in the blood and other important biological processes. The body cannot make iron but, because it is essential for most living organisms, we can get it from many foods. Heme iron, the type most easily absorbed, is found in meat, fish and poultry, while nonheme iron is present in vegetables, pulses and whole grains. Despite this ready availability, iron deficiency is the most widespread nutritional disorder in both developing and industrialized countries. At least 2 billion people—30 percent of the global population—are anemic, according to the World Health Organization. Children and menstruating women, who have the highest iron requirements, are most susceptible. Iron deficiency anemia can also be caused by severe blood loss or medical conditions such as celiac disease. If your iron levels are found to be low, your doctor may prescribe a supplement.

How it works

About 70 percent of the body's iron is found in hemoglobin, which transports oxygen from the lungs to nourish the body's tissues, and in myoglobin, which stores, transports and releases oxygen in the muscles. Iron is also involved in producing ATP (adenosine triphosphate), an energy-bearing molecule found in all living cells.

An iron deficiency saps strength and stamina, affects hair and nails, and makes you vulnerable to infection. Because parts of the brain have a high iron content, attention, memory and learning may be impaired. Research shows that iron supplementation in iron-deficient people effectively restores normal levels, boosting energy, improving mental function and also sports performance.

Safety first *Ingesting high levels of supplemental iron could be dangerous, as excess iron is toxic and the body cannot excrete it. This is particularly important for people with thalassemia who commonly experience iron overload. Iron supplements may cause nausea, constipation and dark stools.*

Where to find *Pharmacies and some supermarkets stock iron tablets. Take only as prescribed by your doctor.*

How to use

To get plenty of iron, eat a healthy diet including good sources of heme iron such as liver, lean red meat and shellfish. Vitamin C, in fruit, juices and vegetables, helps the body absorb more iron, while calcium, tea, bran and unprocessed grains discourage absorption. The US Recommended Dietary Allowance (RDA) of iron for adult men (19+) and both sexes over 50 is 8 mg/day but 18 mg/day for menstruating women and 27 mg/day for pregnant women.

Do not take iron supplements without consulting your doctor. If a blood test confirms a deficiency, your doctor will be able to prescribe an appropriate supplement for your particular needs.

JOURNALING

use for ✓ ***Food intolerances*** ✓ ***Incontinence*** ✓ ***Migraines***

ALL SORTS OF PEOPLE HAVE KEPT JOURNALS, recording details about their lives. These documents provide valuable historical insight and, at times, entertainment. "I never travel without my diary," said 19th-century playwright Oscar Wilde. "One should always have something sensational to read in the train."

Today, psychologists believe there is more to this pastime than pure indulgence. A pen and paper—or computer keypad—may seem like unlikely allies against health problems but research suggests journaling could have a positive impact on well-being and help relieve stress, manage anxiety, solve problems and clarify thoughts. In its simplest form, a date diary can enable you to track the frequency and severity of symptoms, often revealing trends in behavior and triggers that can then be better controlled.

How it works

There is scientific evidence that shows that the act of writing can access the analytical left side of the brain. This removes mental blocks and gives the creative right side of the brain free rein to think and feel. This could help someone gain a better understanding of their personality and offer a clearer view of the world. University of Texas psychologist James W. Pennebaker, PhD, believes that writing regularly can bolster the immune system, help you recover from traumatic events more successfully and ease stress and depression. His research found that those who wrote about past traumatic events for 20 minutes a day, three to four times a week, visited the doctor 50 percent less than those who didn't keep a journal.

People with food allergies or intolerances can record their nutritional intake in a food journal to find out which foods trigger their symptoms. Experts also believe that keeping a food journal may increase weight loss. One study suggested that people who wrote a food journal six days a week lost twice as much weight as those who kept a journal for one day a week or less.

The same principle applies to migraine sufferers and people suffering from incontinence. In fact, the technique can be used for any chronic illness that is puzzling or difficult to resolve. By keeping a regular diary, patterns can be revealed and you can determine which remedies work best for you.

How to use

Food and headache journals need to be filled in daily to be beneficial. Experts recommend that you spend about 20 minutes a day writing a personal journal. Ideally, this should be done in privacy and at a speed that feels comfortable. The entries do not need to be chronological and any topic can be selected. There is no need to show anyone your journal, although allowing a friend or loved one to read certain entries might be easier than voicing it out loud. But there are no rules, other than the ones you choose to impose!

LASER TREATMENT

use for ✓ ***Jaw pain*** ✓ ***Varicose veins*** ✓ ***Warts*** ✓ ***Wound healing***

LASER IS AN ACRONYM FOR "Light Amplification by the Stimulated Emission of Radiation." The invention was first used in industry during the 1960s. Over the next 20 years the technology was refined for a variety of medical purposes.

Since the 1980s, there have been major advances in medical laser technology. Today, a doctor may refer you for laser treatment to alleviate a range of problems, from skin disorders and blood vessel abnormalities to eye surgery. Lasers also have dermatological and cosmetic applications, including depilation (hair removal), stretchmark reduction and tattoo removal. Types of laser treatment include low-level laser therapy (LLLT), laser acupuncture and high-power laser therapy (HPLT).

How it works

There are many types of laser, all capable of emitting concentrated beams of single wavelength light. Lasers enable precision treatments on a target tissue, with minimal impact on surrounding tissue. This is achieved by adjusting the frequency, wavelength, intensity, pulse duration and direction of the laser beams.

Low-level laser therapy

LLLT is increasingly being used in physical therapy, chiropractic and sports medicine, as well as in mainstream medicine. It does not induce heating in tissue like surgical or aesthetic lasers, rather, it works by using low-level lasers—or light-emitting diodes—to alter cellular function. Damaged cells respond better than healthy cells to photochemical reactions, and brief treatments with low-level light are thought to induce a complex chain of physiological reactions that enhance wound healing and tissue regeneration.

LLLT can be used to treat jaw pain, reducing the pain and inflammation, as well as increasing the range of motion to the neck and making it easier to open the jaw wide. High-power laser therapy (HPLT) may also be recommended to treat jaw pain.

Tests suggest LLLT provides short-term pain relief for sufferers of rheumatoid arthritis, osteoarthritis, neck pain and possibly chronic joint disorders. Studies have shown its beneficial use in tooth replantation.

Laser acupuncture

Are you scared of needles but would like to try acupuncture? This could be the answer. As the concentration of light is highest just under the skin, low-level laser beams are used to stimulate acupuncture points. This remedy has been used for soft tissue injuries, pain, wound and bone repair, lymphatic and circulatory disorders. It has also been used to treat addiction, stress and a variety of skin conditions. Laser acupuncture is often used to treat children as it is painless, treatment times tend to be short and it is more acceptable to children than needle acupuncture.

High-power laser therapy

HPLT works through the directed application of heat or "selective photothermolysis." Technicians adjust the frequency of light (photo) to produce heat (thermo) in the area targeted for destruction (lysis). Varicose veins can be treated using this type of laser surgery and a doctor might recommend HPLT, under local anesthetic, to burn off stubborn warts.

Having a laser treatment

Laser treatments are carried out at clinics and in some instances may be done under local anesthetic. Many of the treatments are noninvasive and offer an alternative to taking pharmaceutical drugs.

As a laser cannot penetrate clothing it must be applied directly to the skin; patients say they experience a warm sensation to the skin that is not painful. Most sessions last for just five to 10 minutes, although treatment for varicose veins may take one or two hours. You may need a series of treatments, depending on your condition.

Safety first *LLLT is extremely safe, although it is advised not to stare directly at the laser and to use safety glasses. There are some slight risks associated with laser surgery similar to other forms of surgery such as bleeding, infection and scarring.*

Tell the technician if you are pregnant and mention any medical condition you have and other treatments or medicines you are taking. Laser treatment should be postponed or avoided during pregnancy and while breastfeeding.

Where to find *In many countries, laws are in place to regulate the use of laser equipment. Use a clinic that you have been referred to by a doctor to ensure a high standard of treatment and that the operator is suitably qualified.*

Laser precision

Ordinary or "white" light is made up of all the colors of the rainbow and they all have different wavelengths. Laser machines emit light with a single wavelength and the waves are "coherent," which means that they are all in step with each other unlike the disorderly waves of white light. These features enable laser beams to be directed with high accuracy to a given point.

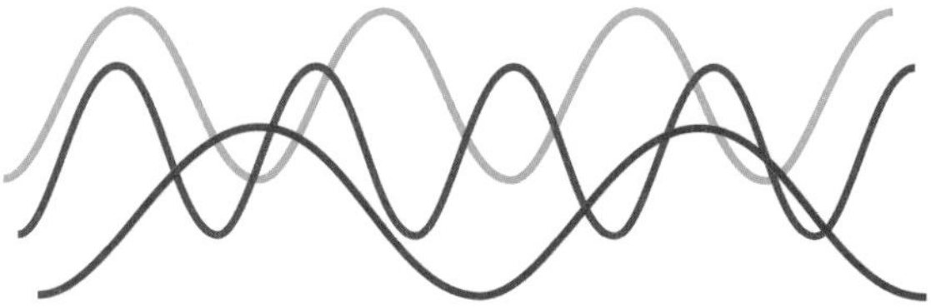

White light
Multiple wavelengths
Noncoherent

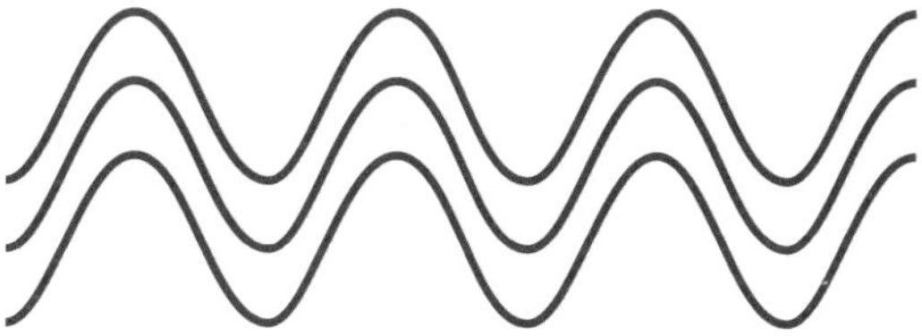

Laser light
Single wavelength
Coherent

LAUGHTER

use for ✓ ***Chronic pain*** ✓ ***Frequent illness***

"A GOOD LAUGH AND A LONG SLEEP are the two best cures for anything," says a traditional Irish proverb. Laughter a remedy? It's no joke! While it can't cure all ills, laughing has many positive benefits—mental and physical. As we all know, a good laugh brings people together, increasing happiness and intimacy. Laughter strengthens bonds, keeps relationships fresh and exciting, and unites people at difficult times. It could also boost your immune system, reduce pain and alleviate stress. Best of all, it's fun, free and the easiest "medicine" to take.

How it works

When we laugh, our body relaxes, relieving physical tension. Laughter also triggers the release of endorphins, the body's natural "feel-good" chemicals. Humor will help to dissolve distressing emotions benefiting our mental health–it is hard to feel anxious, sad or angry when you are laughing.

Laughter increases our intake of oxygen, which stimulates organs such as the heart, lungs and muscles, and improves circulation. Experts believe that laughing has longer-term benefits, too, such as improving our mood, increasing personal satisfaction, relieving pain and strengthening the immune system. When we have positive thoughts, our bodies release brain chemicals that help fight stress and offer relief from various health conditions. Laughing may stimulate the body into producing its own natural painkillers, benefiting those who suffer from chronic pain.

Safety first *While those with heart disease or a hernia should perhaps avoid getting over-excited, people rarely "die laughing."*

Where to find *Visit the American School of Laughter Yoga (www.laughteryogaamerica.com). Laughter Online University (www.laughteronlineuniversity.com/resources) will help you start a community laughter club.*

This was highlighted by Norman Cousins who is considered one of the founders of the field of psycho-neuroimmunology (which investigates the links between the emotions, brain and immune system). In the 1960s Cousins cured himself from painful arthritis by checking out of hospital and checking into a hotel with movies of the Marx Brothers and episodes of *Candid Camera*. In his book *Anatomy of an Illness*, he noted that 10 minutes of genuine belly laughter had an anesthetic effect and provided at least two hours of pain-free sleep.

How to use

There are many ways to share a joke or enjoy a laugh. Watch a funny film or a comedy show, try humorous activities, such as miniature golf or karaoke, or host a games night with friends. Look out for "laughter yoga" and Community Laughter Clubs.

Laughter yoga–described as a complete well-being workout–was devised by Indian physician Dr. Madan Kataria. It combines laughter with yogic breathing to bring about physiological and psychological benefits.

Community Laughter Clubs are based on research that shows it is 30 times easier to laugh in a group than alone. This network of volunteer-run social gatherings gives people the chance to get together to laugh as a form of exercise. Meetings help you to forget your worries, improve communication skills, make friends and much more.

LAVENDER *Lavandula angustifolia, L. officinalis*

use for ✓ ***Anxiety*** ✓ ***Bronchitis*** ✓ ***Cuts and scrapes*** ✓ ***Dementia*** ✓ ***Insect bites and stings***

LAVENDER, A NATIVE HERB OF THE MEDITERRANEAN REGION, is best known for its aromatic purple flowers. But it also has a long history of therapeutic use, being described by medieval herbalist John Parkinson as being of "especially good use for all griefes and paines of the head and brain." Victorian ladies carried hand-sized lavender-filled "swooning sachets" so they could recover from a corset-induced faint.

How it works

Lavender has analgesic (pain-relieving), digestive, sedative, antiseptic, antibacterial, carminative and antispasmodic properties. Its therapeutic benefits are thought to be due to two constituents, linalool and linalyl aldehyde, which counter inflammation, swelling and pain, while protecting against infection.

Lavender is a versatile remedy that can help many minor health ailments, including: insomnia, fatigue, nausea, indigestion, stress-related headaches and migraines. Lavender helps to calm the mind; it may be of benefit in calming the agitation often experienced by people with dementia. Taking a bath scented with lavender oil or misting bedding with lavender water are effective tips for improving sleep quality and duration. Lavender is particularly indicated for a nervous or irritable stomach or bowel as it can help soothe gastrointestinal upsets and reduce excess wind.

Lavender's skin-healing ability makes it a useful remedy for minor cuts, scrapes and burns, as well as itchiness, rashes, herpes, ulcers or shingles. Lavender is a useful gargle and inhalant remedy that can help relieve symptoms of bronchitis, coughs, colds and flu. It may also help relieve asthma, especially if triggered by stress.

Lavender essential oil can be used topically for menstrual cramps, toothache, earache and sore muscles, and as an inhalant for pain and anxiety management during labor and medical or dental procedures and postoperative pain. It may be of assistance for the topical treatment of fungal infections such as candida. It is an effective insect repellent and can be used in both prophylactic and treatment preparations for head lice.

Safety first **Lavender essential oil should not be taken internally.** *People with gallstones or biliary tract obstructions should avoid lavender, as it may stimulate bile secretion. Very occasionally, lavender may cause skin irritation. Do not use lavender if you are allergic to the Lamiaciae family of plants, which includes types of basil, mint and sage.*

Where to find Lavender tea may be purchased in health food stores; lavender essential oil is available in health food stores and pharmacies. Tinctures can be made up by a qualified herbalist.

How to use

Make lavender tea by steeping fresh or dried flowers in boiling water for five minutes. (If purchasing, make sure it is food grade lavender). For topical applications, lavender essential oil is gentle enough to be used neat, massaged into the temples, for example, or in aromatherapy baths, massage oils, ointments, compresses or inhalations. A qualified herbalist can make up a lavender tincture, often in conjunction with other synergistic herbs (such as valerian, for insomnia).

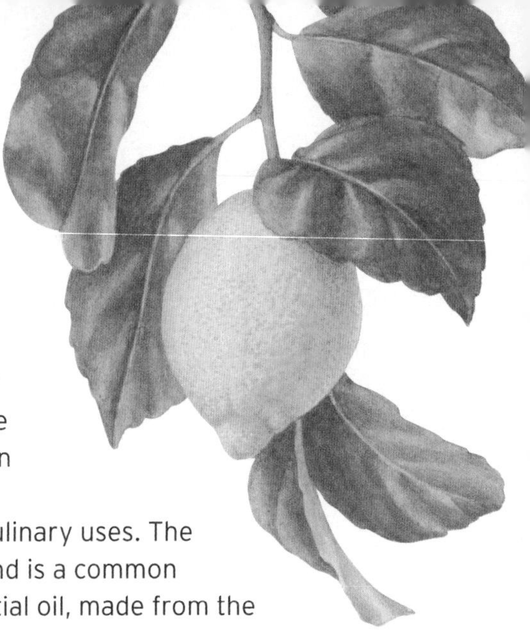

LEMON *Citrus x limon*

use for ✓ ***Bad breath and body odor*** ✓ ***Bronchitis***
✓ ***Colds and flu*** ✓ ***Scalp and hair problems***

DESPITE THEIR SOUR TASTE—a result of citric acid in the juice—the fruit of the small, evergreen lemon tree have many benefits. Thought originally to be a hybrid of the sour orange and citron, the first substantial cultivation of lemons began in Genoa, Italy, in the 15th century.

The juice and zest of this versatile fruit have numerous culinary uses. The juice can also be used as a cleaning agent and deodorizer, and is a common ingredient in cold remedies and hair products. Lemon essential oil, made from the peel, is popular in aromatherapy and as an insecticide.

How it works

Lemon juice contains antioxidants—including vitamin C—that boost the immune system and are believed to improve general health. This explains its traditional use in remedies for colds, coughs and flu.

Lemons have high levels of vitamin C, which the body needs to make collagen. (Lemons and limes were used to prevent scurvy, once the scourge of sailors.) Lemons also contain B vitamins and phosphorus, which may account for why the juice helps to prevent hair damage, promotes hair growth and can be used to treat dandruff.

Studies suggest that the antiseptic properties of lemon essential oil counter a wide range of infections. Added to a carrier oil, it can be massaged onto the skin or scalp to help unblock lymph glands and clear greasy skin and hair.

Safety first **Lemon essential oil should not be taken internally.** *Fresh lemons and lemon juice are nontoxic although lemon juice could exacerbate heartburn or gastroesophageal reflux (GERD). The high acid content in lemons could be bad for teeth if used too frequently, damaging the enamel.*

Always dilute the essential oil in a carrier oil to avoid skin irritation.

Where to find Lemons are available in supermarkets and grocery stores, while lemon essential oil and other products are available in health food stores and pharmacies.

How to use

A tablespoon (15 ml) of lemon juice mixed with a teaspoon (5 ml) of honey in 2 cups (500 ml) of hot water produces a gargle that, when cool, can relieve a sore throat and cold symptoms. Sucking a wedge of lemon or chewing the peel will freshen breath and a lemon mouth rinse is an ally against halitosis. The high acidic content in lemons prevents the growth of bacteria in the mouth.

For use on the hair and scalp, mix lemon juice with olive or coconut oil to promote hair growth, with apple cider vinegar to unblock hair follicles, or with garlic or almond paste to tackle head lice.

Lemon essential oil can be used in the bath for an invigorating dip, but as it can irritate the skin use no more than 2 drops of the oil per bath. It can be bought in lotions or creams to assist with the healing of cuts, boils and minor wounds.

LEMON BALM *Melissa officinalis.* Also called: Bee balm

use for ✓ ***Anxiety*** ✓ ***Dementia*** ✓ ***Herpes***

THIS PERENNIAL HERB FROM THE MINT FAMILY derived its official name from the Greek word for "bee," its tiny white flowers attracting multitudes of the honey-makers. The plant exudes a strong, lemony scent when the leaves are crushed and it produces a relatively expensive essential oil that is valued in aromatherapy for its uplifting and calming qualities.

Lemon balm tea has been used since the Middle Ages to reduce stress and anxiety, and improve sleep. Steeped in wine, it was used to lift spirits, heal wounds and treat insect bites.

How it works

Small laboratory trials suggest that lemon balm contains chemicals that may have antiviral, antioxidant and calmative properties. The leaves of the plant contain terpenes—which play some role in its perceived calming effect—and tannins, which may be responsible for its antiviral properties.

How to use

Lemon balm comes in many forms. It can be bought as a dried leaf, as a tea, in capsules, extracts, tinctures and oils, and as an ingredient in creams and lotions. The herb can also be easily grown.

Fresh cuttings of lemon balm, steeped in boiling water for a couple of hours and then chilled, can be drunk as a tea to help calm shredded nerves. Alternatively, to make lemon balm tea, add 2 cups (500 ml) of boiling water to about 1 oz (25 g) of dried lemon balm leaves and infuse for up to 10 minutes.

Lemon balm is often used along with other herbs, such as German chamomile, fennel and peppermint, to ease an upset stomach and digestive problems such as nausea, bloating, flatulence and infant colic. Tests suggest that taking an extract of lemon balm orally for four months could reduce agitation and improve the symptoms associated with mild to moderate Alzheimer's disease.

Lemon balm may also be helpful in treating herpes. In one study, when a lip salve containing 1 percent lemon balm was applied four times a day to cold sores, healing time was reduced and it might also have helped to prevent the infection from spreading. Another study found that applying a highly concentrated extract of lemon balm cream to oral and genital herpes hastened healing.

When the oil is used in aromatherapy, it is said to lift the mood and relax the body. Mixed with valerian in a tea or capsule, some studies suggest it is an ally against insomnia.

When using lemon balm extract, capsules or any other type of product, follow label instructions or take as professionally prescribed.

Safety first **Lemon balm essential oil should not be taken internally.** *Fresh or dried lemon balm is safe when consumed in food and has been safely used in research for up to four months. When taken as an extract or capsule, it can cause nausea, vomiting, abdominal pain, dizziness and wheezing.*

Lemon balm has not been widely tested during pregnancy or breastfeeding so it is best avoided or used only under medical supervision during these periods.

Where to find *Lemon balm products are available in health food stores, some supermarkets, or from a qualified herbalist.*

LICORICE *Glycyrrhiza glabra*

use for ✓ ***Mouth ulcers*** ✓ ***Skin rashes***

THE DISTINCTIVE SWEET TASTE OF licorice comes from glycyrrhizin, a substance which is 30–50 times sweeter than sucrose. As well as assuaging a sweet tooth, licorice has been valued for its medicinal properties since ancient times.

The licorice plant is native to Greece, Turkey and Asia and the black stuff is extracted from its thick, woody rhizomatous roots. The roots are boiled and most of the water is evaporated off before the extract is sold in solid or syrup form. A staple of traditional Chinese medicine, licorice is commonly added to other herbal remedies to enhance the flavor.

How it works

Numerous potentially healing substances have been identified in licorice, including flavonoids and plant estrogens as well as glycyrrhizin. Two compounds–licoricidin and licorisoflavan–have antibacterial properties that could kill some of the bacteria responsible for dental cavities and gum disease.

Scientists are interested in glycyrrhetinic acid, a derivative of glycyrrhizin, for healing peptic ulcers as it interferes with prostaglandins and encourages digestive mucus production. Applied topically, licorice root extract soothes the skin and makes it less likely to develop rashes and spots by eliminating the bacteria that cause them. Used as an expectorant, licorice can help to treat coughs by expelling mucus.

How to use

Licorice is available dried–for use as a tea–as well as chewable tablets, capsules and as an extract. To treat sensitive skin, mix 5 drops of licorice root extract with water and apply. Leave for 20 minutes and then wash off. In one study, a gel containing 2 percent licorice relieved symptoms of itching, swelling and redness.

Used in the form of a dissolving patch, licorice could reduce the discomfort of ulcers and other mouth sores.

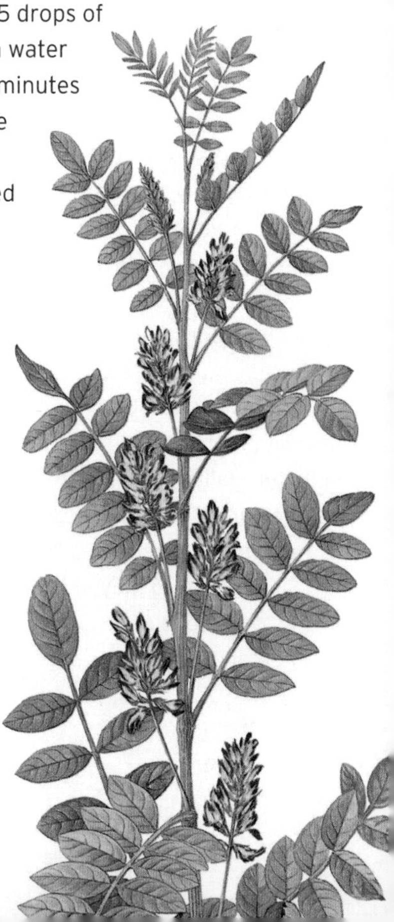

Safety first *Studies have shown that licorice can increase blood pressure or cause muscle weakness and chronic fatigue and it is recommended that people do not consume more than 100 mg of glycyrrhizin a day.*

If you are taking a prescription medicine, check with your doctor before using licorice and do not take licorice while pregnant or breastfeeding.

Where to find *Dried licorice and licorice products are available in health food stores or from a qualified herbalist.*

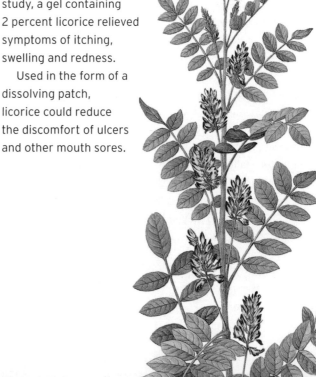

LIGHT THERAPY Also called: Phototherapy, Heliotherapy

use for ✓ ***Eczema and dermatitis*** ✓ ***Jet lag*** ✓ ***Psoriasis*** ✓ ***Seasonal affective disorder*** ✓ ***Sleeping problems***

LIGHT IS CRITICAL FOR OUR HEALTH and well-being. Two hundred years ago, 75 percent of the population worked outdoors; today, less than 10 percent work in natural light. As the brain needs 5000 lux of sunlight to operate correctly, the 400 lux available in an average office falls short and could contribute to light-related health problems. In addition, skin must be exposed to sunlight in order to produce vitamin D.

The right amount of light at the correct time of day ensures your body clock operates normally. Modern living has altered nature's cues, resulting in a dramatic increase in light-deficiency symptoms such as seasonal affective disorder and sleeping problems. Light therapy has been developed as a quick way to restore equilibrium to the body all year round. It is also used to treat certain skin conditions.

How it works

Light therapy can be a valuable tool to rectify a lack of light during the day and therefore restore the balance of melatonin, the hormone that makes us sleepy, and serotonin, a lack of which is associated with depression. A light therapy lightbox mimics daylight without the harmful ultraviolet (UV) rays and timed sessions can be used to treat seasonal affective disorder. It can also fool the body's internal clock into thinking it is a different time of day, which helps frequent travelers to combat jet lag.

Light therapy that includes UV rays is used to treat skin conditions such as eczema and psoriasis. In this case, your doctor will refer you to a dermatologist.

Safety first *This therapy has few side effects, although some people experience mild headaches, nausea, hyperactivity or itchy skin.*

If you want to use a lightbox at home, buy one that is certified as a medical device. Consult your doctor before using if you have an eye problem or are taking antidepressants or medication for epilepsy.

Light therapy has not been widely tested during pregnancy or breastfeeding so it is best avoided or used only under medical supervision during these periods.

Where to find *Your doctor will refer you to a dermatologist, or you can purchase lightboxes from reputable manufacturers online.*

Having a light-therapy treatment

When referred to a dermatologist for light therapy to treat a skin condition, you are likely to need two or three treatments a week. Most people have between 15 and 30 treatments. You might be asked to take a psoralen tablet two hours before your session or take a bath with it added. It might be applied as a cream or gel if the area being treated is small. This is to make your skin more sensitive to UV light. You will have to wear UV protective glasses for 24 hours after taking psoralen as your eyes will be extra sensitive, too.

For the therapy you will be asked to undress, leaving on your underpants. You will be given goggles to wear and might be asked to apply sunscreen to sensitive areas. A test dose of UV light might be given to assess the correct dosage for you. You will then stand in a cabinet containing fluorescent tubes. The first few sessions may only last for a minute, with the time increasing for subsequent sessions.

LOW-FODMAP DIET

use for ✓ ***Flatulence*** ✓ ***Irritable Bowel Syndrome***

DEVELOPED BY RESEARCHERS at Australia's Monash University, this eating strategy eliminates a group of potentially troublesome carbohydrates known as FODMAPs (fermentable oligosaccharides, disaccharides, monosaccharides and polyols). That list may sound exotic, but these compounds are found in everyday foods that contain lactose, fructose, fructans, galactans and sugar alcohols. Certain fruits, vegetables, dairy products and nuts as well as some breads and snack foods contain large amounts of these natural sugars and are considered high-FODMAP foods.

A growing body of research suggests that in some people FODMAPs may linger in the digestive system where they feed bad gut bacteria, leading to gastrointestinal problems including abdominal pain, gas, bloating, flatulence, burping, constipation and/or diarrhea. Saying "no thank you" to high-FODMAP foods can ease symptoms of irritable bowel syndrome (IBS), gas and other digestive complaints that have no apparent cause or cure, experts say. For this reason, low-FODMAP eating is gaining worldwide interest.

How it works

FODMAPs seem to cause behind-the-scenes trouble in two ways. First, they draw extra fluid into the digestive system, which can cause diarrhea. Second, undigested and unabsorbed FODMAPs (especially when eaten in large quantities) may stimulate fermentation by bacteria naturally present in the gut. This fermentation—the same process used to make beer and wine—releases gas that can cause bloating, pain and flatulence.

In one study from King's College London of 82 people with IBS, those who followed a low-FODMAP diet enjoyed significantly more symptom relief than those who followed a standard IBS diet. Eighty-seven percent had less flatulence (compared to 50 percent on the standard diet), 85 percent had less pain (compared to 61 percent on the standard diet) and 82 percent had less bloating (compared to 49 percent on the standard diet).

How to use

Following a low-FODMAP diet is a two-step process. First, you'll eliminate all major, high-FODMAP foods for a trial period of six to eight weeks. Such foods include onions, asparagus, mushrooms, apricots, apples, honey, legumes, rye- and wheat-based baked goods, and most dairy products. If your digestive symptoms improve, you will then reintroduce test foods from each FODMAP category one at a time to see which trigger symptoms. Test foods include milk (for lactose), honey (for fructose), wheat bread (for fructans), lentils (for galactans) and apricots or mushrooms (for sugar alcohols).

You may only react to one FODMAP so the goal is to find the food(s) that you should avoid or limit for the long term. If your symptoms do not ease during the trial period, FODMAPs are probably not the cause.

Safety first *It's wise to work with a dietitian familiar with low-FODMAP diets at first. He or she can help you design a healthy diet during the trial period and, if you find food culprits, suggest alternatives so that you don't miss out on important nutrients.*

Where to find *Read more about this diet strategy on the website of Monash University (www.med.monash.edu/cecs/gastro/fodmap).*

LUTEIN AND ZEAXANTHIN

use for ✓ ***Eye disorders***

AS EARLY AS 1792, SCIENTISTS WONDERED about the bright yellow spot visible during eye exams on the back wall of the human eye. What caused it? Why was it there? Today, opticians have solved the mystery of this yellow dot, called the macula, and know that this is the spot where light is focused when it enters the eye. The surprising hue comes from two antioxidants, lutein and zeaxanthin, that serve to protect the light-sensitive cells.

These sight-saving compounds can reduce the risk of vision-robbing cataracts and age-related macular degeneration and may even offer other health advantages. They are found in leafy green vegetables, egg yolks, corn and some other colorful foods, yet most of us don't get enough from the food we eat and may be missing out on the benefits.

How they work

Lutein and zeaxanthin are carotenoids, which are fat-soluble antioxidants that play a unique role in the body. While there are hundreds of different carotenoids, only lutein and zeaxanthin accumulate in the lens and retina of the human eye. These carotenoids shield the light-sensitive cells in the macula as well as the crystal-clear cells in the lens from damage caused by the sun's high-energy blue light. Research shows that higher intakes of lutein and zeaxanthin can lower the risk for cataracts and age-related macular degeneration and increasing your intake may slow the progression of these eye conditions. Getting plenty of lutein and zeaxanthin as well as vitamin E, another antioxidant, cut cataract risk by 16 percent in a Harvard School of Public Health study of over 23,000 women.

But that's not all. Research suggests lutein and zeaxanthin may also help reduce risk for heart disease and stroke by discouraging the formation of fatty plaque deposits in artery walls. And there's even early evidence that lutein may collect in the skin and help shield cells from the sun's wrinkle-promoting UV rays.

Safety first *These compounds are safe at levels found in carotenoid-rich diets; experts say that up to 25 mg/day has no harmful effects.*

Where to find *Look for lutein and zeaxanthin supplements in supermarkets, pharmacies and health food stores.*

How to use

The American Optometric Association recommends getting 10 mg of lutein and 2 mg of zeaxanthin daily from food or a supplement for optimal vision protection. Good sources include kale, spinach and other leafy greens, bell peppers, egg yolks and corn. Most of us take in just 2 mg of these compounds, combined. Adding a supplement is a safe and effective way to increase your daily intake; take with a meal or fatty foods for best absorption. When using supplements follow label instructions or take as professionally prescribed.

MACA *Lepidium meyenii.*

Also called: Peruvian ginseng

use for ✓ ***Sexual problems***

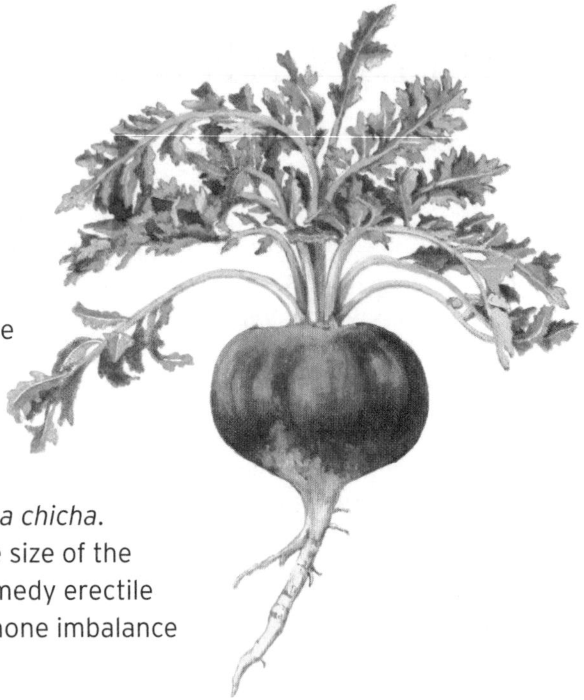

A RELATIVE OF THE RADISH, with an odor similar to butterscotch, maca has been cultivated for at least 3,000 years in the high Andes of Peru and Bolivia. The plant's fleshy root (more correctly, its hypocotyl) is used as a vegetable, for its medicinal properties and reputed aphrodisiac effects. The creamy yellow, red or purple roots are also used in jams and soups. Fermented roots make a weak beer called *maca chicha*.

Maca is claimed to increase energy and reduce the size of the prostate. It may also help people cope with stress, remedy erectile dysfunction, ease joint pain and improve female hormone imbalance and menstrual problems.

How it works

Maca works as an adaptogen, a biological substance that helps the body to adapt to changes and stress. It is also rich in essential fatty acids and amino acids as well as vitamins, minerals and other phytonutrients.

By supporting the endocrine system, adrenal glands and the thyroid, it may aid in the regulation of healthy hormone production. This could provide relief from menopausal and andropausal symptoms, and slow the ageing process by maintaining the correct levels of estrogen, progesterone, testosterone and human growth hormone.

Some studies have shown that maca has a positive effect on sexual dysfunction and sexual desire in healthy menopausal men and women. One study found it alleviated sexual dysfunction caused by the use of medications prescribed to treat depression.

Safety first *Maca has not been widely tested during pregnancy or breastfeeding so it is best avoided or used only under medical supervision during these periods.*

Where to find *Maca root comes in several colors (yellow, red and black). Maca products are available in health food stores.*

How to use

When eaten as a vegetable, maca can be baked, roasted or turned into soup. Maca is available as tablets and capsules or as a powder that can be added to water, juice or smoothies. Follow label instructions or take as professionally prescribed.

MAGNESIUM

use for ✓ ***Cramps, muscle*** ✓ ***Diabetes and insulin resistance*** ✓ ***Fall prevention*** ✓ ***Fatigue*** ✓ ***Osteoporosis***

THIS MINERAL, ESSENTIAL TO THE HUMAN BODY, appears naturally in many foods such as leafy green vegetables, nuts, brown rice, bread (especially whole-grain), fish, meat and dairy foods. An adult body contains about 1 ounce (25 g) of magnesium, of which just over half is found in the bones with most of the rest in soft tissues and 1 percent in the blood. The mineral is essential for bone, protein and fatty acid formation, making new cells, activating B vitamins, relaxing muscles, helping blood to clot and forming adenosine triphosphate (ATP)—the energy the body runs on. The secretion and action of insulin also require magnesium. People most at risk of a deficiency are those with gastrointestinal diseases (such as celiac disease), type 2 diabetes, alcohol dependency and the elderly.

How it works

Magnesium helps turn the food we eat into energy and ensures the parathyroid glands—which produce the hormones important for bone health—work normally. In addition, the mineral activates enzymes and helps to regulate the levels of calcium—as well as copper, zinc, potassium, vitamin D and other important nutrients—in the body. A deficiency in magnesium could cause cells to malfunction resulting in muscle cells contracting and causing cramps or an over response to the stimulation of adrenaline leading to fatigue.

Magnesium supplements can be useful in the treatment of a range of conditions, including high blood pressure, premenstrual syndrome, muscle fatigue, leg cramps and osteoporosis. Studies show that diets containing higher amounts of magnesium are associated with a significantly lower risk of diabetes, possibly because of the role magnesium plays in glucose metabolism. Research also suggests that increasing magnesium intake might increase bone density in postmenopausal and elderly women, and diets rich in the mineral enhance bone health.

Safety first *Taking a high dose of magnesium can cause diarrhea, nausea and abdominal cramping. Do not take magnesium if you have heart block (arrhythmia) or kidney problems.*

Magnesium is said to be safe for pregnant and breastfeeding women when taken orally in the amounts recommended, but only take under medical supervision during these periods.

Where to find *If a deficiency is diagnosed, supplements are available as magnesium oxide, citrate and chloride in tablet form in supermarkets and health food stores.*

How to use

The US Recommended Dietary Allowance (RDA) of magnesium for adult men (19+) is 400 mg/day, rising to 420 mg from 30 years of age. The RDI for adult women is 310 mg/day, rising to 320 mg after age 30. A well-balanced diet should provide all the magnesium you need. The upper limit from supplements is set at 350 mg/day. If taking supplements follow label instructions or take as professionally prescribed.

MANUKA HONEY

use for ✓ ***Bronchitis*** ✓ ***Burns*** ✓ ***Colds and flu*** ✓ ***Cuts and scrapes*** ✓ ***Wound healing***

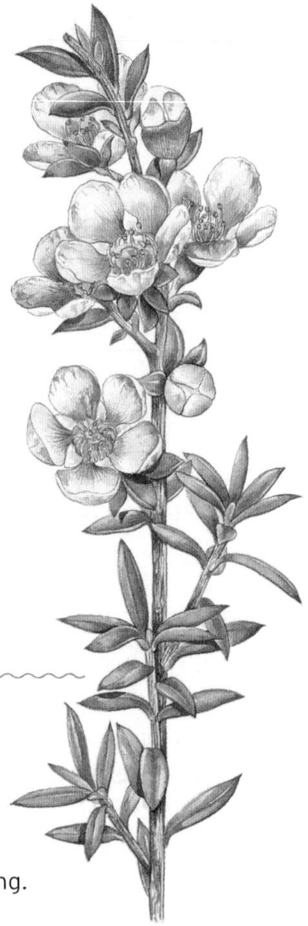

APITHERAPY, OR TREATMENT USING HONEY, has been employed by many different cultures for millennia. It is a popular folk remedy for treating wounds, soothing a sore throat and nourishing dry skin. Today, it is being integrated into modern wound care, and medical grade honey has been available since 1999.

All types of honey have antimicrobial and anti-inflammatory properties, but trials have shown that manuka honey, produced in New Zealand by bees that pollinate the native manuka bush *(Leptospermum scoparium)*, is especially potent. As such it has been formulated into "Medi-honey," which is impregnated into wound dressings and bandages for the treatment of wounds, burns and pressure ulcers. Manuka honey has also been used to treat diarrhea and stomach ulcers.

How it works

All pure honey contains the enzyme glucose oxidase, which releases antiseptic hydrogen peroxide slowly into the body, killing harmful bacteria without damaging soft tissues. In addition, manuka honey offers a nonperoxide activity as the result of methylglyoxal (MG), which greatly enhances the honey's antibacterial properties. Like all types of honey, it has a soothing effect on a throat that's sore due to a virus or from coughing.

Safety first As Clostridium botulinum–*the cause of infant botulism–can be present in any type of honey, only medical grade honey (which has been "pasteurized" to inactivate bacteria spores) should be fed to infants and babies under 18 months old. Avoid honey if you are allergic to pollen.*

Where to find *Manuka honey can be found in health food stores, delicatessens and some supermarkets, or ordered from specialty sites online. Manuka honey dressings can bought in some pharmacies and ordered online. Only buy from producers on the list of UMF licensees, available at www.umf.org.nz/licensees.*

How to use

When buying manuka honey, look for its unique manuka factor (UMF) rating as this corresponds with the concentration of MG. Ratings range from UMF10+ to UMF22+.

Manuka honey can be eaten off the spoon or added to breakfast cereal. To alleviate cold and flu symptoms make it into a hot drink. However, do not mix it with boiling water as this will kill the active enzymes. Add up to 2 teaspoons (10 ml) of manuka honey to a third of a glass of cooled boiled water; to increase its potency, add some lemon juice, too.

Medical grade manuka honey dressings can be applied to external wounds and sores and are particularly good for burns. Dressings are usually changed every 24–48 hours, though can be left in place for longer. If manuka honey is used directly it should be applied every 12–24 hours and covered with sterile gauze or a polyurethane dressing.

MARITIME PINE *Pinus pinaster.* Also called: Cluster pine

use for ✓ ***Asthma*** ✓ ***Tooth and gum disorders***

THIS FAST-GROWING PINE, native to the Mediterranean region, has become naturalized in Australia and South Africa. The impressive tree is widely planted for its timber and ornamental purposes, as well as for the medicinal value.

The supplement Pycnogenol is produced from the pine's bark. It is said to boost the immune system, strengthen blood vessels, act against muscle cramps and fatigue, and protect and rebuild the body's collagen—an important constituent of bone, cartilage, tendons and other connective tissues.

The bark extract has also been used to treat allergies, high blood pressure, osteoarthritis, diabetes, erectile dysfunction and more.

How it works

Pycnogenol contains multiple antioxidants, including high levels of procyanidin that may protect cells from the damage caused by free radicals. It may also have anti-inflammatory properties. Research suggests the extract significantly increases an enzyme in the skin that generates hyaluronic acid, which hydrates skin, helping to remove wrinkles. This makes it a popular antiageing supplement.

How to use

Studies suggest that chewing gum containing Pycnogenol minimizes gum disease and plaque formation on teeth. This is why you may see the extract added to various brands of toothpaste.

Pycnogenol may also assist asthma sufferers. In a recent study more than half the asthma patients who took two 50 mg tablets of Pycnogenol a day for a six-month period saw their condition improve and a study in 2004 showed that the supplement may be useful as an adjunct therapy in the management of childhood asthma.

The supplement can be bought as maritime pine bark extract or, more usually, as Pycnogenol. It is available as capsules, tablets, lotions and in toothpaste. Follow label instructions or take as professionally prescribed.

Safety first *Pycnogenol can sometimes cause dizziness, stomach problems, headaches and mouth ulcers. Follow label instructions or take as professionally prescribed. Do not take for longer than six months.*

Maritime pine has not been widely tested during pregnancy or breastfeeding so it is best avoided or used only under medical supervision during these periods.

Where to find *Find it in health food stores, some supermarkets or online.*

MASSAGE

use for ✓ ***Anxiety*** ✓ ***Cancer support*** ✓ ***Chronic pain*** ✓ ***Cramps, muscle*** ✓ ***Memory problems*** ✓ ***Strains and sprains***

THE WORD MASSAGE COMES FROM the Greek *massein*, which means "to press gently." The Greek gymnasia were famous for their use of massage for athletes, with the Greek physician Hippocrates writing in 400 BC: "The physician must be experienced in many things but assuredly, in rubbing—for rubbing can bind a joint which is too loose and loosen a joint that is too hard." This is as good a general description of massage and its therapeutic qualities as any, and it still holds true today.

How it works

Massage is recommended for relaxing muscles, reducing cramps, easing tension and stimulating blood flow. As well as musculoskeletal applications, the physical contact provided by massage therapy is of great psychological benefit, particularly to infants and the elderly.

Massage relieves anxiety, headaches and back pain; it can ease lower back pain in pregnancy and may also reduce treatment-associated swelling in cancer patients. By inducing a state of relaxation it can counteract stress and so ease stress-related issues such as memory problems.

Common massage techniques include kneading the limbs, pulling gently at the joints, pressing nerve areas or pressure points, stroking and percussing (a technique of tapping on the body with the hands, like mini karate chops). Different remedial massage therapies work in different ways: Some focus on relaxing tense muscles, others aim to stimulate circulation. Allied bodywork therapies, such as the **Feldenkrais Method** *(p. 180)* and the **Alexander Technique** *(p. 115)*, help correct postural imbalances through patterns of movement; **aromatherapy** *(p. 122)* and **acupuncture** *(p. 112)* may also be used in conjunction with massage.

Safety first *Tell the massage therapist if you are pregnant and mention any medical condition you have and other treatments or medicines you are taking.*

Where to find *Ask your doctor for a referral to a massage practitioner. Health spas and beauty clinics of also may offer massage therapy.*

Massage techniques

There are several styles of massage and you should choose one based on what you hope to achieve and your own personal preferences. For example, most people find lymphatic drainage to be relaxing overall, while a Chinese massage is stimulating, but too forceful for some. If you are new to massage, the only way to find out what you like is to try it.

Swedish massage

This system of soft tissue and muscle movement, which uses stroking and pulling manipulation to relax rigid muscle fibers, was developed by Per Henrik Ling in the 19th century. Ling was a physical health enthusiast who also invented vigorous dance exercises performed to music, the forerunner of today's aerobic workouts.

The aim of Swedish massage is to loosen muscular or tissue thickening around joints and so assist in the elimination of waste deposits, such as lactic acid, which build up where blood flow is slow. It is particularly recommended for poor circulation and osteoarthritic pain, and is widely utilized in physiotherapy, especially in assisting patients to regain movement of limbs following surgery, long periods of bed rest or a stroke.

Shiatsu

This Japanese technique of massage and physical manipulation involves the application of pressure, usually through the thumbs, but sometimes the fingers and elbows. Shiatsu is based on Hara massage, which in turn draws on an understanding of the *hara* or spine reflex system and other pressure points in the body.

Shiatsu massage therapists often focus on the face and skull, as this is where the majority of pressure points are found. Shiatsu may be useful for the relief of sinus pain, tension and some types of headaches. A traditional variation is barefoot shiatsu, where the therapist uses their naked feet to apply massage movements and pressure to the patient's body. It is a vigorous technique, and may be useful for people with chronic shoulder or back problems.

Chinese massage (Tui na)

A very deep form of massage, this is based on an understanding of the body's meridian pathways and acupuncture points, with different points being stimulated via strong finger pressure. Very firm rubbing and slapping may also involved, with the aim of restoring circulation and limb movement.

Deep tissue massage

As the name suggests, this is a penetrative form of therapeutic massage that is designed to restore movement to joints and improve blood and lymph circulation to all parts of the body, especially to muscles. Muscles can shrink due to inactivity, accident or poor nutrition. The misuse or nonuse of muscles can also have its origin in psychological issues or past traumas, so deep tissue massage can sometimes result in a strong emotional release as well as a physical response.

Lymphatic drainage

This method is often used in beauty clinics and health spas. It embodies the principle of "ironing out" unaesthetic lumps or fatty deposits on body areas, typically cellulite or fluid deposits. This is done using light, gentle, repetitive massage strokes, often in conjunction with aromatherapy.

A practitioner of lymphatic drainage aims to boost the lymph glands' ability to clear cellular debris, which in turn improves skin tone and condition. It may also be useful for treating lymphodema, the swelling that can develop after a mastectomy or the surgical removal of lymph nodes.

A visit to the massage therapist

The massage therapist will take a detailed case history and note past and present health conditions—for example, some acupressure points in Chinese massage cannot be used on pregnant women. You will then be asked to undress, usually to your briefs, and lie on a massage table covered by towels; or, in the case of shiatsu, possibly on a traditional rush mat on the floor. Whether a massage oil is used depends on the therapist's style and technique. For example, an aromatherapy massage will use a selection of light, scented oils. Other props may include heated volcanic stones and soothing music.

Occasionally, as the massage therapist works on particularly tense spots it may feel a little tender, but generally the experience is relaxing. It is important to communicate with your massage practitioner as to the amount of pressure you prefer and to warn them of any tender spots to either concentrate on or avoid.

MEADOWSWEET *Filipendula ulmaria, Spirea ulmaria.*

Also called: Queen of the meadow

use for ✓ ***Gastroenteritis***

POPULAR FOR CENTURIES IN EUROPE, this wildflower's almond-scented leaves were often strewn on the floors of bedrooms and banquet halls because, in the words of 17th-century British herbalist John Gerard, "the smell thereof makes the heart merrie and joyful and delighteth the senses." Meadowsweet was sacred to the Druids, widely used to flavor honey wine (mead) and beer, and also given to the sick as a remedy for diarrhea and inflammatory conditions.

But it reached new heights as a remedy in 1897 when German chemist Felix Hoffmann synthesized pain-relieving acetylsalicylic acid powder from a chemical called salicin found in its flowers. (Salicylic acid had previously been derived from willow bark, but that form was found to be too irritating to the stomach lining.) Hoffman's employer, Bayer, dubbed the pain-easing compound Aspirin—with the "A" for acetylsalicylic acid (the synthetic version of salicin), "spir" for *Spirea ulmaria* (another botanical name for meadowsweet), and "in" added as a common word ending for medicines of the time. While aspirin is no longer made from meadowsweet, it remains one of the world's most popular pain relievers. Meanwhile, meadowsweet is still recommended by herbalists as a traditional remedy for mild pain, coughs, low-grade fevers and mild diarrhea.

How it works

While few scientific studies of meadowsweet have ever been conducted, in 2013 Irish researchers confirmed that polyphenols extracted from this herb do have inflammation-soothing properties, at least in a test tube. Herbalists suspect that meadowsweet's gentle action against headaches, joint pain and fever are probably due to the natural, aspirin-like salicin it contains. Meadowsweet also has drying, astringent properties that may explain its traditional use for mild cases of stomach flu (gastroenteritis).

How to use

To make meadowsweet tea, steep 1 teaspoon (5 ml) of the dried herb in a cup of just-boiled water for 10 minutes. You may need three to four cups a day to ease pain. Meadowsweet is also available as a capsule and a tincture. Follow label instructions or take as professionally prescribed.

Safety first *Avoid in pregnancy; meadowsweet may trigger uterine contractions. Meadowsweet has not been widely tested during breastfeeding so it is best avoided or used only under medical supervision during this period. Do not use meadowsweet if you are allergic to aspirin or if you are taking aspirin, narcotic pain drugs or salicylates. Use with caution if you have asthma; like aspirin, meadowsweet may exacerbate asthma.*

Where to find *Meadowsweet products and teas are available in health food stores or from a qualified herbalist.*

MEDICINAL MUSHROOMS

use for ✓ ***Cancer support*** ✓ ***Frequent illness*** ✓ ***Warts***

CORNERSTONES OF TRADITIONAL CHINESE and Japanese medicine for thousands of years, four humble-looking fungi have recently claimed the attention of natural healers and scientists alike in the West, for they have the potential to be immune stimulants and even helpers in the fight against cancer. Their names sound exotic, yet hint at the esteem in which they're held in Asia: Maitake *(Grifola frondosa)* means "dancing mushroom" in Japanese because mushroom hunters were said to dance for joy when they found it in times past. The Chinese name for reishi mushroom *(Ganoderma lucidum)* is *lingzhi*, which means "herb of spiritual potency." But are these—along with shiitake *(Lentinus edodes)* and turkey tail *(Trametes versicolor)*—worth taking to bolster your defenses or even battle a tumor? Here's what science says.

How they work

All four of these popular mushrooms contain large, sugar-based molecules called polysaccharides that have demonstrated positive effects on components of the immune system and the ability to stand up to cancer cells—in test tube studies, at least. More recently, preliminary research in people suggests that extracts from some of these fungi may also strengthen and balance immune response and may work alongside conventional chemotherapy drugs, in experimental protocols, to better attack a wide variety of cancers—exciting news in the ongoing quest to find more effective cancer treatments.

In one 2012 review of five well-designed human studies, researchers concluded that adding a reishi extract to chemotherapy or radiation therapy improved effectiveness by 27 percent. Studies of a Japanese maitake extract suggest it also helps, though cancer experts say better research is needed. A turkey tail extract called PSK, along with other treatments, seems to have helped people with cancers of the esophagus, stomach, colon or breast to survive longer. And a polysaccharide from the shiitake mushroom, called lentinan, also seemed to improve quality of life and survival in people undergoing treatment for cancers of the colon, stomach and pancreas.

Safety first *Medicinal mushrooms have not been widely tested during pregnancy or breastfeeding and so are best avoided or used only under medical supervision during these periods. Avoid if you take medications to suppress your immunity. Skip maitake if you take blood glucose–lowering medicines; avoid shiitake if you have a condition called eosinophilia (it could worsen); skip reishi if you have a clotting disorder or low blood pressure.*

Where to find *You may find some of these mushrooms in a supermarket or health food store. You can buy supplements from a qualified traditional Chinese medicine practitioner.*

How to use

In all cases, cancer experts note that medicinal mushrooms cannot replace conventional cancer therapy and should be used by cancer patients under a doctor's supervision. If you would simply like to see if these mushrooms can bolster your immunity to help you fight off frequent illnesses or battle the virus that causes warts, you can try them as a tea, capsule or extract. Follow label instructions or take as professionally prescribed.

MEDITATION

use for ✓ ***Anxiety*** ✓ ***Blood pressure, high*** ✓ ***Cancer support*** ✓ ***Concentration, improved*** ✓ ***Depression*** ✓ ***Heart and circulatory health*** ✓ ***Memory problems*** ✓ ***Phobias***

MEDITATION IS A TERM THAT REFERS to a wide variety of mental techniques that help you relax, focus and experience feelings of inner calm and peacefulness. Regular practice of meditation may result in quite profound experiences of self-realization, awareness and personal development, which is the reason why it is an integral part of many of the world's religions. In India, meditation has been practiced for centuries as part of the yogic tradition as a means of attaining spiritual enlightenment.

How it works

Meditation techniques are simple and easy to learn, and are generally useful for all people as a self-help tool to counter stress and aid relaxation. In particular, meditation has been found to enhance the immune system, improve the circulation of the blood and lower blood pressure, reduce stress, improve mood and assist with pain management, making it particularly relevant as a therapy to be used in conjunction with other treatments for serious ailments, including heart disease, cancer, AIDS, multiple sclerosis, lupus, arthritis and other auto-immune disorders. Meditation may also be employed as part of a holistic program to treat stress-related conditions such as depression, anxiety, sleeping problems or phobias; respiratory problems such as asthma; tension headaches or migraines; or difficulties with concentration or memory.

Australian psychiatrist Dr. Ainslie Meares was among the first to study the effects of meditation on cancer patients, finding that they experienced many positive benefits, notably a significant reduction of anxiety and less pain and discomfort.

Where to find *Check local newspapers and libraries for information about classes. The International Meditation Teachers Association has a web page www.meditationteachers.org.*

One of his patients, Dr. Ian Gawler, purportedly used meditation to cure himself of bone cancer and then went on to establish The Gawler Foundation as the world's largest cancer support group that advocates meditation in the treatment of serious disease. Similarly, Dr. Dean Ornish of the University of California recommends regular meditation as part of any medical program to combat heart disease.

Meditation techniques

There are many schools and methods of meditation from autogenic training to Zen. All are concerned with clearing the mind so that a state of relaxation can be reached. There are many ways of achieving this from counting the breath to repetition of a mantra. Even simply taking a walk in the countryside with a clear intent can be a form of meditation.

Simple meditation

Focusing on a symbol (such as a mandala), an object (a candle flame, a crystal or a picture) or a rhythmic sound (such as a mantra, chanting, peaceful music or one's breathing pattern) can assist in letting go of distractions and focusing the mind. Lighting a candle or burning calming aromatherapy oil blends also help to create a peaceful atmosphere that is conducive to meditation and can act as focal points for the meditation practice itself.

continued on page 236

Mandala meditation

The word mandala is from the Sanskrit language and can be loosely translated to mean "circle." It represents wholeness, and has been embraced by Eastern religions. Buddhist monks make intricate sand mandalas in a meditative ritual, while "yantras" have their roots in ancient Indian Vedic culture. They are designed to be gazed at and contemplated during meditation. The Sri Yantra, a modern version of which is shown below, is one of the oldest mandalas known. Gazing at the mandala and its complex patterns helps to still the mind.

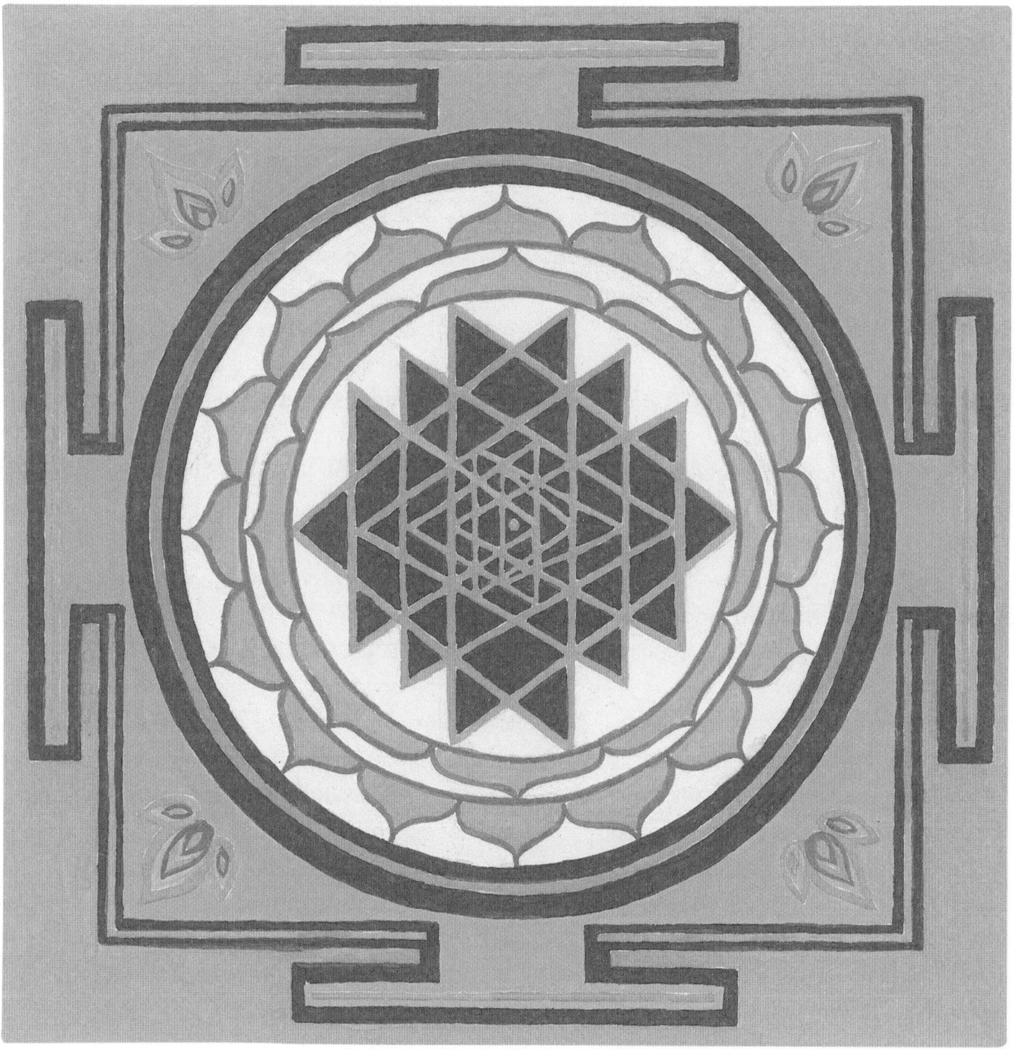

MEDITATION *continued*

Transcendental meditation

The Indian spiritual teacher Maharishi Mahesh Yogi brought this form of meditation to the West during the 1960s, when he became well known for attracting celebrities such as the Beatles. Transcendental Meditation (TM) involves relaxing totally and concentrating on repeating a personal mantra (given to you by a teacher) so as to become emptied of all unnecessary information and achieving a state of "pure being." Students are taught the technique over a series of lessons.

TM has been shown to heighten creativity and perceptual ability, and to decrease high blood pressure significantly. In 2013 a report by the American Heart Association stated that TM should be considered as a therapeutic tool for preventing and treating high blood pressure.

Autogenic training

This is the term given to a meditation technique based on a method of medical self-regulation developed in the 1920s by German neurologist Dr. Johannes Schulz. The word comes from the Greek for "coming from within." Schulz drew on research into the healing benefits of hypnotic suggestion and developed a set of standard exercises, designed to bring about a state of deep relaxation.

By silently repeating one of six affirmations—such as "My heartbeat is calm and regular" or "My forehead is cool"—the individual is able to bring about the corresponding physical sensation in the body. Specific health conditions that may respond to autogenic training include stress-related ailments, insomnia, depression and anxiety, as well as breathing difficulties such as asthma. Indigestion and irritable bowel syndrome are also said to respond to the therapy.

Autogenic training is usually taught in small groups over several weeks, focusing on one affirmation at a time until all six have been mastered and the students can then practice on their own. At first the training is done in quiet rooms with subdued lighting, but with practice the technique can be used in any stressful situation such as a traffic jam or while waiting for a business meeting.

Mindfulness meditation

This concept comes from Zen Buddhism and refers to a condition of detached awareness and consciousness. An old Zen saying is: "When I eat, I eat; when I sleep, I sleep." It refers to the conscious act of staying in the present moment.

Most of us spend our time thinking about past mistakes or traumas or worrying about future events. It is these thoughts that cause us the most distress. Letting go of our attachment to this pattern of thinking and focusing instead on the present moment, brings relief from anxiety and worry.

The technique is easy to use and involves learning how to open up and to be aware of what is happening around you right now, in the present moment. The person focuses on the events, sensations, feelings, thoughts, sounds and smells—in an objective, non-judgmental way. Practicing the technique during times of stress can offer instant relief.

Regular practice is best

Being able to slow down and settle a "busy brain" is a common problem for many people starting any meditation technique. Meditating at the same time and for a similar duration each day is advisable, but not essential. TM practitioners sit for around 15–20 minutes twice a day. However, benefits can be experienced with as little as 10 minutes of meditation a day. Anything is better than nothing, and it is more important to practice regularly. Meditating in groups is another popular approach.

MELATONIN

use for ✓ ***Cancer support*** ✓ ***Jet lag*** ✓ ***Seasonal affective disorder*** ✓ ***Sleeping problems***

MELATONIN IS A HORMONE PRODUCED in the brain by the pineal gland. Its secretion is triggered by the absence of light, peaking around the middle of the night and declining again as daylight returns. Supplements can help with certain conditions but you should check with your doctor fist to see if it is suitable for your needs.

How it works

Melatonin helps to regulate the body's "circadian rhythms," the internal biological clock that ensures we are mentally and physically alert during the daylight hours and at rest during the night. If melatonin production is inadequate or disrupted—which can happen with increasing age, shift work or international travel—taking a melatonin supplement can help restore normal circadian rhythms.

Safety first *Melatonin should not be used long term or in high doses except under medical supervision. It is not suitable for women who are pregnant or planning to conceive, and its safety for children and breastfeeding women has not been established.*

If you are taking prescription medicines, do not take melatonin unless advised to do so and supervised by your doctor.

Side effects may include drowsiness, nausea, headaches and dizziness. If symptoms occur, discontinue use and seek medical advice. Caution is advised when driving or operating heavy machinery.

Where to find *Look for melatonin supplements in health food stores and pharmacies. In some countries they are available only with a doctor's prescription.*

Since it's a hormone, melatonin also has numerous other functions in the body. For example, it may exert a number of potentially cancer-fighting effects, including helping to protect against free radical damage and inhibiting the growth of tumor cells.

How to use

If you suffer from sleeping problems, taking melatonin may help you fall asleep more quickly, wake up less frequently during the night, and stay asleep longer. To prevent or treat jet lag, take melatonin before bedtime in your destination time zone, ideally for several days before traveling.

When combined with exposure to light in the morning, taking melatonin in the afternoon may help improve moods in most people with seasonal affective disorder; however, some patients respond better to morning doses.

Studies combining melatonin with standard cancer therapies suggest it may improve survival rates and reduce the adverse effects of treatments such as chemotherapy and radiotherapy in some patients. Talk to your doctor about whether melatonin is suitable for you, and do not use it in place of standard therapies. Follow label instructions or take as professionally prescribed.

MILK THISTLE *Carduus marianus.* Also called: St. Mary's thistle

use for ✓ ***Cancer support*** ✓ ***Gall bladder problems*** ✓ ***Gastroenteritis***

MILK THISTLE IS "THE" LIVER HERB, beloved by herbalists throughout the centuries. In the same family as the stately globe artichoke, the young leaves and stems of the milk thistle may be eaten in salads. However, it is the seeds of this plant that are used medicinally and some of its traditional applications are being backed up by science.

How it works

Milk thistle contains the antioxidant and anti-inflammatory agent silymarin along with other phytochemicals that protect liver cells from damage. The protection afforded by milk thistle covers damage from free radicals during day-to-day metabolism as well as industrial toxins and other toxic substances including alcohol. Studies have shown that milk thistle can even protect the liver against the long-term damage caused by chemotherapy drugs.

Many diseases that damage the liver, including hepatitis, cause a hardening or fibrosis of the tissue, which can impair liver function. Milk thistle has been found to reduce this fibrosis as well as repair liver damage and help liver cells regenerate. Milk thistle has also been found to protect Kupffer cells against damage. Kupffer cells are specialized immune cells found in the liver that destroy bacteria, and basically clean up the surrounding tissue.

Milk thistle should be thought of for any liver-related conditions including hepatitis, cirrhosis, non-alcoholic liver disease and fatty liver disease. There is evidence it may help protect against certain cancers including liver, bowel, skin and prostate. Milk thistle has also been shown to be helpful in the treatment of diabetes, raised cholesterol, gall bladder disease and gastroenteritis.

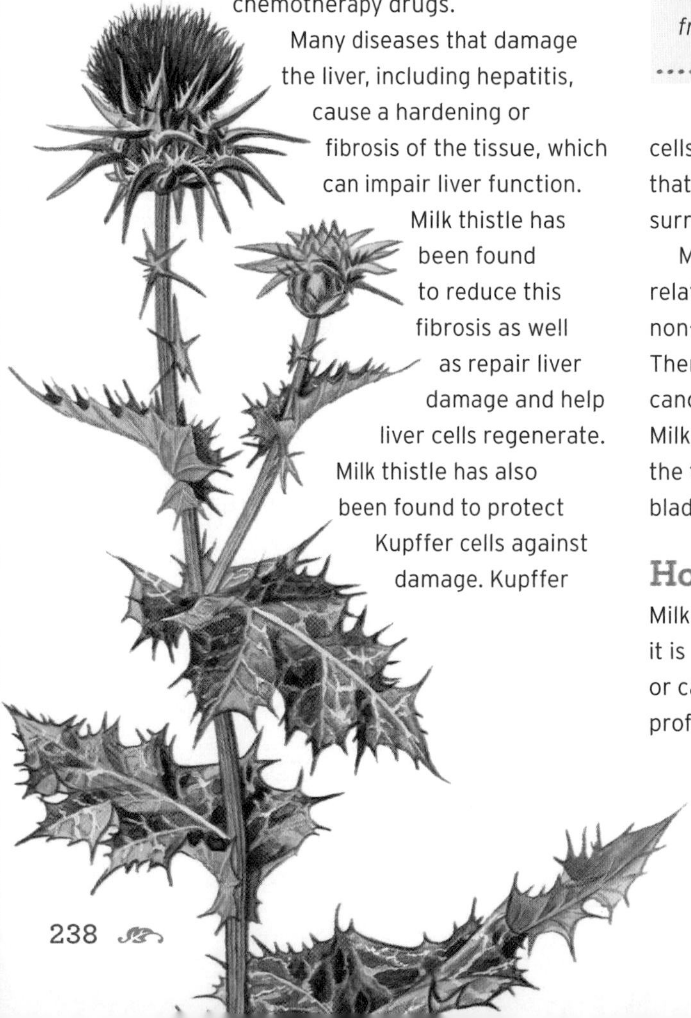

Safety first *Milk thistle is a very safe herb, it can even be used by pregnant and breastfeeding women. The only consideration with milk thistle is that it may hinder iron absorption from food. If you are prone to iron deficiency anemia, don't take milk thistle with iron-rich meals.*

Where to find *Milk thistle supplements can be found in health food stores and supermarkets or from a qualified herbalist.*

How to use

Milk thistle seeds can be made into a tea, although it is more customarily used in fluid extract, tablet or capsule form. Follow label instructions or take as professionally prescribed.

MULLEIN *Verbascum thapsus*

use for ✓ ***Bronchitis***

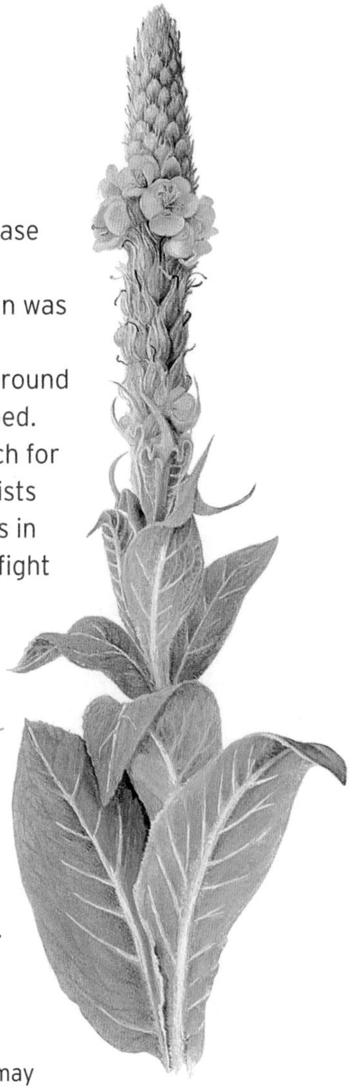

HUNDREDS OF YEARS AGO, THIS HARDY PLANT was widely used to ease bronchitis, coughs and even tuberculosis and leprosy. Native American healers brewed mullein-leaf tea for coughs and colds. In England, mullein was fed to cattle to treat breathing problems, too.

Today, mullein grows so widely and so readily in fields and on open ground in North America and Europe that it's considered a noxious, invasive weed. But as pharmaceutical researchers return to Mother Nature in the search for novel antimicrobial compounds, mullein is getting a second look. Scientists at Ireland's Cork Institute of Technology have been studying compounds in the herb in the hope that there may be something with the potential to fight dangerous, antibiotic-resistant tuberculosis. But research is in its early stages. For now, herbalists say mullein is best used for the relief of sore throats and chesty coughs associated with colds and bronchitis.

How it works

Mullein contains compounds called saponins—natural foaming "detergents" that help loosen mucus for easier removal when you cough. Saponins can also have bacteria-fighting abilities. Mucilage in mullein soothes irritated tissues, while another mullein constituent, verbascoside, acts as an anti-inflammatory, according to Italian researchers. In laboratory studies, mullein extracts have also demonstrated antiviral properties, researchers from Canada's University of British Columbia report.

How to use

This herb is most often taken as a tea and you may find it as an ingredient in herbal blends for sore throats. Use herbal tea bags or steep 3–4 teaspoons (15-20 ml) of loose, dried mullein leaves in a cup of just-boiled water for 10–15 minutes. Strain and sip. Enjoy one or two cups a day.

Safety first *Mullein seeds contain a potentially toxic substance called rotenone; it's best to use just the leaves for tea.*

Where to find *Mullein tea is available in health food stores or from a qualified herbalist.*

MULTIVITAMINS

use for ✓ ***Cramps, muscle*** ✓ ***Eye disorders*** ✓ ***Inflammatory bowel disease*** ✓ ***Natural fertility management*** ✓ ***Shingles***

YOUR BODY REQUIRES MANY NUTRIENTS in order to function properly, but is able to produce only a small proportion of them, with the remainder coming from your diet. Though a well-balanced diet should be able to provide you with all the vitamins and minerals you need, at certain times and for certain conditions, taking a multivitamin and mineral supplement (a "multi") can be helpful.

How they work

Multis contain small quantities of a wide range of nutrients and are intended to overcome any dietary shortfalls that may occur. They typically include a broad spectrum of vitamins and minerals, sometimes along with other ingredients such as herbs and essential fatty acids. It is best to take a multi with natural rather than synthetic forms of nutrients and you can expect to pay more for quality products such as those prescribed by practitioners.

Some multis are specially formulated for specific health concerns. Examples include B-complex formulas to support the body during times of stress, preconception multis to ensure optimal nutrition in a woman's body at the time of conception, pregnancy and breastfeeding formulas to support the nutritional requirements of both mother and baby, and antioxidant formulas to support the cardiovascular system, eyes or brain.

Safety first *Multis should not replace a balanced diet. Most people can safely take multis at recommended doses, but talk to your doctor beforehand if you are taking prescribed medicines or have been diagnosed with cancer, hemochromatosis or a bleeding disorder. You should also talk to your doctor about your multivitamin use before undergoing medical tests or surgery.*

Where to find *Multivitamins are available in pharmacies, health food stores, supermarkets and from natural health practitioners.*

How to use

Taking a multi may be advisable if you or your doctor are concerned that you lack certain food groups or nutrients, or require additional nutritional support due to your individual health needs.

Women who are pregnant or planning to conceive should consider taking a multi containing high levels of folic acid, as well as iron, iodine, omega-3 fatty acids and other nutrients required for fetal development.

People with recurrent diarrhea, shingles or post-herpetic neuralgia may benefit from taking a multi to offset the nutritional deficiencies that can be associated with these conditions.

People with or at risk of age-related macular degeneration (AMD) may benefit from the long-term use of an antioxidant formula containing carotenoids, vitamins C and E, zinc and selenium. This combination of nutrients has been shown to delay the progression of AMD.

For muscle cramps, take a multi or vitamin B-complex supplement, ideally one that includes magnesium, deficiency of which can cause muscle spasms and cramps.

MUSIC

use for ✓ ***Anxiety*** ✓ ***Blood pressure, high*** ✓ ***Chronic pain*** ✓ ***Sleeping problems***

IF YOU'VE EVER FELT YOUR SPIRIT SOAR when you listened to a beloved hymn, felt love rekindle when a song from your courting days plays on the radio or relaxed to the soothing slow movement of a symphony, you've experienced the health benefits of music firsthand. Now, medical science is revealing the long-hidden reasons for music's mind-body benefits. It turns out that listening to your favorite tunes, playing an instrument and singing (yes, even if you can't carry a tune) all have positive effects.

In fact, the evidence is so strong that music's health benefits are no longer simply seen as a nice bonus from time spent crooning with a local choir. Music therapy, tailored to specific needs, is becoming a widespread, integrative-medicine prescription to help ease pain, insomnia, anxiety and even control blood pressure.

How it works

Listening to favorite musical selections trimmed blood pressure four points (on par with cutting back on salt or increasing weekly exercise) in an Italian study of 59 people with high blood pressure. Why? It could be that simply relaxing helps switch off the body's stress response; breathing calmly to a slow, steady beat may also explain the effect. In fact, a 2012 study from Sweden found that relaxing with music was more effective in lowering stress hormones than resting in silence.

In the US, a Seattle study of 78 people with generalized anxiety disorder found that music eased anxiety as effectively as a massage or "thermotherapy" treatment. And getting lost in a melody blunted sharp pain in a University of Utah study, in which brave volunteers listened to music while receiving brief electric shocks to their fingertips. Researchers think that music may have helped by distracting or relaxing the participants.

In another study, relaxation is probably the reason why older people with insomnia fell asleep faster, slept longer and reported that they enjoyed deeper sleep when they listened to a 45-minute recording of soothing melodies at bedtime.

Safety first *Listening, singing and playing an instrument are very safe.*

Where to find *Music's healing benefits are as close as your CD collection or the playlist in your smart phone. You can also purchase recordings aimed at improving sleep and achieving other health goals online or at some natural healing shops.*

How to use

Music seems to help most when you choose styles, songs and artists that you personally enjoy, and that hold your attention while allowing you to breathe calmly and relax. Set aside time to listen when you can sit or lie down comfortably without being disturbed. But don't stop at listening. There's growing evidence that singing with others improves immune function and emotional health—and even some hints that singing or playing a wind instrument could tone throat muscles to reduce snoring! Dancing to music also has profound benefits that combine the relaxing effects of music with physical and social activity.

NASAL IRRIGATION

use for ✓ ***Allergies*** ✓ ***Hay fever*** ✓ ***Sinusitis*** ✓ ***Snoring***

ACCORDING TO AYURVEDA, India's traditional medical system, the nose is the doorway to the brain. Life energy or *prana* enters the body through breath taken in by the nose, and any excess of bodily *doshas* (the body's three basic biological elements, *vata*, *pitta* and *kapha*, which need to be in balance) are also eliminated via the nose. Therefore, cleanliness of the nose is of vital importance. Nasal cleansing is one of the six *shad kriyas*, or classical purification techniques, practiced in yoga.

How it works

The aim of nasal irrigation is to assist the elimination of waste products from the nose, nasal passages and sinus cavities. Practiced daily, this easy hygienic exercise helps counteract the effects of pollution, dust and pollen. It is beneficial for asthma, allergies, sinusitis, hay fever, snoring, colds or flu; it may be of particular benefit to people who are exposed to conditions that predispose them to nasal problems such as those who fly frequently, work in dehumidified surroundings, or are exposed to dust, mold or workplace chemicals.

Where to find *You may be able to buy a neti pot from a yoga school. Some health food stores stock them, too. Squeeze bottles or bulb syringes are available in pharmacies. An Ayurvedic practitioner may perform other forms of nasal cleansing therapy, or nasya, including inserting powdered herbs, ghee or oil.*

How to use

Mix 1/2 teaspoon (2 ml) of sea salt in a cup of lukewarm water. Place it in a ceramic or brass neti pot, which is the small, spouted pot used to administer the flush. Leaning over a sink, tip your head far to the left, so your ear is parallel to the floor, and hold your breath. Use the neti pot to pour water into the right nostril and out of the left. The objective is to let the liquid flow freely through in a thin stream, not spill out of your nose; it takes practice, so go slowly. Blow the nose gently and repeat on the other side.

Daily practice is recommended as a preventive lifestyle measure; it may be repeated several times a day during acute episodes of sinusitis or hay fever. An alternative to a neti pot is a squeeze bottle or bulb syringe, which can be used to deliver liquid into one nostril at a time.

NEEM *Azadirachta indica*

use for ✓ ***Insect bites and stings*** ✓ ***Tooth and gum disorders***

THE NEEM TREE IS ONE OF THE SACRED TREES of India, where it has long played a central role in village life and Hindu religious practices. Its medicinal properties have been recognized for at least 4,000 years and it is used to treat such a wide variety of ailments that it is sometimes even referred to by the name the "village pharmacy."

How it works

More than 60 different compounds have been identified in neem trees, but it has not been determined which ones contribute to the plant's therapeutic effects. Traditionally, the bark and leaves of the neem tree have been applied to a wide range of skin conditions (including cuts, rashes and chicken pox) and are also sometimes taken internally. The twigs are prized for their antiseptic properties and used to brush the teeth and gums, and have been shown to remove plaque as effectively as normal toothbrushes. The ground seeds and their oil are used as a natural pesticide.

How to use

For the treatment of gingivitis (gum disease), rinse with a neem mouthwash twice daily for three weeks while continuing to maintain good oral hygiene by brushing and flossing your teeth. In one clinical study, doing so was found to be as effective as a standard mouthwash used to treat gum disease, but had fewer side effects.

To prevent mosquito bites, apply insect repellent containing neem oil according to the manufacturer's directions. To treat head lice, wash the hair and scalp with neem shampoo according to the directions on the label. Bedding that has been infested with lice, fleas, bed bugs or dust mites can also be washed with neem products.

Safety first *Topical and internal use of neem should be avoided during infancy, childhood, pregnancy and breastfeeding, as safety during these times has not been established.*

Do not take neem if you have been diagnosed with diabetes, liver disease, thyroid disease or any form of cardiovascular disorder.

Allergic reactions to neem products sometimes occur. If affected, discontinue use and seek medical advice.

Where to find *Mouthwashes, toothpastes, insect repellents and products to aid the management of head lice and dust mites are available in health food stores and pharmacies.*

NETTLE *Urtica dioica.* Also called: Stinging nettle

use for ✓ ***Hay fever*** ✓ ***Prostate problems***

IRONICALLY—GIVEN ITS STINGING LEAVES—nettle has long been a herbal remedy for relieving pain and inflammation. It is rich in iron, explaining the traditional use of young nettle shoots in a detoxifying tonic to "cleanse the blood" in spring. Today, it is best known as a treatment for enlarged prostate, hay fever and joint pain.

How it works

Nettle has antiallergenic, anti-inflammatory, diuretic, tonic and astringent (tightening) properties. It contains plant sterols, including beta-sitosterol, which is thought to be involved in the herb's ability to treat an enlarged prostate. Nettle may work in several possible ways: It may interfere with the enzymes necessary for prostate cell growth, plus, it may decrease activity in prostate cell receptor sites that would otherwise respond to growth hormones.

While the precise mode of its action appears complex, it is widely used in Europe to treat an enlarged prostate, often in conjunction with **saw palmetto** *(p. 278)*. Research has shown that nettle extracts significantly reduce symptoms of benign prostatic hypertrophy (BPH) with similar effects to the drug finasteride.

Safety first *Fresh nettle will sting. Occasionally, nettle extracts can cause mild gastrointestinal upsets or an allergic skin reaction and nettle may reduce blood glucose and blood pressure. Medical advice should be sought if taking nettle with prescription medications including finasteride and antidiabetic or antihypertensive medications.*

Where to find *Nettle supplements and teas are available in health food stores and pharmacies. A qualified herbalist can prescribe a tincture or ointment made with nettle and other synergistic herbs.*

Being beaten with stinging nettle stems was once considered a cure for arthritis and rheumatism; interestingly, taking nettle extracts may indeed help relieve inflammation. It is thought to work by damping down the production of cytokines, which cause inflammation. Nettle may also be of assistance in reducing hay fever symptoms, possibly by increasing production of interleukin-2 and T-cells, which control the allergic response.

Given its high content of iron, vitamin C and chlorophyll, nettle is a helpful remedy for anemia, and may be helpful for people experiencing heavy menstrual bleeding or chronic nosebleeds.

How to use

Nettle is available dried or fresh (for use as a tea), as a tincture, or as a freeze-dried extract in tablet or capsule form. Follow label instructions, or take as professionally prescribed.

A rinse made from cold nettle tea may counteract an itchy scalp, or be used topically for inflamed skin conditions, such as eczema, hives and rashes, and as an astringent poultice for varicose veins.

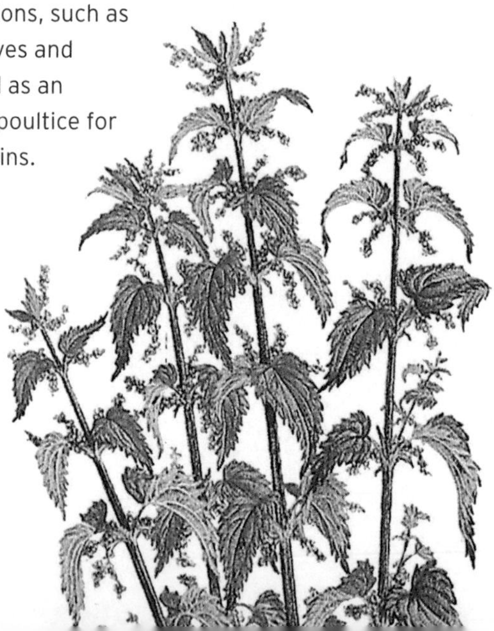

NIACIN

use for ✓ ***Acne*** ✓ ***Cholesterol, high***

NIACIN IS ALSO REFERRED TO AS NICOTINIC acid, vitamin B_3 and nicotinamide. You obtain niacin from dietary sources such as meat, brewer's yeast, legumes and peanuts. In addition, your body can produce it from the amino acid tryptophan, which is found in dairy products and other foods.

How it works

Niacin is required for the activity of more than 50 enzymes. Among other functions, it is essential for releasing energy from carbohydrate foods, regulating blood glucose, repairing the DNA in cells and is involved in the production of sex hormones.

Safety first *High doses of niacin can cause uncomfortable flushing, which may be avoided by using a slow release formulation or increasing the dosage slowly over four to six weeks and/or taking aspirin at the same time. Liver inflammation can sometimes occur with high-dose niacin therapy and is more likely with slow-release forms so careful monitoring by your doctor is required when high doses are used.*

Do not take niacin alongside cholesterol-lowering medications unless advised to do so and supervised by your doctor as dangerous interactions may occur in some circumstances.

Where to find *Supplements are available in health food stores and pharmacies, although some are only available on prescription.*

Nicotinamide gels for topical use are available in pharmacies.

How to use

The US Recommended Dietary Allowance (RDA) of niacin is 16 mg/day for adult men (19+), and 14 mg/day for adult women, increasing to 18 mg/day during pregnancy and 17 mg/day while breastfeeding. When taken as nicotinic acid, the upper level of intake for adults is set at 35 mg/day.

Under medical supervision, high doses of niacin (but not nicotinamide) can help to lower total and LDL cholesterol ('bad" cholesterol) and raise HDL cholesterol ('good" cholesterol). Take according to your doctor's instructions.

When applied to skin with moderately severe acne twice daily for eight weeks, a gel containing 4 percent nicotinamide reduced the quantity and severity of acne lesions. It appears to be particularly beneficial for acne sufferers with oily skin.

NIGELLA *Nigella sativa.* Also called: Black seed, Black cumin

use for ✓ ***Eczema*** ✓ ***Fungal infections*** ✓ ***Hair loss*** ✓ ***Hay fever*** ✓ ***Headaches***

NIGELLA HAS BEEN USED AS BOTH a food and a medicine since ancient times. It is referred to in the Bible and the writings of Hippocrates, Dioscorides and the Persian medical philosopher Avicenna. It takes its name from the Latin word niger, which means black, and is also known by the names black seed and black cumin.

Nigella is particularly prized in Unani Tibb (a form of traditional medicine practiced in the Arab world and parts of Africa and Asia), because the Prophet Muhammad is quoted as saying: "The black seeds are the remedy for every disease except death."

How it works

Nigella has traditionally been used to treat an extensive range of health problems, including respiratory conditions, digestive troubles, skin problems, allergies and blood disorders. Although more clinical studies are required before nigella's effects in humans are fully understood, many of these traditional uses are supported by research. Studies have shown that nigella and its active constituents have widespread physiological effects, including (among others) antioxidant, antibacterial, antifungal and antidiabetic properties. Nigella may also help to stimulate the immune system.

The oil from the seeds is rich in unsaturated fatty acids, which may contribute to some of nigella's therapeutic effects.

Safety first *Unless advised to do so by your doctor, do not take nigella in medicinal quantities if you have an immune-system or bleeding disorder, low blood pressure, low blood glucose, or are taking prescribed medicines. It is also unsuitable for women who are pregnant, breastfeeding or trying to conceive.*

Avoid nigella if you are allergic to the Ranunculaceae family of plants, which also includes buttercups, aconites and anemones.

Where to find *Nigella oil, liquid and capsules are available in health food stores.*

How to use

Taking nigella seed oil may help aid the management of some types of allergies, including hay fever and eczema. For example, in hay fever sufferers it has been shown to relieve sneezing and a runny, blocked or itchy nose when taken for at least two weeks.

The oil can be taken as a liquid or in capsules, and has also traditionally been rubbed into the skin of the affected area to assist with conditions such as fungal infection, hair loss, stomach upset, chesty cough and headache. Follow label instructions or take as professionally prescribed.

NUTS

use for ✓ ***Eye disorders*** ✓ ***Heart and circulatory health***

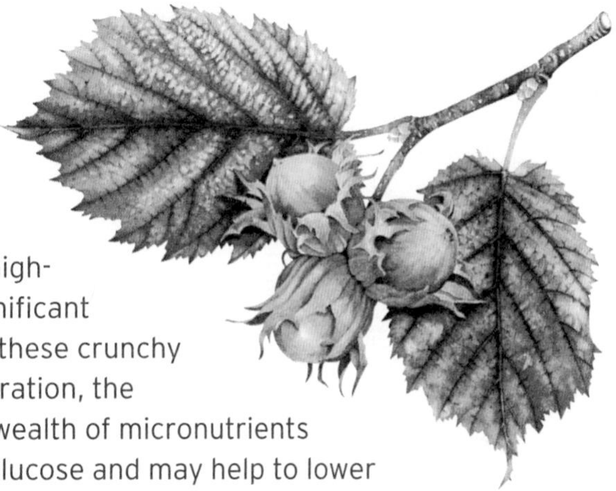

GO AHEAD—INDULGE. Once dismissed as just a high-energy snack food, research shows nuts pack significant health benefits. True, the high fat content makes these crunchy nuggets high in calories. But when eaten in moderation, the satisfying "good" fats plus fiber, protein and the wealth of micronutrients in nuts offer benefits for your heart, your blood glucose and may help to lower your risk of fatal cancers. Adding nuts to your diet can even help with weight control.

How they work

Only vegetable oil ranks higher than nuts as a source of good-for-you monounsaturated fat—the plant-based fat shown in a series of Spanish studies to discourage the accumulation of body fat at the waist. In a 2013 study from Spain's Universitat Rovira i Virgili that followed 7,216 people for several years, those who ate three 1-ounce (28 g) servings of nuts weekly were 55 percent less likely to develop fatal heart disease or cancer than those who rarely or never had nuts. Other studies have linked regular nut consumption with a lower risk for diabetes, high blood pressure and high cholesterol, too.

Oleic acid, a type of monounsaturated fat, may be one reason. This fat becomes part of healthy cell walls, allowing cells lining blood vessels to relax and letting muscle cells more readily absorb blood glucose. Monounsaturated fats also help bolster levels of "good" HDL cholesterol while lowering LDLs. Meanwhile, the omega-3 fatty acids and high levels of cell-protecting antioxidants found in walnuts make this particular nut especially heart-healthy and have been shown in studies to reduce heart-threatening LDL cholesterol.

Nuts offer a big weight-loss advantage in a small package, too. Researchers at Purdue University report that people ate less in the hours after a nut snack—compensating for 55 percent of the calories in walnuts, 50–100 percent from almonds and 60–95 percent from peanuts. The good fat in nuts may explain why eating one handful a week was associated with a 40 percent lower risk for vision-robbing age-related macular degeneration in one Harvard study, too.

Safety first *Avoid if you have nut allergies.*

Where to find *Look for nuts in supermarkets and health food stores.*

How to use

Enjoy a small handful of nuts—22 almonds, 14 walnut halves, 18 cashews, 20 pecan halves, 18 peanuts, 20 hazelnuts or 47 pistachios—several times a week to get their health benefits. Avoid added calories and sodium by skipping nuts that are oil-roasted, salted or candied. Half of the health-protecting antioxidants in nuts are found in their papery skin; so when possible, eat that, too. Storing nuts in the fridge helps to keep them fresh and prevents the oils in them from going rancid.

continued on page 248

NUTS *continued*

Nutrient-packed

Nuts are the embryos of trees and other plants and as such contain everything the plant needs to grow. That's good news for us since it means that they are full of beneficial phytochemicals. Nuts are a great source of protein, "good-for-you" polyunsaturated and monounsaturated fats and many other nutrients.

Macadamia

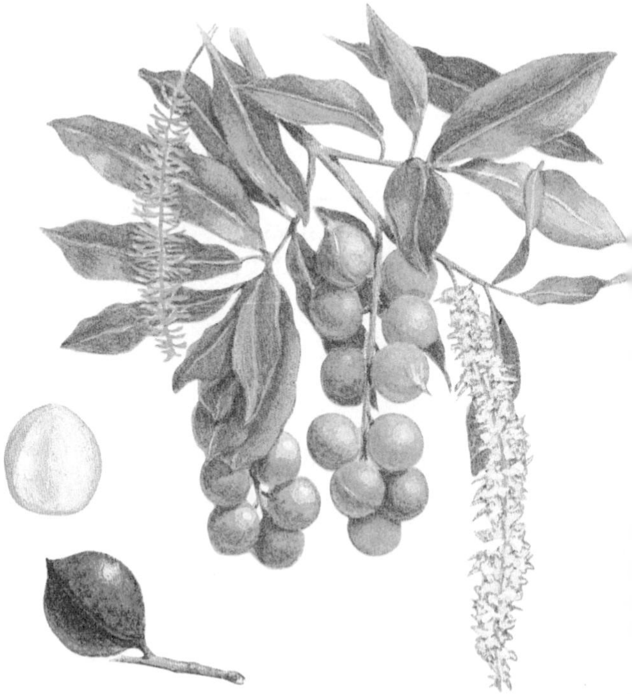

Almonds

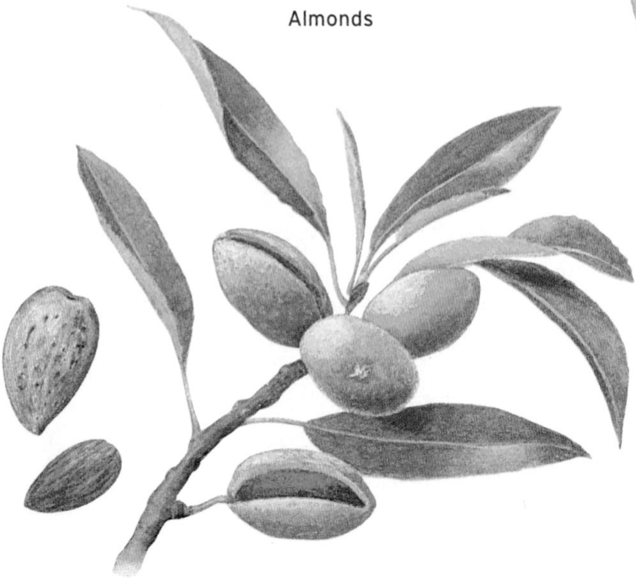

Walnuts

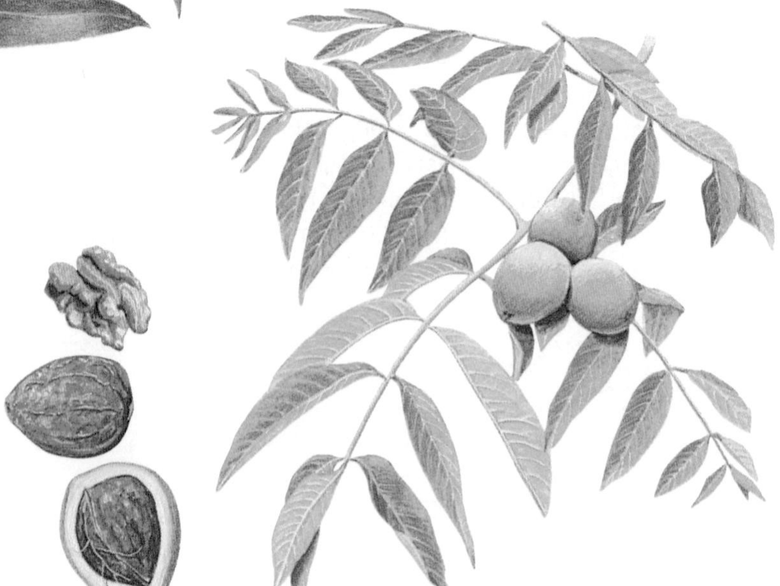

OLIVE OIL

use for ✓ ***Heart and circulatory health*** ✓ ***Scalp and hair problems***
✓ ***Stroke prevention*** ✓ ***Tinnitus***

OLIVE OIL HAS A REPUTATION AS A "SUPERFOOD," yet before 1958, this delicious golden-green fat was found mostly in the kitchens and on the tables of cooks from Italy, Greece and Spain. American biologist Ancel Keys first highlighted olive oil's amazing health benefits, with a groundbreaking research study that tied the Mediterranean diet (heavy on the olive oil) to better heart health. Today, the benefits of the good-for-you monounsaturated fats and antioxidants in olive oil reach beyond arteries and heart health.

How it works

Recent studies show that using olive oil as your preferred fat (instead of butter or most other vegetable oils) can reduce the risk for fatal heart disease by 28–44 percent and cut stroke risk by 41 percent. Good fats in olive oil help lower levels of heart-threatening LDL cholesterol, bolster levels of heart-friendly HDL cholesterol, improve blood pressure and also seem to help the body process blood glucose in a healthier way. Meanwhile, olive oil has a long history of use as a beauty product and as a home remedy for a range of conditions including removing bugs from ears and loosening ear wax.

Safety first *Olive oil is generally safe to use. Do not use olive oil in the ear if there is any concern about a ruptured ear drum.*

Where to find *Look for olive oil in the supermarket. For eating, choose extra virgin olive oil; it has the highest levels of cell-protecting polyphenols.*

How to use

Aim to include 1–2 tablespoons (15-30 ml) of olive oil in place of other fats in your daily diet. Some experts recommend using extra virgin olive oil "raw" (uncooked) over salads, vegetables and as a dip for bread. (The smoke point of olive oil–the point at which the oil begins to break down, losing its nutritional value–is relatively low compared to other oils.) For ear-wax removal, place 3–4 drops of olive oil in the affected ear two or three times a day for up to two weeks. The wax will often come out by itself. (Use loose cotton wool in your ears to avoid oil drips.)

To soothe a dry, itchy scalp (and deep-condition your hair), carefully warm olive oil on the stove. Remove from the heat and make sure the oil is not too hot then use a kitchen pastry brush to apply it to your scalp. Comb the oil through your hair, then wrap your hair in a shower cap and cover with a towel. After 15–30 minutes rinse out the oil, then shampoo and condition as usual.

OMEGA-3 FATTY ACIDS

use for ✓ ***Asthma*** ✓ ***Cancer support*** ✓ ***Cholesterol, high*** ✓ ***Dementia*** ✓ ***Depression*** ✓ ***Diabetes and insulin resistance*** ✓ ***Eye disorders*** ✓ ***Heart and circulatory health*** ✓ ***Psoriasis*** ✓ ***Rheumatoid arthritis***

THE THREE MOST IMPORTANT omega-3 fatty acids are alpha-linolenic acid (ALA), eicosapentaenoic acid (EPA) and docosahexaenoic acid (DHA). Dietary sources of ALA include walnuts, flaxseed oil (linseed oil), canola oil and soybean oil. EPA and DHA are predominantly obtained from oily fish and other seafood, and to a lesser extent can be produced in the body from ALA. Research suggests that many people don't eat enough foods that are rich in omega-3s and consequently may benefit from taking supplements containing fish oil or other sources of omega-3 fats.

How they work

Omega-3 fats are involved in a wide range of physiological activities, including muscle function, reproduction, growth and development. They also trigger anti-inflammatory activities and play a structural role in the cell membranes, especially those of the eyes, brain and nervous system.

How to use

Oily fish, such as salmon, sardines and mackerel, are the best dietary sources of omega-3s. Nutritionists recommend eating two or three servings of oily fish per week. Supplements are available as capsules and liquids made from fish, krill, calamari (squid) and flaxseed oils. Follow label instructions or take as professionally prescribed.

Consuming high levels of omega-3s has been shown to lower the risk of heart problems and stroke. Among other effects on the cardiovascular system, omega-3s lower triglycerides and high blood pressure, help maintain heartbeat regularity, and improve the blood vessels' ability to relax and open. In people with diabetes, they may reduce elevated triglycerides and increase levels of HDL ("good") cholesterol.

Omega-3s have protective effects against age-related macular degeneration, dry eye syndrome, dementia, depression and some forms of cancer. They may also help to reduce the risk of inflammatory conditions such as asthma, psoriasis and rheumatoid arthritis (RA). In people with RA, high doses of omega-3s can reduce pain, the number of tender joints, and the duration of morning stiffness. In psoriasis, they help to relieve itching, redness and skin scaling, and improve quality of life when taken in conjunction with standard topical treatments.

Safety first *If you have a bleeding disorder, are taking anticoagulant or blood-thinning medications, or plan to have surgery, do not take omega-3 fatty acids unless supervised by a doctor.*

If you are allergic to seafood, do not take omega-3 supplements from seafood sources.

Omega-3 supplements sometimes cause mild gastrointestinal symptoms such as burping, loose bowel movements and halitosis.

Where to find *Buy fresh fish in supermarkets and supplements in health food stores and pharmacies. Some fish (typically larger predatory fish) can be contaminated with mercury and other toxins and are best avoided by children and pregnant women and consumed only in small amounts by others—follow the advice of your local health authority.*

OSTEOPATHY

use for ✓ ***Headaches*** ✓ ***Jaw pain*** ✓ ***Neuralgia***

THE DISCIPLINE OF OSTEOPATHY was founded by an American doctor named Andrew Taylor Still in 1874. Like **chiropractic** *(p. 152)*, the therapy focuses on the relationship between the structure of the body and the way that it functions. Osteopathy focuses on the interconnectedness of all the different organs, bones and joints of your body.

How it works

The goal of osteopathic treatment is to bring all elements of the musculoskeletal system into alignment. The aim is to restore mobility, blood flow and the functioning of the lymphatic system, providing optimal conditions for the body to heal itself.

Most of the scientific evidence supporting osteopathy is for the use of spinal manipulation in conditions associated with musculoskeletal tension and misalignment. There is some evidence to support its use for headaches (especially those caused by musculoskeletal issues in the head and neck) and jaw pain, as well as sciatica, carpal tunnel syndrome and other forms of neuralgia.

A visit to the osteopath

After taking your case history, your osteopath will use their hands to feel the bony and soft tissues of your body and identify any areas of restriction or impairment. You will be required to remove your outer clothing and may be asked to lie on a therapy couch for the duration of the treatment. The subsequent treatment may then incorporate massage, mobilization of restricted joints, spinal manipulation, physical therapy, and education about changes to your posture, exercise routine or diet that would be beneficial for your health.

Mobilization and spinal manipulation may involve gentle touch, passive movement (in which the practitioner moves your body into certain positions without your active involvement), active movement (in which you move your body yourself) and/or firm thrusts to release restricted joints and free up movement and circulation in the affected area.

Mild, transient pain may be experienced during or after an osteopathic treatment, but usually diminishes over the next few hours or days.

Safety first *Tell the osteopath if you are pregnant and mention any medical condition you have and other treatments or medicines you are taking.*

Where to find *To find a qualified osteopathic practitioner, visit the American Osteopathic Association (www.osteopathic.org) or get a referral from your doctor or local health clinic.*

PASSIONFLOWER

Passiflora incarnata

use for ✓ ***Sleeping problems***

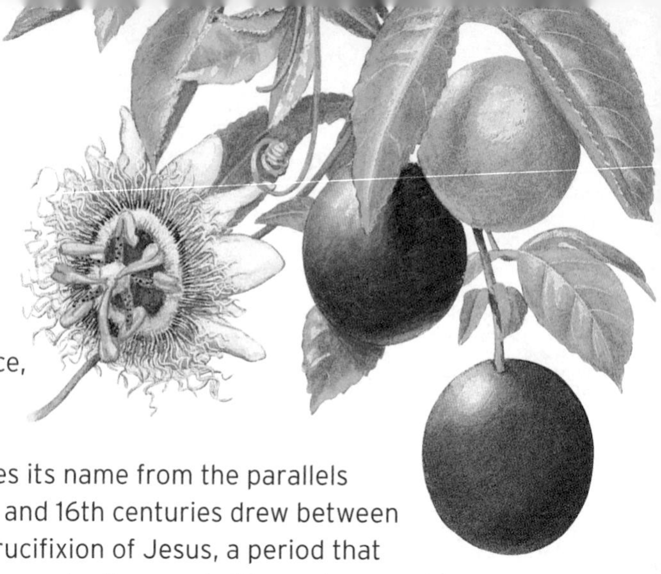

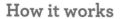

PASSIONFLOWERS HAVE A DISTINCT appearance, with prominent stigmas and anthers encircled by a ring of blue or purple filaments, which are in turn surrounded by white petals. The plant takes its name from the parallels that Spanish Christian missionaries from the 15th and 16th centuries drew between these and other structures of the plant and the crucifixion of Jesus, a period that is referred to as the *Passion of Jesus Christ*. For example, the purple filaments are said to represent the crown of thorns worn by Jesus, while the three stigmas and five anthers respectively symbolize the three nails of the cross and the five wounds he sustained.

How it works

While it's not entirely clear how passionflower works, research suggests that its antianxiety and sedative properties may be at least partially due to effects on the brain chemical gamma aminobutyric acid (GABA, the most important of the body's brain chemicals that have inhibitory effects on the nervous system) or its receptors.

How to use

Passionflower has traditionally been used for the treatment of sleeping problems and other conditions associated with nervous tension such as anxiety. When used for sleeping difficulties, passionflower can be taken at or before bedtime as a tea, tablet or herbal liquid. Preliminary clinical research suggests that when taken daily for a week, an evening dose of passionflower helps to improve sleep quality.

For the treatment of anxiety, passionflower is usually taken in multiple doses throughout the day, usually as a tablet or herbal liquid. Clinical studies indicate that it may be beneficial for many different forms of anxiety, including generalized anxiety disorder, presurgery anxiety and (when taken with prescribed medication and under medical supervision) the nervous and mental symptoms that sometimes occur during withdrawal from opiates.

In many instances, passionflower is taken in combination with other herbs used to relax the nervous system such as valerian and hops. Stress-relief formulations often include these herbs alongside passionflower. Follow label instructions, or take as professionally prescribed.

Safety first *If you are taking any sedative, antidepressant or antianxiety medication, do not take passionflower unless advised to do so by your doctor. Passionflower has not been widely tested during pregnancy or breastfeeding so it is best avoided or used only under medical supervision during these periods.*

Where to find *Passionflower products are available in pharmacies, health food stores and from a qualified herbalist. Some health food stores also sell passionflower tea.*

PELVIC FLOOR EXERCISES

use for ✓ ***Incontinence***

ATTACHED TO YOUR PUBIC BONE in front and your tailbone at the back, your pelvic floor is a strong yet flexible muscular hammock that helps support and control your bladder, bowels and reproductive organs. Ageing, hormonal changes, a pulled muscle, abdominal surgery and childbirth can weaken or overly tighten your pelvic floor resulting in a range of disorders including incontinence, chronic constipation and pelvic pain issues including pain with sexual intercourse, vulval pain and interstitial cystitis.

Research shows that home exercises (and sometimes, treatment by a pelvic floor physical therapist) are effective, easing nearly 60 percent of serious bladder pain and about 50 percent of vulva pain, reducing or eliminating incontinence up to 85 percent of the time and even helping to ease lower back pain when regular care (such as stretching exercises and ultrasound treatment) wasn't enough. Preventive measures may help you avoid problems, but don't assume that this means just doing tightening exercises (also known as Kegel exercises after the obstetrician who developed them). Pelvic floor experts say relaxing these muscles is more important for some women. Read on to learn how to check your muscles and exercise them properly.

How they work

Through targeted exercise or relaxation, you can strengthen or loosen the muscles in your pelvic floor. Your pelvic floor muscles may be too weak or loose if you have "stress incontinence"–you leak sometimes when you laugh, sneeze, cough, jump or get up from a chair. One way to check your pelvic floor strength is to try to completely stop your urine stream while you urinate. This will help you identify the correct muscles to exercise and if you can't stop your urine, it means your muscles are weak and you would benefit from strengthening exercises. (Stopping your urine is recommended as a check and not as a regular exercise.)

On the other hand, your pelvic floor may be too tight if you have frequent constipation, if you have to push to urinate or have a bowel movement or if you have pelvic pain. In this case relaxation exercises and targeted physical therapy may help.

A new understanding of pelvic floor disorders is emerging whereby experts are discovering that other ailments can have a direct impact on the functioning of the pelvic floor. Discomfort and inflammation caused by other medical conditions that affect pelvic organs–such as endometriosis, irritable bowel syndrome and even bladder infections–can create additional tension in pelvic floor muscles. In turn, this tension can intensify the pain of the original

Safety first *If you have pelvic pain or another ongoing problem that seems related to your pelvic floor, ask your doctor about a referral to a specialist physical therapist for an examination and possible treatment.*

Where to find *You can practice pelvic floor exercises at home. You can also find tools online aimed at helping you perform strengthening exercises correctly, such as weights and electronic biofeedback devices.*

continued on page 254

PELVIC FLOOR EXERCISES *continued*

medical condition in a vicious cycle of increasing pain. Relaxation exercises targeted at the pelvic floor can go a long way to reducing the added discomfort.

Pelvic floor disorders aren't just a problem for women. Men experience them, too, often as a result of an injury, surgery or heavy lifting at work or at home. Still, they are more common in women, and largely associated with pregnancy, childbirth and gynecological surgery such as a hysterectomy. Pregnancy and childbirth increase the risk of a pelvic floor disorder by 50 percent with one child, and triple for women who have had three children.

How to do the exercises

To strengthen weak pelvic floor muscles, sit or lie down in a quiet place. Inhale, tightening the muscles around your urethra, vagina (for women) and rectum. Hold for 10 seconds, then relax completely as you exhale. Repeat up to 10 times daily.

To reduce or prevent tightness in the pelvic floor, try this relaxation exercise. As you sit, stand or lie down in a quiet place, relax your body while breathing calmly for a minute or so. Then take a deep breath; as you exhale, imagine your pelvic muscles relaxing and dropping (similar to the feeling when you begin to urinate). Don't push. Repeat 10 times.

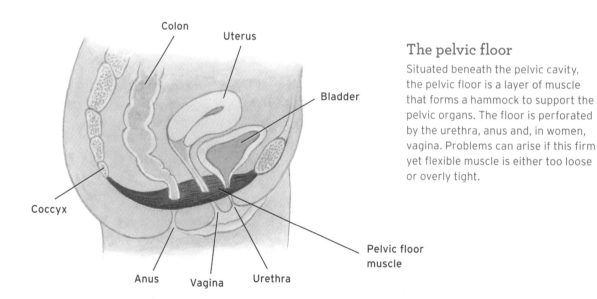

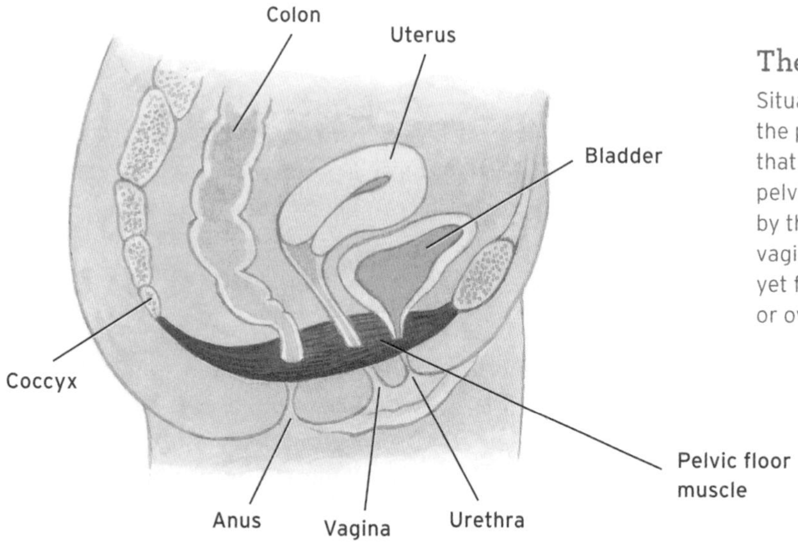

The pelvic floor

Situated beneath the pelvic cavity, the pelvic floor is a layer of muscle that forms a hammock to support the pelvic organs. The floor is perforated by the urethra, anus and, in women, vagina. Problems can arise if this firm yet flexible muscle is either too loose or overly tight.

PEPPERMINT *Mentha x piperita*

use for ✓ ***Bad breath and body odor*** ✓ ***Bronchitis*** ✓ ***Cancer support*** ✓ ***Colds and flu*** ✓ ***Concentration, improved*** ✓ ***Fatigue*** ✓ ***Gall bladder problems*** ✓ ***Headaches*** ✓ ***Indigestion*** ✓ ***Menstrual problems***

PEPPERMINT IS A HYBRID OF THE HERBS spearmint and watermint that was first cultivated near London in 1750. A popular culinary and medicinal herb, its prime therapeutic benefit lies in its ability to ease digestive complaints. It is also a useful inhalant remedy for respiratory problems and has a wide variety of other applications.

How it works

Peppermint contains a volatile essential oil that contains the active ingredients menthol and menthone, which have antiseptic, antispasmodic, digestive, antibacterial, and mildly analgesic (pain-relieving) and sedative properties.

Peppermint has specific effects on the digestive tract and colon, stimulating secretion of gastric juices and bile and helping to expel gas. It blocks contractions of the muscles in the gut wall and thereby eases spasms and griping pain. It is therefore useful for indigestion, nausea, flatulence, bloating, cramping, inflammatory bowel disease and irritable bowel syndrome (IBS). A *British Medical Journal* study concluded that peppermint oil was a more effective treatment for IBS than either antispasmodic medications or a fiber-rich diet.

Peppermint may be helpful in treating gallstones by relieving bile-duct spasm and increasing bile flow. It is also a useful remedy for coughs, colds, headaches, lethargy, anxiety, menstrual cramps, bad breath and burping. An inhalation may benefit a blocked nose or sinusitis.

Diluted and applied topically, the oil may cool and soothe skin irritations such as bites or stings, rashes or minor burns. Applying peppermint oil to the temples can relax muscles, decrease tension, improve concentration and relieve a headache. In one study, it was found to be as effective as paracetamol.

Safety first **Peppermint essential oil should not be taken internally, other than in the dosages in the enteric-coated form.** *Peppermint should be avoided during pregnancy. Do not give peppermint to children under five. Do not use if you are allergic to the Lamiaceae family of plants, which also includes basil, lavender, rosemary and sage.*

Where to find *Peppermint tea and essential oil are available in health food stores; the essential oil and enteric-coated capsules are found in pharmacies; a tincture may be made up for you by a qualified herbalist.*

How to use

Peppermint may be taken as a tea, a tincture, or in enteric-coated capsules, which ensure the oil bypasses the stomach where it can cause irritation and is released in the intestine to relieve irritable bowel symptoms. Follow label instructions or take as professionally prescribed. The essential oil may be used in aromatherapy treatments and inhalations.

PERILLA *Perilla frutescens.* Also called: Shiso, Beefsteak plant, Chinese basil

use for ✓ ***Allergies*** ✓ ***Hay fever***

THE LEAVES AND STALKS OF PERILLA are a popular salad ingredient in Japanese cuisine and are also used to wrap sushi and to color and flavor the pickled plums called umeboshi. The medicinal use of perilla can be traced to ancient China (where it was used as an antidote to fish and crab poisoning). From there it spread to Japan and was incorporated into several of the traditional herbal formulas known as Kampo medicines, which are still in use today. Research studies are starting to back up the herb's reputation as an antiallergy agent—in laboratories and animals, at least.

How it works

Perilla has demonstrated antiallergenic effects in a number of research studies, which indicate that the component rosmarinic acid (also found in rosemary) is responsible for much of its therapeutic benefit. It appears to be particularly relevant to type-1 hypersensitivities (allergies that cause an immediate reaction, rather than a delayed one). However, most scientific research to date has been conducted in laboratories or on animals, and additional clinical studies will be needed before perilla's effects on humans are fully understood.

Safety first *Perilla leaves are considered safe to use in food, but if used directly on the skin it can cause a rash or allergic reaction.*

Perilla has not been widely tested during pregnancy or breastfeeding and so it is best avoided or used only under medical supervision during these periods. Do not use perilla if you are allergic to the Lamiaciae family of plants, which also includes mint, lavender, basil, rosemary and sage.

Where to find *Buy the leaves from Asian grocery stores. The supplements are available in health food stores and from natural health professionals, usually in combination with other antiallergy herbs.*

How to use

Perilla can be bought as leaves for culinary use, and as capsules, tablets and extracts. Choose a product standardized for its content of rosmarinic acid. The supplements are predominantly used for the treatment of hay fever and other allergies. Follow label instructions or take as professionally prescribed.

In one small clinical study, patients with mild seasonal hay fever who took perilla supplements standardized for rosmarinic acid for three weeks were less likely to experience allergy symptoms such as itchy, watery eyes and an itchy nose than those who took a placebo supplement. Their nasal secretions also indicated decreased levels of allergic activity in their bodies.

PET THERAPY

use for ✓ ***Anxiety*** ✓ ***Depression***

THEY'RE CUTE AND OFFER UNCONDITIONAL LOVE. But these are not the only attributes of domestic pets. Research is revealing that companion animals offer big mind-body health benefits to those lucky enough to spend time in their company. Here's the latest on how pet therapy can help you feel better.

How it works

Experts aren't certain why pets have such positive effects on our health, but they've documented many benefits that offer clues. Spending just five minutes with a therapy dog reduced levels of the stress hormone cortisol for 20 health professionals in one Virginia Commonwealth University study. And University of Missouri aging experts say caring for a pet can increase levels of oxytocin, prolactin and norepinephrine, "feel-good" hormones related to joy, nurturing and relaxation. This can certainly ease anxiety and may help give your mood a lift if you have depression.

As well as unconditional love, companion animals provide us with a routine, activity (someone's got to walk the dog) and social interaction—it's natural to chat with friends, neighbors and even strangers about a beloved pet. No wonder a 2011 Miami University study found pet owners to have higher self-esteem and be less lonely than pet-less people.

In another study, dog owners were 54 percent more likely to get recommended amounts of physical activity (30 minutes most days of the week) simply because they walked their four-footed friends regularly. A pet in the house can also help lower your blood pressure and cholesterol levels and reduce your risk for becoming overweight. These effects may be due to petting and stroking your animal's fur, which reduces stress and, in the case of weight loss, simply because having a pet makes you more active.

Safety first *Select a pet according to your preferences and to avoid dander allergies.*

Where to find *Buy your pets from a reputable breeder. A local vet will be able to provide a recommendation. Otherwise, spend time with "borrowed" pets. Ask your doctor where you can access specially trained therapy dogs.*

Getting some pet therapy

If you own a pet, spend time with it—stroking, playing, walking and just enjoying its company. If you or a loved one are spending time in a hospital or nursing home, ask if there's a therapy dog that could pay a visit or an animal-assisted therapy program you can take advantage of. Choose a pet that suits your circumstances: Cats need little exercise and make good companions while dogs need regular daily exercise. If you are unable to keep a pet where you live, consider "pet sitting" for neighbors or walking a neighbor's dog.

Even low-maintenance and "virtual" pets can have benefits. Just gazing at fish swimming in a tank before a dental procedure has been found to reduce pain and lower blood pressure.

PILATES

use for ✓ ***Back and neck pain*** ✓ ***Bursitis and tendonitis***

IF THE WORD "PILATES" CONJURES images of people exercising on equipment that looks like it was cobbled together with old bed springs (among other odd pieces), you're right! The German-born developer of this popular exercise technique, Joseph Pilates, was working in England as a self-defense instructor for Scotland Yard detectives when the First World War broke out in 1914. He was interned during the war, and spent his time refining and teaching his personal fitness regimen—an eclectic mix of yoga, Zen and ancient Greek and Roman exercise.

Late in the war, Pilates was transferred to the Isle of Man as a caretaker for sick and injured internees. There, he rigged up exercise equipment using hospital beds and springs. Today's Pilates equipment uses the same principles: spring tension, straps for hands and feet and supports for back, neck and shoulder, all designed to hold and challenge the body. Pilates later moved to the US, where his method became popular among dancers and slowly gained an international following.

How it works

Pilates routines focus on core strength, stability, flexibility, posture and muscle control. Research suggests it may have special benefits for people with back and neck pain. In several studies, regular Pilates sessions for six to 12 weeks proved superior to home stretching exercises or to inactivity for easing aches and reducing disability. In a Turkish study, women with fibromyalgia got relief after taking three Pilates classes a week for 12 weeks. The therapy may also ease pain and improve mobility for people with bursitis and tendonitis.

Safety first *Pilates is considered safe for most people. Moves can be customized and studios usually offer classes for beginners and for advanced students. Tell the instructor if you are pregnant and mention any medical condition you have.*

Where to find *Pilates studios are easy to find through local information sources such as libraries and health clinics...or visit the United States Pilates Association website at www.unitedstatespilatesassociation.com.*

A Pilates session

The "roll down—roll up" exercise on the opposite page is a typical example, but it's best to learn Pilates in a class or through one-on-one instruction. The exercises require precision and control. Routines are performed on a thick mat as well on specialized Pilates equipment such as the "Reformer"—the machine originally made from a hospital bed!

You'll need to wear comfortable exercise clothing and expect a hands-on experience; a good Pilates instructor will correct your technique by gently adjusting your position with his or her hands.

ROLL DOWN–ROLL UP

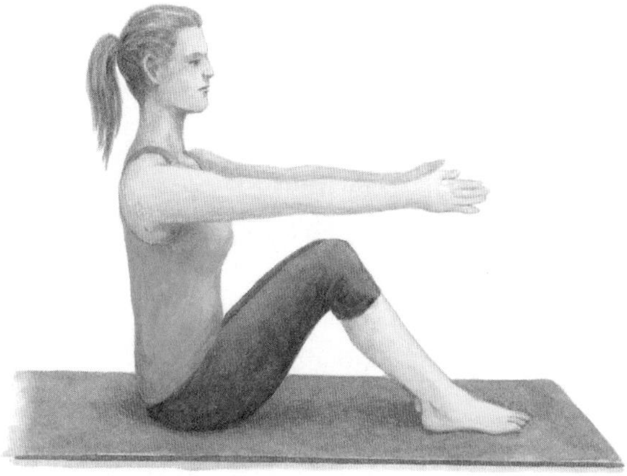

STEP 1 Sit tall on the mat with your knees drawn up, feet flat on the floor in front of you and arms outstretched.

STEP 2 Breathe out as you begin to roll down, curling your lower back in a C shape and drawing your navel to your spine. Keep your feet firmly planted as you roll slowly all the way down. Rest your arms by your sides.

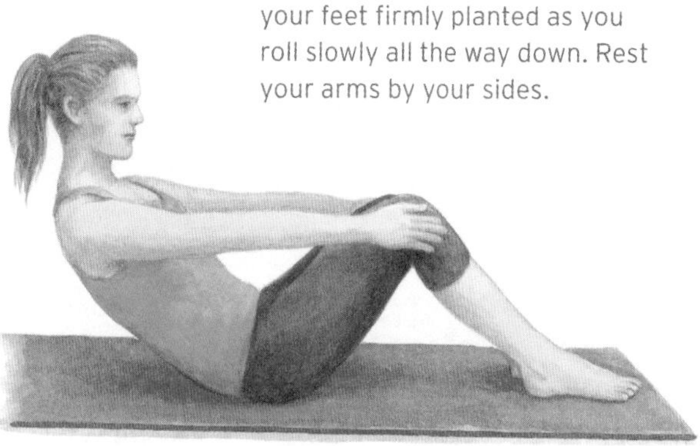

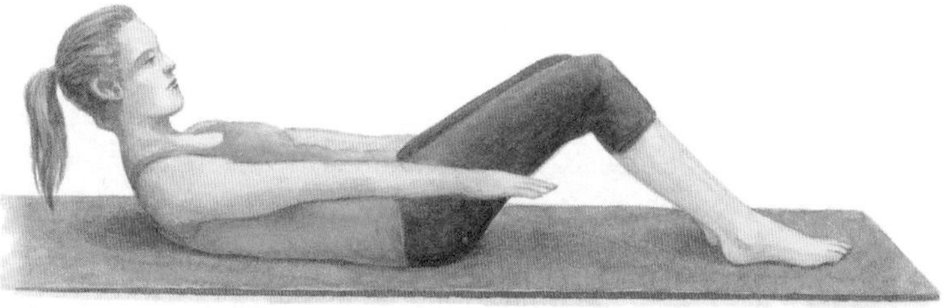

STEP 3 Take a deep breath, filling your lungs and expanding your back. Exhale as you peel yourself off the floor, rolling up as you rolled down, arms outstretched by your sides. Keep your chin tucked in and lift your head first, drawing navel to spine.

STEP 4 Reach your arms forward to rest on your feet and use those hollowed abdominals to hold you in a C curve. Then inhale and lift up from the base of your spine to take up your original position. Do this three times.

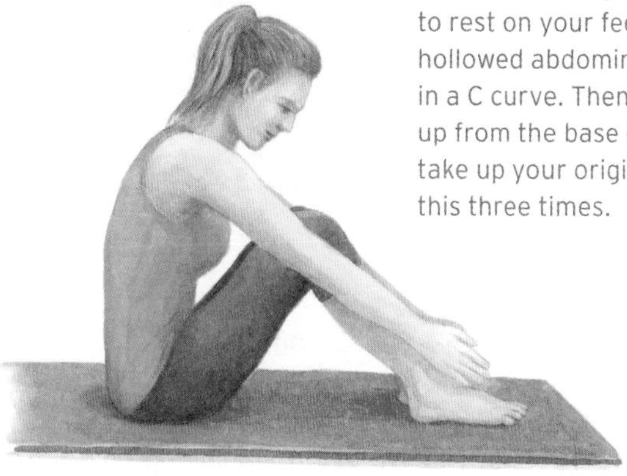

POTASSIUM

use for ✓ ***Cramps, muscle*** ✓ ***Kidney stone prevention***

POTASSIUM HELPS MAINTAIN THE BODY'S water balance, and is required for the healthy functioning of the kidneys, muscles and nerves. It helps to regulate the heartbeat and blood pressure, and is involved in the removal of toxins from the body.

In many countries, the average daily consumption of potassium is lower than recommended, which can increase the risk of health problems such as high blood pressure and stroke. However, in most circumstances it is preferable that you increase your potassium intake by eating more fruits and vegetables such as bananas, apples, oranges, dried apricots, tomatoes and leafy green vegetables, rather than by taking supplements.

How it works

Potassium is an important component of the body fluids and adequate levels must be present in the body to maintain fluid balance and prevent dehydration. It is required for muscle contraction, the conduction of nerve impulses, the maintenance of the heart rhythm and blood pressure, and the balance of acidity and alkalinity in your body.

Potassium levels can be reduced due to poor diet, vomiting, diarrhea, profuse perspiration or the use of certain medications, leading to muscle cramps, weakness and heart problems.

Safety first *Most people don't need to take potassium supplements in quantities greater than those used in multivitamins unless advised to do so by their doctor.*

If you have any form of renal impairment or are taking prescribed medicines, do not increase your intake of potassium except under the advice and supervision of your doctor.

In many instances, increased potassium should be accompanied by a decrease in sodium consumption, ideally to below 2,000 mg/day.

Where to find *Find potassium-rich fruits and vegetables in supermarkets. When required, buy potassium supplements from pharmacies.*

How to use

It's best to get all your potassium needs from your diet. For US adults (19+) an adequate intake (AI) of potassium has been estimated at 4,700 mg/day for men, and 4,700 mg/day for women. In people with high blood pressure, increasing potassium intake may lower blood pressure. Raised consumption of potassium may also have other benefits for heart and cardiovascular health, including reducing stroke risk by as much as 24 percent.

Some medicines (including diuretics sometimes prescribed for blood pressure) can deplete potassium levels, causing muscle cramps. If you are concerned your medication may be contributing to muscle cramps, talk to your doctor, who can determine whether additional potassium is warranted.

If you have a history of calcium oxalate kidney stones, taking a potassium-magnesium citrate supplement could reduce the risk of recurrence by as much as 85 percent. Talk to your doctor to find out whether these supplements are suitable for you.

No upper limits of potassium intake from dietary sources have been established.

PROBIOTICS

use for ✓ ***Bad breath and body odor*** ✓ ***Celiac disease*** ✓ ***Colds and flu*** ✓ ***Constipation*** ✓ ***Diarrhea*** ✓ ***Eczema and dermatitis*** ✓ ***Flatulence*** ✓ ***Food intolerance*** ✓ ***Frequent illness*** ✓ ***Fungal infections*** ✓ ***Gastroenteritis*** ✓ ***Hemorrhoids*** ✓ ***Hay fever*** ✓ ***Inflammatory bowel disease*** ✓ ***Tooth and gum disorders***

DEEP IN YOUR DIGESTIVE SYSTEM, over 100 trillion "good" bugs are hard at work right now digesting the food you eat and converting it into beneficial compounds. This collection of bacteria, known as your microbiome, represents 10 times the total number of cells in your whole body. A growing pile of cutting-edge research suggests that this all-natural "zoo" has a profound effect on your health, promoting good digestion, fighting infection, reducing toxicity, tamping down inflammation and keeping body tissues in good condition.

How they work

Probiotics are collections of beneficial bacteria that can be ingested to improve health. Playing host to plenty of "friendly" bacteria in your gut enables the food you eat to be turned into the nutrients you need including vitamins B and K as well as folate. Good bugs also keep "bad bugs" in check by displacing them, using up their food supply and producing compounds called bacteriocins that limit their growth.

There's evidence that a healthy colony of good bugs within your gut can help protect you from stomach ulcers and gastric flu, lower your odds for urinary tract infections, guard against diarrhea brought on by antibiotic use, boost immunity and even protect against skin, tooth and gum problems caused or worsened by infections and inflammation. In one review of 14 studies, researchers found that taking probiotics reduced the number of colds slightly and led to milder upper respiratory problems.

Meanwhile, there's recent evidence that having a mix of good bacteria on board can help you to control your weight. In a 2014 Canadian study of 125 overweight women, those who took a daily probiotic supplement while following a reduced-calorie diet lost about 10 pounds (4.4 kg) in 12 weeks-compared to about 6 pounds (2.6 kg) for those who dieted but received a placebo. The probiotic pills contained the *Lactobacillus rhamnosus* species, which researchers say is similar to types found in yogurt containing live, active cultures. In another study from Stanford University, probiotics helped people lose more weight after gastric bypass surgery.

Good bugs may even affect your mind. A 2013 report in the journal *Biological Psychiatry* says there's early evidence that they may help improve stress response and boost mood. And they aren't just in your gut. Researchers are currently at work on mouthwashes and lozenges that may one day be used to restore good bacteria in your mouth to promote fresh breath and fight gum disease.

How to use

It's smart to know that your own collection of good bacteria can become depleted by stress, a diet that's low in produce and whole grains, or when you take bacteria-menacing medications such as antibiotics (which wipe out beneficial bacteria while attacking the harmful kind). What's the best way to foster your own personal colony of "friendly" bacteria? One approach is to start with food—then add supplements to address specific situations.

Introduce good bacteria into your digestive system by regularly consuming yogurt or kefir (a fermented milk drink) with live active cultures. You could also try other fermented foods like sauerkraut, kimchee and miso. Look after the good bacteria

continued on page 262

PROBIOTICS *continued*

you've already got by eating foods that contain "prebiotics." These are compounds, such as fructo-oligosaccharides, that the good bacteria feed on. You'll find them in bananas, asparagus, onions and garlic; also, dandelion greens, Jerusalem artichokes and jicama. There are prebiotics in barley, berries, tomatoes, honey and beans, too.

Probiotic supplements include those proven to help guard against antibiotic-related diarrhea such as *Saccharomyces boulardii, Lactobacillus acidophilus, L. casei, L. rhamnosus GG, L. reuteri* and *L. acidophilus*. Taking a supplement aimed at replacing bacteria wiped out by antibiotics may be a good idea if you're using an antibiotic for more than five to 10 days, if you develop diarrhea while using your antibiotic, or if you've had antibiotic-associated diarrhea in the past.

Experts recommend taking a probiotic for no longer than one or two weeks. Follow label directions for the right dose; this can range from one billion to 10 billion colony-forming units (CFU)—the amount contained in a capsule or two. Store your supplements as directed since the bacteria within have to be alive, or freeze-dried, when you take them. Some require refrigeration and many must be kept away from high heat and excess moisture.

Safety first *Probiotics, in food and supplements, are considered safe. But be cautious with young children, the elderly and anyone with weakened immunity.*

Where to find *Foods containing probiotics, as well as supplements, are available in supermarkets and health food stores. Fermented foods, such as kefir, sauerkraut and kimchee, can be made at home with the right starter cultures.*

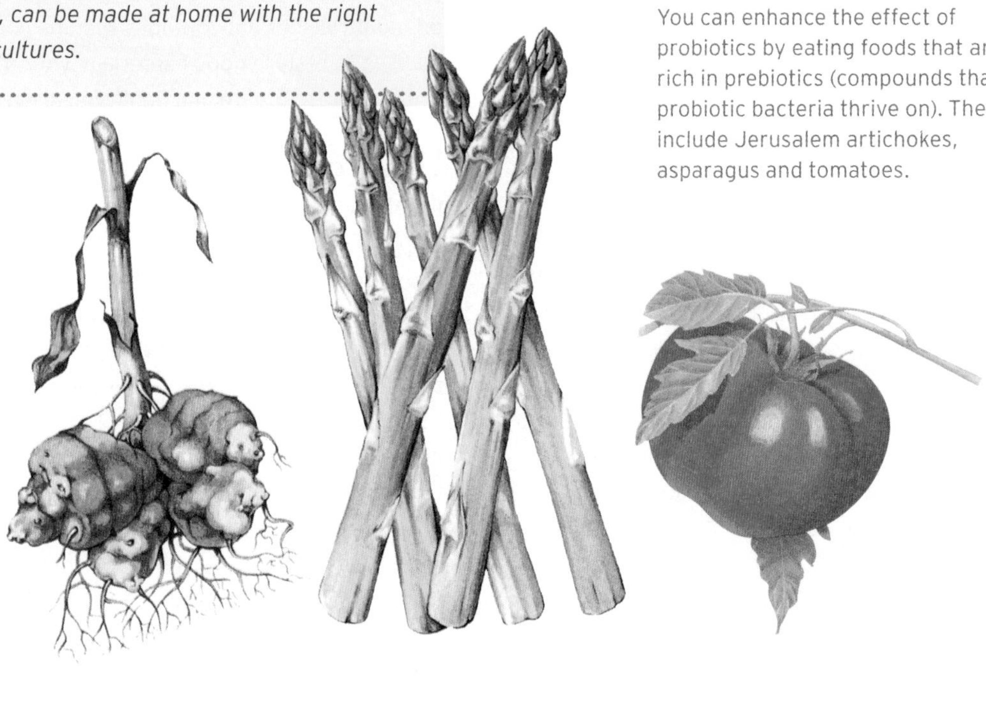

Feeding the good bugs

You can enhance the effect of probiotics by eating foods that are rich in prebiotics (compounds that probiotic bacteria thrive on). These include Jerusalem artichokes, asparagus and tomatoes.

PROPOLIS

use for ✓ ***Fungal infections*** ✓ ***Mouth ulcers*** ✓ ***Tooth and gum disorders***

PROPOLIS IS A RESIN PRODUCED BY BEES, made from beeswax, other bee secretions and the buds and sap of certain trees, including conifers and poplars. Bees use propolis to seal and sterilize the hive, and to boost their immune systems.

Propolis has long been prized by humans for its anti-infective properties, and its medicinal use can be traced back to the ancient Greeks and Assyrians. The ancient Egyptians even used it in the mummification process.

How it works

Laboratory studies have shown that propolis has potent antimicrobial actions against a wide range of microorganisms including those that cause fungal infections, respiratory tract infections and dental cavities. It also has anti-inflammatory and antioxidant effects, and when applied topically, may help to hasten wound healing.

Safety first *Do not use propolis if you are allergic to bees, bee products (including honey), Balsam of Peru, conifers or poplar. Other allergy-prone individuals should also use it with caution, as cross-sensitivity may occur.*

Sensitization to propolis may occur after repeated use, and adverse reactions including skin rash and contact dermatitis can occur. If you think you are having a reaction, discontinue use immediately, and seek medical advice.

Where to find *Propolis products are available in health food stores and some pharmacies.*

How to use

Propolis is available as a resin, liquid and capsules. It is also formulated into mouthwashes, gargles and toothpastes. For the treatment of tooth and gum disorders, fungal infections of the mouth, and to inhibit plaque formation, use a propolis mouthwash twice daily. The resin may also be applied directly to affected areas of the mouth. Research suggests that using propolis extract in conjunction with conventional dental treatment for chronic periodontitis is more effective than the standard treatment alone.

If you have recurrent mouth ulcers (recurrent aphthous stomatitis), taking propolis capsules may help to reduce the frequency of outbreaks.

Topical applications of propolis may also be beneficial for herpes infections and to promote wound healing. Follow label instructions or take as professionally prescribed.

PSYLLIUM *Plantago ovata, P. psyllium, P. arenaria, P. ispaghula*

use for ✓ ***Cholesterol, high*** ✓ ***Constipation*** ✓ ***Diabetes and insulin resistance***
✓ ***Diarrhea*** ✓ ***Hemorrhoids*** ✓ ***Heart and circulatory health***
✓ ***Irritable bowel syndrome***

EACH PSYLLIUM PLANT PRODUCES up to 15,000 seeds, which are the richest known grain source of soluble fiber, most of which is concentrated in the husks. The name is derived from the Greek word *psylla*, which means flea, a reference to its diminutive size, also reflected in its traditional English name, fleaseed.

How it works

The therapeutic effects of psyllium occur because the soluble fiber it contains forms a thick, mucilaginous gel when it comes into contact with water or other fluids. When consumed, the gel moves through the digestive tract, where its bulk and absorbent characteristics have a number of beneficial effects. As well as forming stools that are soft and easy to pass, the soluble fiber in psyllium slows down the absorption of glucose and so helps to regulate blood glucose levels. It also helps to lower cholesterol, in part by binding to it and promoting its excretion in the faeces.

Safety first *Always take psyllium with a couple of glasses of water or juice; do not take it dry. Some people experience abdominal discomfort when initially taking psyllium. This can be minimized by starting with a low dose and building up to the recommended dose over time.*

Take psyllium at least two hours after taking prescribed medicines and any supplements, as it may interfere with their absorption.

Do not take psyllium if you have a bowel obstruction, colonic impaction or gastro-intestinal stenosis.

Where to find *Psyllium products are available in supermarkets, health food stores and pharmacies.*

How to use

Psyllium increases faecal bulk, softens hard stools and eases their passage through the bowel, relieving constipation and associated conditions such as hemorrhoids and constipation-dominant irritable bowel syndrome. It can also add firmness to stools that are too loose, and decrease the frequency of bowel motions in diarrhea.

Psyllium lowers total and LDL ("bad") cholesterol, but does not appear to affect triglycerides or HDL ("good") cholesterol. Other benefits of psyllium for heart health include the ability to enhance weight loss by helping to create sensations of fullness, as well as improving blood glucose levels in people with diabetes and insulin resistance.

Psyllium husks come as a powder to add to water or in capsules. Follow label instructions or take as professionally prescribed.

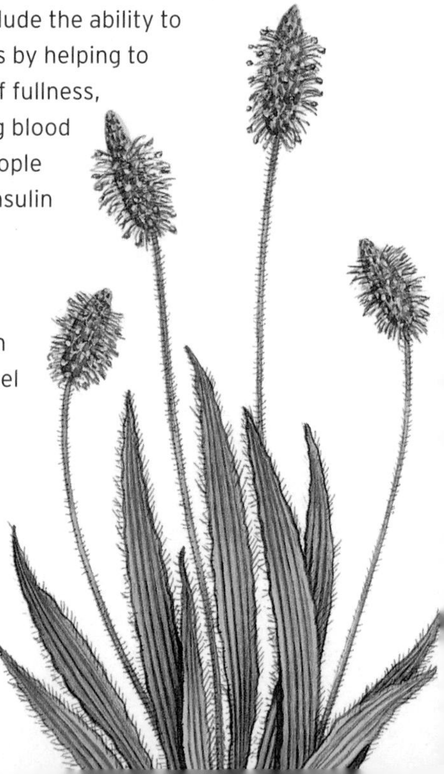

PYGEUM *Pygeum africanum*

use for ✓ ***Prostate problems***

IN THE 18TH CENTURY EUROPEAN TRAVELERS to Africa were introduced to the bark of a tall, mountain-loving evergreen called inyazangoma-elimnyama by the Zulu people. Its claim to fame: a cure for the bladder discomforts of "old man's disease," or as it is more correctly termed, benign prostatic hyperplasia (BPH). Today, the reddish-brown bark of *Pygeum africanum* is widely used to ease BPH, the common, noncancerous prostate-gland enlargement that causes urine retention, slow flow and nighttime visits to the bathroom.

While this herbal remedy has a good safety record, the tree it comes from has not always been safe. Overharvesting of bark in the wild killed tens of thousands of these handsome trees annually in the 1990s; pygeum became an endangered species in 1998. Since then, international trading of this popular remedy is now monitored under the Convention on International Trade in Endangered Species of Wild Fauna and Flora.

How it works

Pygeum contains inflammation-soothing compounds called phytosterols as well as ursolic and oleanic acids that reduce swelling. These and other active constituents reduce bladder sensitivity (which reduces urination urges) and help the bladder to empty more efficiently.

In a 2002 review of well-designed studies of pygeum for BPH, researchers from the Minneapolis Veterans Affairs Center for Chronic Disease Outcomes Research noted that studies show men who used it were twice as likely to get relief, when compared to men who received a placebo. Nighttime urination episodes fell by 19 percent, urine retention dropped by 24 percent and peak urine flow increased by 23 percent.

How to use

Pygeum is sold as powdered bark, in capsules and as a liquid extract. For symptoms of BPH, experts recommend choosing a product that is a lipophilic extract standardized to contain 14 percent triterpenes and 0.5 percent n-docosanol. It is also an ingredient in some combination herbal formulas for prostate health. Follow label instructions or take as professionally prescribed.

Safety first *Pygeum is considered safe for most men for use for up to one year (the length of the longest research study). Occasional side effects include diarrhea, constipation, dizziness, gastric pain and visual disturbance.*

Where to find *Look for pygeum in health food stores or buy from a qualified herbalist.*

QIGONG

use for ✓ ***Blood pressure, high*** ✓ ***Cancer support*** ✓ ***Depression*** ✓ ***Fall prevention***

USED IN CHINA FOR THOUSANDS OF YEARS to boost fitness and stamina, qigong is a collection of flowing, dance-like exercises that combine breathing, meditation and specific postures to strengthen your life force or *qi* (pronounced *chee*). It is common to see hundreds of older adults practicing qigong early in the morning in parks throughout China—and for good reason. Similar to **tai chi** *(p. 290)*, this gentle exercise has proven mind-body benefits.

How it works

By combining calm, controlled breathing with gentle exercise and mindful concentration, qigong reduces stress and improves physical fitness. Traditional practitioners would say that this time-tested practice has more profound effects by improving the flow of life energy (*qi*) through the body. Recent research reveals a wide range of benefits, including improved strength and stamina, reduced risk of falling, improved mood and physical function in arthritis sufferers, better immunity and relief from depression and anxiety. People with fibromyalgia may experience reduced pain and fatigue, while cancer survivors and those undergoing cancer treatment have reported less anxiety and tiredness after practicing qigong. It has also been associated with better breathing, strength and quality of life for people with chronic obstructive pulmonary disease (COPD), improved sleep, reduced blood pressure and more.

Safety first *Qigong is very safe and people of all ages and fitness levels can benefit. But it is worth checking first with your doctor if you are pregnant or have a serious medical condition.*

Where to find *Look for qigong classes in your community and for videos and DVDs online.*

Qigong exercises

Qigong routines are simple, gentle and flowing—like a slow-motion dance. "Feeling the flow of *qi*" on the opposite page is good for relaxation. However, to gain the most benefit from qigong, it is best to learn in a class or from a video or DVD. Every exercise incorporates three elements: posture, breathing techniques and mental focus on the movement of *qi* through the body.

FEELING THE FLOW OF *QI*

BREATH, MOVEMENT AND *QI* Stand erect but relaxed with your feet pointing forwards and knees slightly bent. Relax your shoulders and let your arms hang by your sides (1). Imagine that your feet are rooted into the earth. Now position your hands as if cradling a ball and rest them in front of your body about three finger widths below your navel (2). This region is your *Dantian*, the place where *qi* is stored in the body. But according to qigong, *qi* is all around us and we can connect with the abundant *qi*. Taking a slow, deep breath in, begin to raise your hands. Imagine you are pulling *qi* up from the earth through your legs and body (3). Keep moving your hands to chest height then turn palms so they face the ground (4). Breathing out slowly, lower your hands and imagine the *qi* going back down through your body. Pause when your hands are level with your *Dantian* (5). Repeat the up and down movement several more times, focusing on feeling the *qi* moving through your body.

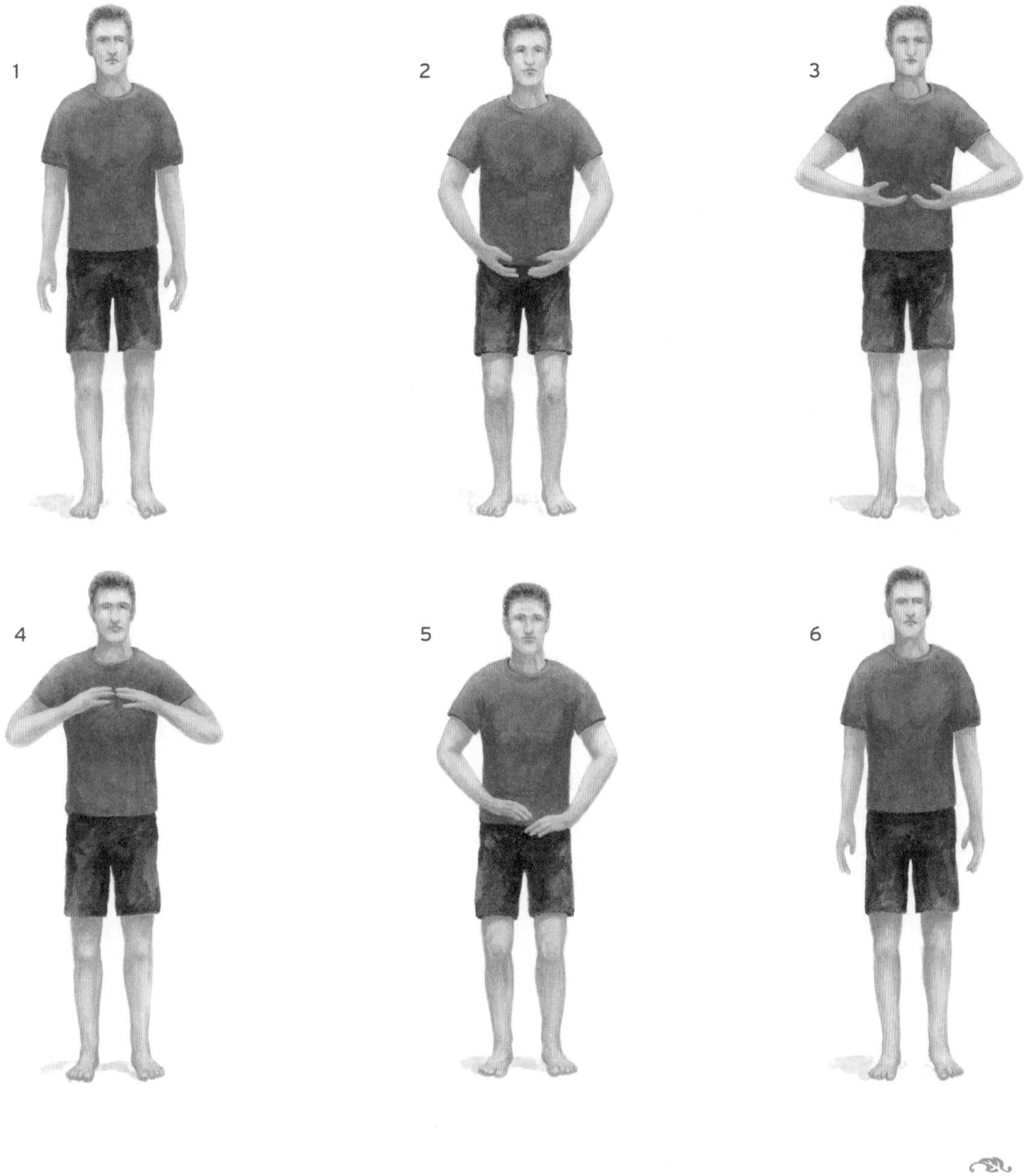

RED YEAST RICE

use for ✓ ***Cholesterol, high***

A TRADITIONAL INGREDIENT IN PEKING DUCK, red rice vinegar and other Chinese delicacies, red yeast rice has also emerged as a popular—and controversial—alternative remedy for high cholesterol. Made from a strain of yeast called *Monascus purpureus* that's grown on rice and then pulverized, red yeast rice (RYR) has been used in traditional Chinese medicine for more than 1,000 years to improve digestion and vitality.

In the late 1970s, pharmaceutical researchers made an amazing discovery: A compound in red yeast rice called monacolin K was identical to lovastatin, a cholesterol-lowering medication then in development. Cholesterol-clobbering statins hit the market in the late 1980s and have become one of the world's blockbuster drugs, while red yeast rice has been relegated to a dietary supplement that naturally contains varying amounts of a pharmaceutical drug.

How it works

Monacolin K works like other statins to reduce cholesterol by blocking a liver enzyme called HMG-CoA reductase that controls cholesterol production in the body. In studies using supplements with standardized levels of monacolin K, red yeast rice has been shown to reduce levels of heart-threatening LDL cholesterol by 10–33 percent in eight to 12 weeks. But because RYR supplements contain an ingredient that's classified as a drug, the US Food and Drug Administration (FDA) in 2007 ordered three supplement purveyors to stop marketing red yeast rice products containing monacolin K.

The FDA cited concerns that monacolin K could cause the same serious, though extremely rare, side effect as lovastatin: muscle damage leading to kidney problems. RYR is still available as a food and as supplements although the quality of supplements and levels of monacolin K vary widely.

Safety first *Talk to your doctor before taking RYR and skip it if you're pregnant or breastfeeding or have kidney or liver disease. Do not use if you're taking cholesterol-lowering medications, the antibiotics erythromycin and Biaxin, the antidepressant Serzone or medications to suppress immunity or fight fungal infections.*

Where to find *RYR is sometimes sold in health food stores or you may need to ask your doctor to prescribe it.*

How to use

RYR is sold in capsules and also as an extract called xuezhikang. While studies continue to show that RYR supplements can reduce cholesterol, it's important to know that RYR contains a natural form of a statin drug and it is best to find a brand with standardized levels. If you decide to use red yeast rice, tell your doctor and see your doctor if you notice any unusual muscle aches, pains or fatigue.

RELAXATION

use for ✓ ***Anxiety*** ✓ ***Asthma*** ✓ ***Blood pressure, high*** ✓ ***Eye disorders*** ✓ ***Frequent illness*** ✓ ***Headaches*** ✓ ***Heart and circulatory health*** ✓ ***Inflammatory bowel disease*** ✓ ***Jet lag*** ✓ ***Neuralgia*** ✓ ***Phobias*** ✓ ***Sleeping problems*** ✓ ***Stroke prevention*** ✓ ***Tinnitus***

STRESS IS A NORMAL REACTION TO ANY real or perceived threat that activates the ancient "fight-or-flight" response. A certain amount of stress is necessary for an active life as it motivates us and stimulates creativity and learning. However, when stress becomes overwhelming, or is continuous with no relief, it can be harmful to our health and well-being. Learning how to relax can be a useful tool to alleviate stress and associated symptoms such as anxiety, sleeping problems and chest pain. Regular relaxation can even help boost your immune system, bolstering your resilience to illness.

How it works

Collapsing in front of the TV after a hard day does little to reduce the damaging impact of stress. To achieve this, it is essential to activate the body's natural relaxation response. Most relaxation techniques use the breath to balance the mind and body and involve slow, deep breathing, which helps to lower blood pressure and promote feelings of calm. When under stress, our mind races and we tend to take shallow breaths, not utilizing the full capacity of the lungs. Deep, abdominal breathing allows the lungs to be completely filled and emptied with each breath, providing more oxygen to the body and removing the waste products of metabolism. This full and efficient oxygen exchange slows the heart rate and stabilizes blood pressure, while also serving to quiet the mind.

Some techniques work by focusing on each muscle and consciously relaxing it. Other techniques evoke the power of the mind such as guided visualization. This is similar to inducing a vivid daydream and is a variation on meditation. It employs the senses to take you to a calm and peaceful place in which you can let go of tension and anxiety.

Relaxation techniques

Consider your specific needs when choosing a relaxation technique: what you are comfortable doing, your fitness level and how you react to stress. Pick a technique that suits your lifestyle. If you become angry or agitated when you are stressed try something that soothes the emotions such as deep breathing or guided imagery. If stress leaves you depressed or withdrawn, stimulate your nervous system through rhythmic exercise.

Mind-body systems like **qigong** *(p. 266)*, **Tai chi** *(p. 290)* and **yoga** *(p. 316)* may be particularly helpful. **Meditation** *(p. 234)*, including a practice called "mindfulness" that aims to change the way we think about experiences, is another well-known route to relaxation. Even simply sitting down and listening to a favorite piece of **music** *(p. 241)* can help reduce stress.

Breathing techniques

There are several breathing techniques that can be used to relieve anxiety and help you relax. Diaphragmatic, or abdominal breathing, is done with one hand on the chest and the other on the stomach, either lying on your back or sitting comfortably. Take a deep breath in through the nose, feeling your stomach moving out against one hand and stretching the lungs. Tighten your stomach muscles, letting them fall inward as you exhale through pursed lips, the hand on your chest remaining still. Practice this for five to 10 minutes three or four times a day.

continued on page 270

RELAXATION *continued*

As well as relieving stress, it helps to strengthen the diaphragm, which could alleviate chronic obstructive pulmonary disease and improve heart health. Another breathing technique, the Papworth method, has been used to reduce symptoms of anxiety and asthma. The technique emphasizes breathing through the nose and developing a breathing pattern to suit a particular situation.

A third breathing technique, the Buteyko method, is said to relieve the symptoms arising from anxiety (and many other health problems). The strategy involves specialized breathing exercises, which are taught through classes over four to five days.

Guided imagery

Directed by a coach, therapist or even a recording, you will be encouraged to breathe deeply while focusing on pleasant, positive images that replace negative thoughts. It can be tried anywhere that you can sit or lie comfortably and close your eyes. Guided imagery—or visualization—uses the power of the imagination. It is based on the idea that our body and mind are connected. So, if we use all our senses our body will respond as if what we are imagining is real. So if we imagine, for example, that we are on a tropical beach, this could induce a relaxed state that helps us to calm our emotions and thoughts. The technique has been used to reduce blood pressure, achieve goals, such as losing weight or quitting smoking, to manage pain and promote healing.

Safety first *No known risks are associated with relaxation techniques, apart from falling asleep—so don't attempt any while driving or operating heavy machinery.*

Where to find *Check online for more information about relaxation techniques. For methods that involve a therapist, seek out one that is qualified via your country's register of accredited practitioners. To find a registered Buteyko practitioner, contact the international Buteyko Institute of Breathing and Health (www.buteyko.info). The Biofeedback Certification International Alliance (www.bcia.org) oversees standards for this technique.*

Progressive muscle relaxation

This is a two-step process during which you systematically tense and relax different muscle groups in the body. Most methods start at the feet and work upward toward the face, although this is not essential.

Wearing loose clothing and sitting comfortably, spend a few minutes breathing deeply to relax. Then, slowly tense the muscles in, say, your right foot, squeezing them tightly and holding for a count of 10. As you allow your foot to relax, focus on the tension flowing away. Then begin again with your left foot, moving gradually up through the body. Allow about 15 minutes to complete this exercise. This technique is thought to alleviate a number of ailments, including ulcers, insomnia and hypertension.

Biofeedback

Used by therapists to help stroke victims regain movement and anxious clients to relax, biofeedback is also used to treat migraines, disorders of the digestive system, Raynaud's disease and incontinence. During a session, electrodes attached to the skin send signals to a monitor, which beeps, flashes or displays an image when your heart and breathing rate, blood pressure, skin temperature, sweating or muscle activity increase, signifying stress. The therapist will suggest relaxation exercises to reduce these bodily reactions, giving you instant feedback on the screen so that your body learns how to relax. Each session lasts about 30 minutes and benefits are usually noticed within 10 sessions or fewer.

ROSE HIPS *Rosa* spp. Also called: Rose haws, Rose heps

use for ✓ ***Osteoarthritis*** ✓ ***Rheumatoid arthritis***

ONCE ITS STUNNING BLOOMS HAVE faded, the rose bush has more to offer in the form of its fruits, or "hips." The plump red seedpods make an ornamental feature in the garden and can be used to make jam, wine and tea. They also have a long history of medicinal applications based on their high vitamin C content and other active constituents.

How they work

Rose hips have long been used to treat colds and flu symptoms and are a common ingredient in herbal tonics, used during illness and convalescence to speed recovery. These nutritional pods are said to contain more than 60 times the amount of vitamin C found in the equivalent amount of citrus fruit, although some of this goodness can be lost when the hips are processed.

Safety first *Some mild side effects could result from the taking of rose hips, including constipation or diarrhea, nausea, heartburn, stomach cramps or headaches. Taking rose hips has not been widely tested during pregnancy or breastfeeding so they are best avoided or used only under medical supervision during these periods. Avoid if you have an allergy to roses or plants of the Rosaceae family.*

Where to find *Available in a garden near you every autumn, rose hips can also be bought as a powder or as dried fruits from a qualified herbalist. In tablet form or as a tea they can be found in health food stores.*

In addition to vitamin C, the fruits contain polyphenols, anthocyanins and a special lipid called galactolipid, which has anti-inflammatory actions and is thought to relieve joint inflammation and reduce joint damage in arthritis sufferers. In trials, a standardized powder made from the wild dog rose *(R. canina)* was found to be effective in relieving pain resulting from osteoarthritis and rheumatoid arthritis. Other studies have found that the hips can reduce the production of an enzyme responsible for the breakdown of cartilage.

How to use

Most tests into the effectiveness of rosehips in natural remedies involve the use of rosehip powder produced from *R. canina*. Follow label instructions or take as professionally prescribed. Rose hips can also be used in teas, jams, jellies and soups. Great care must be taken in the preparation of rose hips, as many of the valuable nutrients can be destroyed during drying and processing.

ROSEMARY *Rosmarinus officinalis*

use for ✓ ***Colds and flu*** ✓ ***Memory problems***

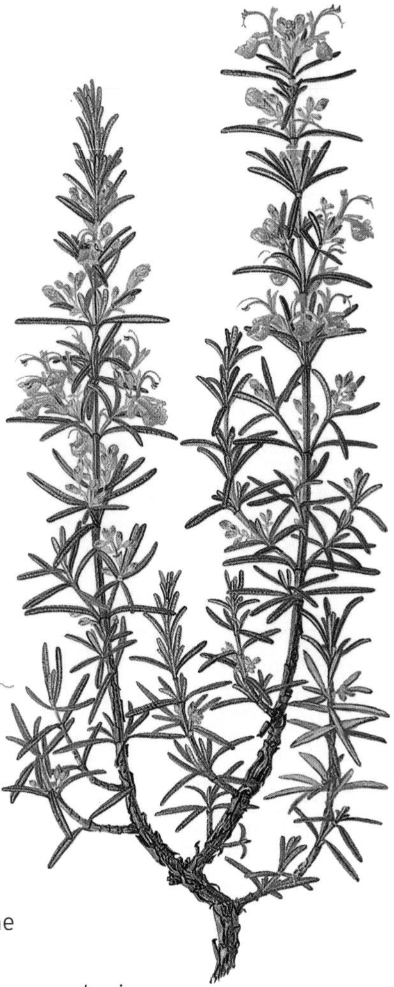

"THERE'S ROSEMARY, THAT'S for remembrance; pray, love, remember." So said Shakespeare's Ophelia, mourning the loss of her love in *Hamlet*. The Tudors were confident that this woody, perennial herb with needlelike leaves and small white, pink, purple or blue flowers enhanced the memory. Modern research concurs. In tests, patients who inhaled rosemary essential oil significantly increased their chances of remembering things. Their ability to do mental arithmetic also improved and they appeared more alert.

Other traditional uses include relieving indigestion, treating bronchial infections and as a general tonic. An aromatic member of the mint family, rosemary is a staple on the herb rack and is used to flavor lamb, chicken, game, fish and bean dishes or bread.

How it works

Compounds in rosemary have been shown to improve long-term memory by inhibiting enzymes that would normally block certain brain functions. Studies have also found that people left in a rosemary-scented room had higher levels of 1,8-cineole in their blood, a chemical that has been shown to have anti-inflammatory and analgesic (pain-relieving) properties as well as improving the memory.

The herb may also improve brain function by stimulating healthy blood flow to brain tissue and cleansing the blood. And rosemary is said to prevent the degradation of acetylcholine, a brain chemical that maintains proper memory and cognitive acuity.

Safety first **Rosemary essential oil should not be taken internally.** *Fresh or dried rosemary is safe to eat in food or as a tea. Taking large amounts of rosemary can cause stomach upset, vomiting and interact with medications.*

The herb has not been widely tested during pregnancy or breastfeeding so it is best avoided or used only under medical supervision during these periods.

Do not use rosemary if you are allergic to the Lamiaciae family of plants, which includes basil, mint, lavender and sage.

Where to find *Rosemary is easy to grow or buy it fresh or dried in the supermarket. Rosemary essential oil and extract are available in health food stores or from a qualified herbalist.*

How to use

Rosemary leaves can be eaten fresh or dried in a multitude of dishes. It can be taken as a tea after steeping a teaspoon (5 ml) of dried herb in boiling water for 10 minutes. Drink up to three times a day.

A few drops of rosemary essential oil can be used in a burner and inhaled gently. Rosemary extract is also available as capsules. Follow label instructions or take as professionally prescribed.

SAGE *Salvia officinalis.* Also called: Garden sage, Common sage

use for ✓ ***Memory problems*** ✓ ***Menopausal symptoms***

ACCORDING TO 17TH-CENTURY HERBALIST Nicholas Culpeper: "Sage heals the memory, warming and quickening the senses." This plant has a long history of use in both the kitchen and medicine cabinet. It has been used since ancient times to treat snakebites, increase a woman's fertility and even to ward off evil.

Sage has long been considered to have healing properties. In Austria, it was traditionally chewed or drunk as tea to treat disorders of the mouth, respiratory tract, gastrointestinal tract and skin. Modern research suggests it can be used as an antiperspirant or antifungal agent, antibiotic, astringent and more.

The strongest active constituents—including the anti-inflammatory compounds cineole, borneol and thujone—are found in sage essential oil, while the leaf also contains tannic acid, flavonoids, glycosides and estrogenic substances, which could regulate hormonal change and ease the night sweats associated with the menopause.

How it works

Much like rosemary, to which it is related, sage has long been believed to boost memory. Now these properties are being researched to see whether the herb could be used as a treatment for Alzheimer's disease or dementia. In tests, it was demonstrated that sage inhibits an enzyme called acetylcholinesterase, which breaks down acetylcholine, a brain chemical that has an important role in memory.

Research has shown that sage has benefited women experiencing light or infrequent menstruation, or who are failing to menstruate at all, due to its estrogenic activity. The herb's estrogenic substance is thought to constitute up to 2 percent of the dried plant. Sage's antihydrotic, or antiperspirant, action is a useful ally against night sweats suffered by women during the menopause.

How to use

Sage is usually used as fresh leaves or in tablet or capsule form. It is also available as dried leaves, liquid extracts or as a tea. Follow label instructions or take as professionally prescribed.

Safety first **Sage essential oil should not be taken internally.** *Most providers suggest taking a sage supplement internally for no more than two to four weeks at a time. Check with your doctor.*

Sage has not been widely tested during pregnancy or breastfeeding so it is best avoided or used only under medical supervision during these periods.

Do not use sage if you are allergic to the Lamiaciae family of plants, which also includes basil, mint and lavender.

Where to find *Sage is easy to grow or you can buy the herb in supermarkets. Supplements and sage essential oil are available in health food stores or from a qualified herbalist.*

ST. JOHN'S WORT *Hypericum perforatum*

use for ✓ ***Depression*** ✓ ***Eczema and dermatitis***

A NATIVE OF EUROPE, THIS HERB is named after St. John the Baptist as it is usually in bloom on his birthday, June 24. The yellow-flowering wild herb has been taken medicinally and applied to wounds since ancient times. In the Middle Ages, it was used for casting out evil spirits: "St. John's wort doth charm all the witches away, if gathered at midnight on the saint's holy day," begins one old English poem. Still renowned for its positive effect on mood, the herb is widely used to treat mild depression. Scientific research supports this and some other traditional uses.

How it works

Preparations of St. John's wort are generally standardized to include its two most active ingredients, hypericin and hyperforin. Like some common antidepressant medications, both substances appear to boost levels of certain neurotransmitters, chemicals that relay signals in the brain, by preventing nerve cells from reabsorbing them. Low levels of neurotransmitters such as serotonin are thought to be one factor that triggers depression. A 2008 *Cochrane Review* of 29 trials involving 5,489 patients found that St. John's wort was superior to a placebo treatment for patients with major depression and as effective as standard antidepressants with fewer side effects.

Constituents such as hypericin and hyperforin also have an anti-inflammatory, antioxidant and antibacterial action. In scientific research, topical preparations of St. John's wort have shown promise in the treatment of atopic dermatitis, and also burns, bed sores and other wounds.

How to use

Taken internally, St. John's wort is generally used to treat mild depression, seasonal affective disorder (SAD) and anxiety. It is available as capsules, tablets, in liquid extract form or as a tea.

St. John's wort creams and lotions are available for topical use. In all forms, follow label instructions or take as professionally prescribed. St. John's wort preparations can differ in their activity and it is best to take standardized preparations to treat depression. Check with your doctor.

Safety first *Consult your doctor before using St. John's wort if you are taking any other medications as the herb is known to interact with many pharmaceuticals. It can enhance the effect of antidepressants and reduce the efficacy of other medicines including statins, antihistamines, oral contraceptives, blood thinners such as warfarin, as well as HIV and antipsychotic medications. Creams and lotions can make the skin more sensitive to the sun.*

Where to find *St. John's wort products are available in health food stores, some pharmacies or from a qualified herbalist.*

SALT WATER

use for ✓ ***Bad breath and body odor*** ✓ ***Cuts and scrapes***

SALT IS A MINERAL SUBSTANCE composed mainly of sodium chloride, and it is essential for human life. There is evidence of salt processing dating back around 6,000 years, and it is almost certainly the oldest and most commonly used food seasoning as well as being an important means of preserving fresh produce.

The modern diet often contains more salt than we need. This can raise our blood pressure and puts us at increased risk of health problems such as heart disease and stroke. World Health Organization guidelines suggest adults should consume less than a teaspoon (no more than 5 g) of salt a day. Although salt has a bad name in dietary terms, it remains a useful natural remedy when dissolved in water and used topically.

How it works

Gargling salt water helps to wash away mucus that protects bacteria and many bacteria, especially *Streptococci* and other mouth-dwelling organisms, are sensitive to salt, which damages or destroys them by drawing out their water content leaving them dehydrated. This makes salt a useful ally against gum disease and the bad breath that goes with it.

Salt water is a natural disinfectant, making it an excellent short-term treatment for wounds in the mouth and a useful alternative to commercial mouthwashes, many of which contain high levels of alcohol. Salt's antibacterial and disinfectant properties also mean it is a useful ally against the harmful bacteria that cause infection in cuts, wounds, animal bites and burns.

Regular salt scrubs will prevent body odor by neutralizing odor-causing bacteria on the skin, while an isotonic saline solution that has a similar concentration of salt as body tissues can be used to rinse the mouth, eyes or wounds without irritating sensitive or exposed tissue.

Safety first *A saltwater mouthwash can disguise chronic bad breath but it is important to consult a dentist if the problem continues. Salt water should not be used as a mouthwash for long periods as its high acidity level can damage tooth enamel. If cuts and wounds do not start to clear after three days of cleaning with salt water, consult your doctor.*

Where to find *Salt is sold in supermarkets. Sterile isotonic saline solutions are sold in pharmacies and health food stores.*

How to use

To treat small wounds, bathe in a warm, saltwater solution of 2 teaspoons (10 ml) of table salt to 4 cups (1 L) of water. Alternatively, apply a warm, wet cloth soaked in the solution for 20 minutes three times a day. This will help keep the wound clean and clear mild infections.

To prepare a saltwater mouthwash or gargle, add 1/2 teaspoon (2 ml) of salt to a glass of warm water. A salt scrub to treat body odor is easy to make and it can rejuvenate tired skin. Pour a good, cold-pressed vegetable or nut oil over a cup of natural sea salt and then add 5 drops of a favorite essential oil such as lavender or rose oil. Apply to the skin in the shower, using a gentle circular motion, then rinse off.

SAMe (S-adenosylmethionine)

use for ✓ ***Depression*** ✓ ***Osteoarthritis***

SAMe IS A SUBSTANCE THAT IS FOUND naturally in all cells in the body. It is formed from the amino acid methionine, found in protein-rich foods. The key to its usefulness is that it is one of the best "methyl donors," meaning that it easily donates its methyl group to other molecules—an important step in numerous reactions in the body.

How it works

The process of methylation, whereby a SAMe molecule donates its methyl group to other substances, is involved with reducing inflammation and protecting against free radical damage, especially in the brain and joints. SAMe is thought to improve memory, and so may be of benefit to Alzheimer's patients. Research also suggests a link between low levels of SAMe and increased likelihood of neurodegeneration in patients with Parkinson's disease. According to a *Clinical Chemistry* study, brain power is improved when levels of SAMe are higher.

Research generally supports SAMe as a safe and effective antidepressant with few side effects, and one that starts to work quickly, usually within a week. A review from the University of Pittsburgh suggested that, along with omega-3 fatty acids, SAMe was an effective remedy for some forms of depression. Another review, published in the *American Journal of Psychiatry*, found it a valuable adjunct therapy for patients with major depressive disorders who had not responded to serotonin reuptake inhibitor medication. A *Journal of Clinical Psychopharmacology* study showed that antidepressant medications were of greater benefit when combined with SAMe than when used alone.

SAMe also helps regenerate and protect cartilage and so may be beneficial for disorders of the joints and connective tissues, including osteoarthritis and fibromyalgia. One study, published in the *American Journal of Medicine*, found that SAMe was as effective as ibuprofen in treating symptoms of arthritis such as morning stiffness, pain during movement and swelling. SAMe may also protect liver function: Not only does it help decrease blood alcohol levels by inducing liver enzymes, but high SAMe levels have also been linked with a lower incidence of a variety of liver disorders.

Safety first *Occasionally, high doses of SAMe may result in nausea or gastrointestinal upset. Although SAMe is considered safe and has no known side effects, if you have been diagnosed with severe depression or bipolar disorder, do not cease taking prescribed medication or start to take SAMe in conjunction with other antidepressant medications without consulting your doctor. SAMe has not been widely tested during pregnancy or breastfeeding so it is best avoided or used only under medical supervision during these periods.*

Where to find *SAMe supplements are available in pharmacies, health food stores or from a qualified naturopath.*

How to use

SAMe is available in tablet or capsule form. It is often sold in formulations where it is combined with vitamins B_6 and B_{12} and folic acid, which are thought to have synergistic effects. Follow label instructions, or take as professionally prescribed.

SAUNA

use for ✓ ***Heart and circulatory health***

"SAUNA" IS THE ONLY FINNISH WORD to have made it into everyday spoken English. Promoted as a form of relaxation, meditation and physical cleansing, this relaxing bathing ritual has been performed across Finland for thousands of years. A sauna is a small, wooden room that produces dry heat up to 158°F (70°F). Modern saunas use either a small stove that heats a pile of rocks that, in turn, heat the air inside the sauna or special infrared heaters that produce far infrared radiation.

How it works

Sitting in the heat of a sauna, the body quickly sets about controling its temperature. The heart begins to beat a little faster, while the blood vessels and capillaries dilate bringing blood to the surface of the skin (so you appear flushed) and you begin to sweat. During a 15–30 minute session a person will shed about 4 cups (1 L) of sweat.

Sweating, like urinating, is a form of excretion, ridding the body of waste and toxins. When the body sweats deeply, the skin is cleansed and dead skin cells are replaced. The production of sweat also flushes bacteria out of the epidermal layer and sweat ducts.

Research has shown that having a sauna is good for your heart and circulation, too. During a sauna the cardiovascular system is given a gentle workout and peripheral blood vessels are dilated and flushed without the buildup of metabolic waste products that occurs with other forms of exercise. Researchers in Japan found that patients with congestive heart failure who took a sauna regularly showed a significant decrease in blood pressure and their heart's ability to pump blood improved, as did their tolerance to exercise and oxygen uptake.

Other conditions that could benefit from a sauna are chronic fatigue, mild depression, rheumatoid arthritis, musculoskeletal pain and skin conditions.

How to use

Naked is best, although a towel or swimsuit can be worn. Before entering the sauna, take a shower to remove any chemicals from your skin, then towel yourself dry. Ensure you are well hydrated before you start, and take water in with you. It is also recommended to use a towel to absorb sweat during the sauna so that any toxins excreted are removed and not reabsorbed.

Expose your body to the rigors of saunas slowly, and always come out when you feel you've had enough. You can gradually build up the length of time you stay in with each visit.

Following your sauna, either cool down rapidly by jumping into a cold pool, which will send your circulation into overdrive, or take it more slowly with a warm shower. Then rest and drink some water. Repeat this sequence two or three times each session. The cycle of heating and cooling encourages the body's own natural ability to regulate temperature and immune response.

Safety first *Fluid depletion can be damaging for certain people. Consult your doctor before taking a sauna if you have kidney problems, high or low blood pressure or have a history of fainting. Women who are pregnant or menstruating and children under 14 years of age are advised not to use a sauna. Jumping into a pool of freezing water following a sauna could be dangerous for anyone with a heart condition.*

Where to find *Many spas, health clubs and sports centers have sauna facilities.*

SAW PALMETTO *Serenoa repens, Sabal serrulatum*

use for ✓ Hair loss ✓ Prostate problems

SAW PALMETTO IS A SLOW-GROWING, clumping shrub with palmate leaves and reddish-black fruits. An excellent host plant for butterflies, birds and other wildlife, the plant has many uses in traditional medicine. Native Americans used its fruits for food and to treat urinary and reproductive system problems, while the Mayans drank an extract as a tonic.

Today, saw palmetto extract—which is produced from the fruit—is best known for decreasing the symptoms of an enlarged prostate, a condition known as benign prostatic hypertrophy (BPH), and treating certain types of prostate infection. Among other things, it is sometimes used to treat baldness, colds and coughs, chronic bronchitis and migraines.

How it works

A number of studies have shown that men with enlarged prostates who took saw palmetto noticed an improvement in symptoms. It reduced the need to urinate at night and improved urinary flow. This may be due to the fact that the extract counteracts the effects of male hormones. By blocking a key enzyme, it prevents testosterone being turned into dihydrotestosterone, the androgenic hormone thought to cause prostate enlargement. Saw palmetto may also act as an anti-inflammatory agent, and there is some evidence that it works by shrinking the lining that puts pressure on the tubes that carry urine, rather than reducing the size of the prostate.

The antiandrogenic properties of saw palmetto extract has also led to its use as a treatment for androgenic alopecia—hair loss and baldness in men and women.

Safety first *The mild side effects associated with taking saw palmetto include nausea, stomach pain, bad breath, constipation and diarrhea. The extract should not be taken by women using birth-control pills—as it decreases estrogen levels in the body—or by those on anticoagulant medications, as it might further slow blood clotting.*

Saw palmetto has not been widely tested during pregnancy or breastfeeding so it is best avoided or used only under medical supervision during these periods.

Where to find *Saw palmetto is available in health food stores or from a qualified herbalist.*

How to use

Saw palmetto comes as dried berries, capsules, tablets, tinctures and extracts. To treat BPH, it is best taken as a liposterolic extract in capsules or in tablet form. Look for extracts standardized to contain 85–95 percent fatty acids and sterols. For bald patches it can be taken as a capsule or used topically. It could take several months to notice any change. In both cases follow label instructions or take as professionally prescribed.

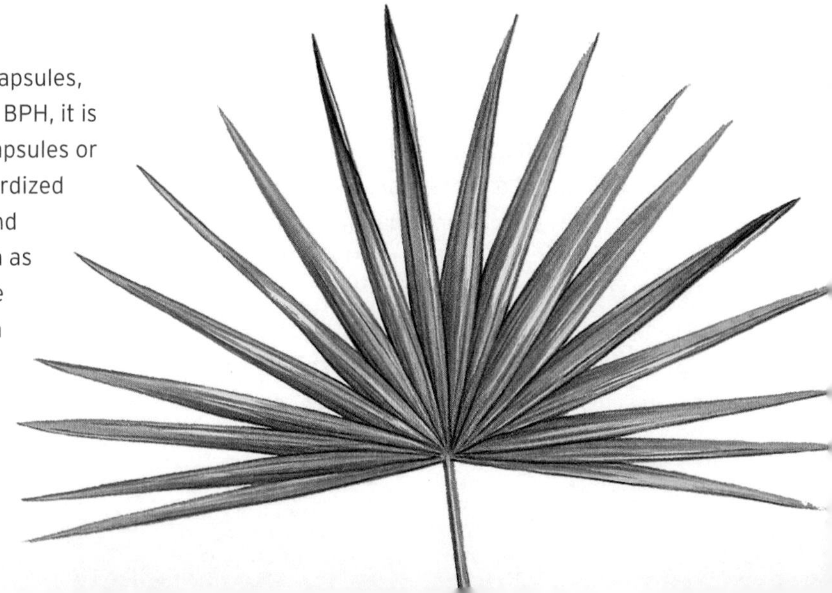

SENNA *Senna alexandrina, Cassia angustifolia, C. acutifolia*

use for ✓ ***Constipation***

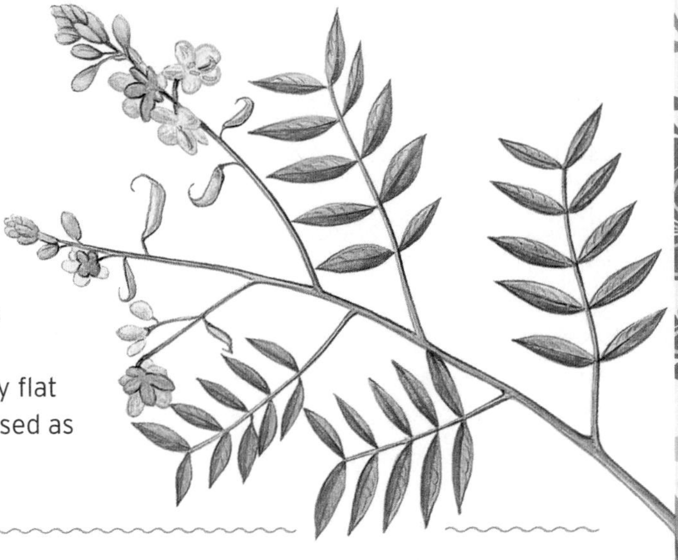

A MEMBER OF THE LEGUME or pea family, sennas form a large group of flowering plants that includes herbs, shrubs and trees. *Cassia acutifolia* has small, yellow flowers followed by flat papery pods. Its leaves and pods have been used as an effective laxative since the 10th century.

How it works

Senna contains sennosides that stimulate the nerve endings in the walls of the large intestine, increasing the frequency and strength of bowel muscle contractions. This increased action helps to move the contents of the bowel toward the rectum, from where they can be expelled.

Known as a stimulant laxative, sennosides are activated by the natural bacteria found in the colon, so the remedy will not start acting until it reaches this part of the gut. A significant number of clinical trials have shown that senna-based products offer gentle but effective relief from the effects of constipation by improving the movement through the large bowel. As a result it is often recommended as a nonprescription laxative.

Safety first *The side effects associated with taking senna include diarrhea, bowel problems, heart and kidney problems, coloration of the feces and urine, and stomach cramps. Senna tea should not be taken for more than seven days consecutively, and is not suitable for children. Senna has not been widely tested during pregnancy or breastfeeding and so it is best avoided or used only under medical supervision during these periods.*

Where to find *Senna products can be found in health food stores and pharmacies. Senna is also found with other ingredients in many commercial laxative products.*

How to use

Senna can be taken in liquid form or as tablets. Follow label instructions or take as professionally prescribed. A bowel movement should occur within six to 12 hours of taking the remedy.

The herb is also available as a tea. It can be bought as tea bags, in loose-leaf form or as pods. To make a tea using leaves, steep 2 teaspoons (10 ml) of senna in a cup of boiled water for about 10 minutes or for 10–12 hours in cold water. To make tea using pods, put three to six pods in a glass of water and leave to infuse for 10–12 hours. When ready, strain and drink. Using cold water reduces the amount of resin in the tea, thereby reducing the chances of abdominal cramping. Drink one cup a day, preferably at bedtime so relief occurs in the morning.

As the tea doesn't have a particularly pleasant flavor, some people mix it with a second type of tea before steeping or add another ingredient such as fresh grated ginger.

SILICA

use for ✓ ***Hair loss*** ✓ ***Nail problems*** ✓ ***Osteoporosis***

WE REQUIRE ONLY SMALL AMOUNTS of this trace mineral (an oxidized form of silicon), which is found in the body's structural tissues: arteries, tendons, skin, bones and cartilage. A well-balanced diet that contains plenty of fresh produce, nuts and grains (including oats, barley and brown rice) should provide all the silica we need. However, to boost these levels it can be taken as a supplement derived from bamboo, green vegetables or the herb horsetail. Silica is traditionally taken to strengthen bones, hair and nails, and to reduce hair loss.

How it works

Silica's vital role in the body is to repair collagen, the main structural protein in skin and connective tissues. This can boost hair production, strengthen nails and improve skin quality—especially as we age and skin loses its elasticity.

Silica is also closely involved with the way calcium is utilized in the body. It is essential for turning calcium into bone. Case studies have shown that taking a silica supplement can boost calcium absorption into the bones by up to 50 percent. When there is a lack of silica and the body is unable to store calcium in the bones, calcium can build up in the joints (where it can cause osteoarthritis), the kidneys (where it could form stones) or the artery walls, leading to arteriosclerosis.

Silica can help to alleviate the symptoms associated with osteoporosis by strengthening the connective tissues found in joints, improving flexibility, reducing swelling and ensuring calcium is absorbed and utilized correctly. Silica also helps to ensure there's a healthy balance between calcium and magnesium in the body, which, in turn, aids hormonal balance.

It is thought that silica may impede the body's absorption of aluminium—a risk factor that has been linked to Alzheimer's disease.

Safety first *Because silica contains thiaminase, an enzyme that destroys thiamine (vitamin* B_1*), taking it for long periods could result in a deficiency in this vitamin. It has also been linked with excessive urination and kidney problems and should not be taken for prolonged periods without professional advice.*

Silica has not been widely tested during pregnancy or breastfeeding so it is best avoided or used only under medical supervision during these periods.

Where to find *Silica occurs naturally in fresh produce, nuts and grains. Silica supplements are available in health food stores.*

How to use

It's best to get silica from food, and a healthy diet should provide all you need. Silica supplements are available in tablet or powdered form. Follow label instructions or take as professionally prescribed. When taking silica as a supplement, adults are advised to take no more than 20–30 mg/day.

SLEEPING STRATEGIES

use for ✓ ***Anxiety*** ✓ ***Concentration, improved*** ✓ ***Depression*** ✓ ***Fatigue*** ✓ ***Frequent illness*** ✓ ***Jaw pain*** ✓ ***Jet lag*** ✓ ***Seasonal affective disorder***

WE ALL NEED SLEEP: ENOUGH SLEEP, and at the right time. Why, though, is a question that intrigues scientists, as the amount of energy we actually save during eight hours under the duvet is minimal. It turns out that sleep does much more than simply allow our body to rest. The brain never entirely switches off and it appears to do some crucial "housekeeping" while we drift off into dreamland. Though scientists are still exploring the mysteries of sleep, what is certain is that sufficient sleep is vital for our mental and physical health and well-being. Sleep helps our brains to function properly and improves our ability to learn.

A lack of sleep can affect our quality of life—and even our safety. The 1989 Exxon Valdez oil spill off Alaska, the Challenger Space Shuttle disaster in 1986 and the Chernobyl nuclear accident in 1986 were attributed to human errors in which sleep-deprivation played a role. Studies have shown that sleep deficiency can alter activity in specific parts of the brain, making it harder to make decisions, solve problems or cope with life's stresses and strains. In extreme cases, it has been linked to depression and suicidal thoughts.

How they work

We spend roughly a third of our lives asleep and there is no denying that we feel revitalized after a good night's rest. In part, this is due to the fact that sleep enables the body to repair itself and replenish energy supplies after an active day. In addition, research shows that human growth hormone and melatonin are secreted during sleep, which are important for healthy growth in children and for the repair of muscle and other tissues in adults.

Humans, on average, stay awake for 16 hours and then sleep for eight at night. However, individual sleeping patterns vary widely from person to person and are influenced by environment, habit and hereditary factors. There are various internal mechanisms that govern our sleep patterns: When we need sleep, they make us feel sleepy; when we have slept enough, they act to wake us up. An example is the chemical adenosine, which accumulates in the brain while we are awake, making us feel sleepy, then decreases when we are asleep. Caffeine blocks adenosine receptors, which is why drinking coffee is not advised before bedtime.

The various physiological processes that regulate sleeping patterns follow a 24-hour cycle known as the "circadian rhythm." Sleep cycles are determined by the timing of exposure to light and dark, exercise, eating and cognitive and social activity and are controlled by a part of the brain called the suprachiasmatic nucleus. Disrupting this rhythm—jet lag is one thing that will do this—can leave us feeling tired, unwell and struggling to concentrate.

The sleep cycle

Sleep occurs in a recurring cycle of 90–110 minutes and is divided into two phases: non-REM and REM sleep. REM stands for "rapid eye movement" and refers to the flickering movements of the eyes during this phase of sleep. This is the phase when we dream. The non-REM phase begins with "light sleep," when we are still half awake but muscle activity slows. Stage two, about 10 minutes later, is "true sleep" and it lasts about 20 minutes, during which our breathing pattern and heart rate slow. Stages three and four are "deep sleep": Breathing and heart rate are lowest

continued on page 282

during stage three, before we enter the rhythmic breathing and limited muscle activity of stage four. A period of REM sleep follows before the cycle begins again at stage one.

It seems that the deep sleep part of the cycle is the most important as it is the phase our body first catches up on when sleep deprived. REM sleep is important, too, and studies have shown that if REM sleep is disrupted one night, the following night the sleeper will experience more bouts of REM sleep in order to "catch up."

How to get a good night's sleep

It is generally recommended that adults need around eight hours of sleep a night while infants need 14–15 hours. If you feel like you are not getting enough, here are some strategies you can try.

Bedtime habits

Getting into a good bedtime routine helps you wind down and prepare for sleep. It trains the brain to become familiar with sleep and wake times, as well as setting our internal clocks. It might involve reading a book or listening to music, a warm bath, relaxation exercises, or writing a list of things to do tomorrow.

Environment

Your bedroom should be a relaxing environment. So no TVs, computers, loud music, bright lights—or anything else the body might find stimulating. A comfortable bed and good-quality mattress can, according to research, give us an extra hour's sleep a night. Exposure to bright light during the night can turn off melatonin production so if you need to go to the bathroom in the middle of the night it is best to use low-powered orange or red night lights.

A bedroom should be dark, tidy, smell fresh and be at a temperature of between 64°F and 75°F (18°C and 24°C). Buy curtain liners if the outside light is bright and consider double-glazing—or earplugs—if the area where you live is noisy.

Keep track

If you struggle to sleep, experts recommend keeping a sleep diary (see Journaling, *p. 215*). This will help to identify lifestyle habits that contribute to your insomnia. Include such information as: sleeping times; how long it took to get to sleep; how many times you woke during the night; how much caffeine you consumed during the day; and whether you are sleepy or fall asleep during the day, and so on.

Stay cozy

According to Swiss researchers, you are more likely to fall asleep quickly if your hands and feet are warm. This is because as we approach the threshold of sleep, the body's temperature regulation system redistributes heat from our core to our extremities—so invest in some bedsocks or a hot-water bottle.

Calming remedies

There are a number of herbal remedies, too, designed to aid relaxation and sleep. **Valerian** *(p. 300)* capsules, **chamomile** *(p. 147)* tea or placing a few drops of **lavender** *(p. 219)* oil on your pillow may help.

The power nap

Daytime snoozes can be one way to cheat sleep deprivation. According to experts, a 20-minute catnap increases alertness and motor-learning skills while longer naps of up to an hour improve decision-making skills. A study by NASA into tiredness in pilots and astronauts found that their performance improved by 34 percent and their alertness by 100 percent following a 40-minute power nap.

Safety first *Sleep is a priority and a lack of it will affect your health and well-being. So if sleep continues to evade you, seek advice from your doctor. People with a sleep disorder may be referred to a sleep clinic or center.*

SOCIAL CONTACT

use for ✓ ***Anxiety*** ✓ ***Dementia*** ✓ ***Depression***

AS THE BEATLES SO MEMORABLY PUT IT, "I get by with a little help from my friends," which study after study confirms. People with good social relationships tend to enjoy better mental and physical health, and live longer. By contrast, social isolation may be one of life's biggest health risks, according to a 2010 analysis of 148 studies involving more than 300,000 people. The risk is comparable to smoking or being an alcoholic and more dangerous than inactivity or obesity, say the researchers from Brigham Young University.

How it works

From childhood onwards, loving relationships and friendships make us feel good. We are instinctively, innately sociable. One intriguing US study suggests that, even when faced with danger, a woman's hormones encourage her to "tend and befriend"—nurturing and creating social networks to protect herself and her offspring. The more usual male reaction to danger is "fight or flight."

For both sexes, establishing good social relationships has measurable physical and mental benefits throughout life. Friendly interactions calm and relax the body, for instance, by decreasing the release of adrenal hormones that make the heart beat faster. Such effects increase both a sense of well-being and actual well-being because our bodies function better when we're not under stress.

Studies suggest that people with supportive friends and family have fewer heart attacks and suffer fewer mental problems. The physical and mental stimulation of an active social life may also protect against Alzheimer's disease and other dementias in older age. Even those who suffer cognitive loss are not unhappy if their social networks remain strong, according to a recent large international survey.

Safety first *Meet people in person rather than online. A recent US study suggests that interacting indirectly on social networks such as Facebook can undermine well-being.*

Where to find *Check bulletin boards and the local press for activities, clubs and volunteering opportunities.*

How to use

Modern technology can help you keep in touch with far-flung family and friends but face-to-face contact is also crucial. "The very best thing that can happen to people is to spend time with other people they like," says Dr. Daniel Kahneman, a Nobel Prize-winning psychologist. So make time to drop in on your friends. If it's difficult to get out, invite them over.

To build a local social network, seek out clubs, groups or physical activities that interest you. Alternatively, become a volunteer—having a sense of purpose and performing a service can be especially rewarding. According to a 2013 US study, this produces so-called "eudaimonic" happiness, which not only protects against depression but also boosts the immune system.

SOUTH AFRICAN GERANIUM

Pelargonium sidoides. Also called: Umckaloabo

use for ✓ ***Bronchitis***

IN 1897, CHARLES HENRY STEVENS marketed his "Stevens Cure" in Britain as a treatment for tuberculosis, the main ingredient of which was South African geranium root. When antibiotics became readily available half a century later it fell out of favor, but geranium root remains popular today as a supplement, taken to treat bronchitis as well as sinusitis, sore throats, tonsillitis and the common cold. In Germany, it is an approved medication for the treatment of acute bronchitis.

This member of the Geraniaceae family is native to coastal regions of South Africa, where it is known as Umckaloabo—which, in the Zulu language, translates as "heavy cough," indicative of its traditional application. The plant has narrow, deep-red flowers and large, heart-shaped leaves. Today, it is grown on specialized farms in the country using ecologically friendly cultivation methods to produce a root extract, called EPS 7630, under which it is sometimes marketed.

How it works

There is evidence that South African geranium has antibacterial properties that work against strains of multiresistant *Staphylococcus aureus*, which are frequently found in the respiratory tract and on the skin. Research suggests that the supplement works by killing bacteria or preventing them from attaching to surfaces within the body. It is thought that the supplement might also enhance the body's natural response to infection.

How to use

South African geranium is sometimes sold as EPS 7630, *Pelargonium sidoides* or Umckaloabo. It is most commonly taken in tablet form. It is also available as oral drops, sometimes marketed as Umckaloabo extract, which can be added to water or juice and taken between meals. Follow label instructions or take as professionally prescribed.

Safety first *Most people can take South African geranium supplements safely for periods of up to two weeks, although in some cases it has caused allergic reactions and stomach upsets. As the extract might cause the immune system to become more active it could increase the symptoms associated with auto-immune conditions such as multiple sclerosis, lupus and rheumatoid arthritis. Check with your doctor before use.*

South African geranium has not been widely tested during pregnancy or breastfeeding and so it is best avoided or used only under medical supervision during these periods.

Where to find *The supplement can be found in health food stores and some pharmacies.*

SOY

use for ✓ ***Cholesterol, high*** ✓ ***Menopausal symptoms*** ✓ ***Osteoporosis***

FOR MILLENNIA, SOY HAS BEEN A CORNERSTONE of the Asian diet. Unlike most other plant foods, it is extremely rich in protein and over the past 50 years, scientists have come to recognize its important medicinal value, too. Research in Asian populations first suggested that it could help reduce menopausal symptoms, protect against heart disease and osteoporosis, and possibly reduce the risk of certain hormone-related cancers. Clinical studies are confirming some of these findings and identifying the most helpful constituents.

How it works

When eaten daily, soy has been shown to help lower "bad" LDL cholesterol, the type that clogs arteries and triggers cardiovascular problems, by up to 10 percent. It may also help raise "good" HDL cholesterol levels. This is probably due to a combination of constituents, including proteins, fiber and estrogen-like isoflavones, rather than a single nutrient.

Some studies suggest that upping your intake of isoflavone-rich soy foods can reduce menopausal symptoms such as hot flashes. Soy may also help combat or protect against osteoporosis. In one US study, post-menopausal women who took soy protein with 90 mg of isoflavones daily for six months showed significant gains in spinal bone density. A more recent review of studies suggests that while soy may help strengthen the spine, it has no effect on hip, neck or thighbone density.

How to use

Soy beans make a great snack boiled or steamed as edamame. Soy is also available in the form of tofu or tempeh, for use in savory or sweet dishes. Around 3½ ounces (100 g) of firm tofu supplies about ½ ounce (13 g) of soy protein, more than half the daily amount shown to lower LDL cholesterol by 6 percent in those with mildly raised levels. One soy burger contains about ½ ounce (13 g) soy protein as does a glass of soy milk. Changing your diet so that you replace fattier animal foods with soy products is likely to enhance the cholesterol-lowering effect.

It is best to choose organic soy products as other soy products are likely to contain genetically modified soy beans and have higher pesticide residues. For soy supplements, follow label instructions or take as professionally prescribed.

Safety first *Soy products are very safe. However, consult a doctor before eating more soy if you are taking thyroid medication, as it can alter the medication's effects. If you are taking zinc, iron or calcium supplements, do so two hours before or after eating soy as it may reduce their absorption.*

Where to find *Soy products are available in supermarkets and health food stores, which also stock soy supplements.*

STRETCHING

*use for ✓ **Back and neck pain** ✓ **Chronic pain** ✓ **Cramps, muscle** ✓ **Osteoarthritis***

WATCH A CAT OR DOG GET UP after sleeping—stretching is often its very first action. We do it, too, after sleep or following a long drive or flight. It's a natural, pleasurable way to relieve the stiffness caused by being confined to one position for long periods. Regular stretching keeps muscles strong and flexible. It relieves cramps and is often prescribed for back or hip pain. Many relaxation techniques also include some form of muscle stretching and releasing to reduce the strain that nervous tension puts on various parts of the body.

How it works

While bones, joints, tendons, ligaments and muscles all make up the musculoskeletal system, it is only muscles that give us the ability to move. When you stretch, the muscle fibers elongate bit by bit to their maximum resting length; further stretching then exerts tension on the surrounding tendons and ligaments. The whole process helps to realign fibers, increases flexibility and encourages healing of any damaged tissue.

Muscle cramps may be caused by injury, poor physical condition or the tightening of tendons that often occurs in older age, and stretching the affected area can help to relieve the pain and prevent further spasms. Stretching can help ease back and neck pain and other types of chronic pain such as joint pain associated with osteoarthritis.

Safety first *Stretching cold muscles can be harmful; warm them first with low-intensity exercise. Don't bounce when you stretch as that can cause muscle tears. Always stop before stretching becomes painful.*

Where to find *Your doctor or physiotherapist can suggest stretches best suited to your activity or physical condition. Your doctor might refer you to a pain clinic, which can recommend particular stretches to help certain conditions.*

How to use

Regularly stretching all the main muscle groups will help you keep flexible as you age. To avoid strains, injuries and cramps, never stretch cold muscles. Either warm up and stretch, or stretch after exercise when the muscles are still warm. Specific stretches may be prescribed for back or joint pain or recuperation from an operation or illness.

To treat a cramp, massage the area, then stretch. For a calf cramp, put your weight on the affected leg and bend the knee. If you cannot stand, sit with the leg straight out in front of you and pull your toes toward you. This also relieves cramps in the back of the thigh. For a front thigh cramp, stand on your other leg with your hand against a firm post or chair, then bend the affected leg, take hold of your foot or ankle and pull it toward your buttocks.

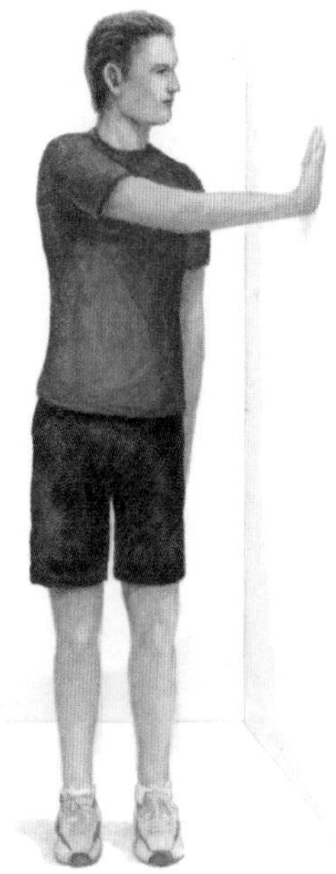

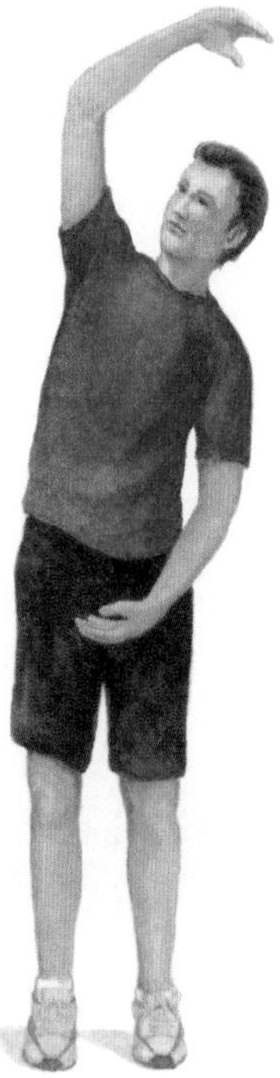

Chest and shoulders

For chest and shoulders, stand at right angles to a wall. Reach across to press against the wall. Make sure you're close enough to do this without leaning your body. Keeping your hips facing forwards, twist your torso towards the wall to feel a stretch in the back of your shoulder. Hold for 15 seconds then swap sides.

Side stretch

For a side stretch, stand with feet roughly shoulder-width apart and raise your right arm. Relax your left arm in front of you. Gently lean to the left, curving your right arm over your head, palm down. Stop when you feel a pull from hip to shoulder. Hold for 15 seconds then straighten. Repeat on the other side.

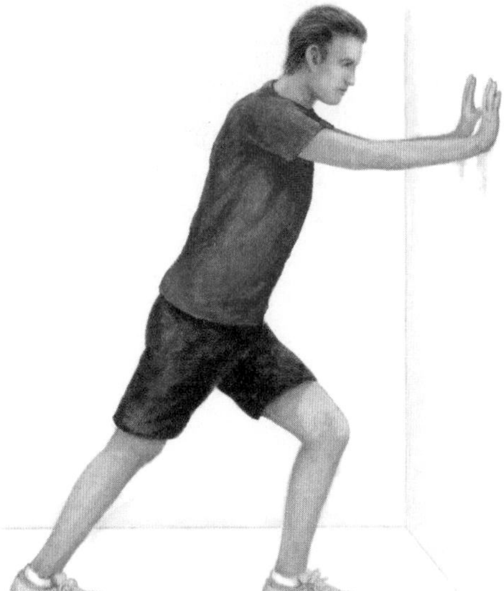

Calf stretch

For calves, stand arm's length from a wall and brace yourself with your palms flat against it. Step back with your right leg and lean gently in, bending the left leg at the knee, while keeping both heels firmly on the floor and making sure that your back and right leg remain straight. Press against the wall until you feel a stretch in your right calf and hold for 15 seconds. Push yourself upright and repeat with the other leg.

continued on page 288

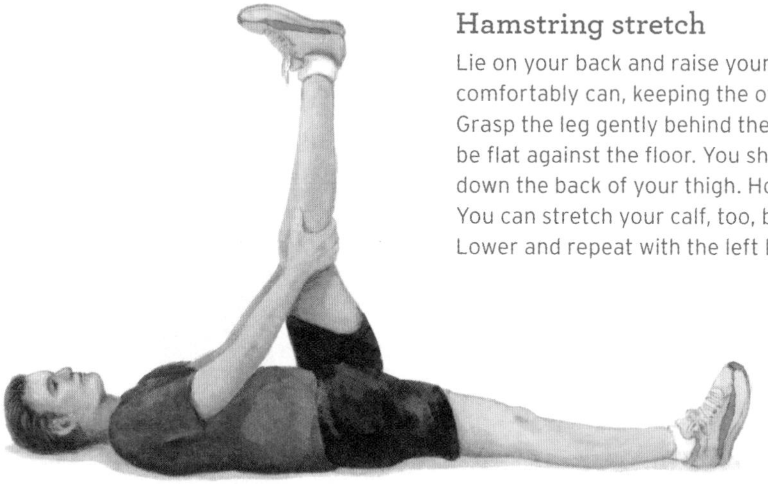

Hamstring stretch

Lie on your back and raise your left leg as high as you comfortably can, keeping the other leg on the floor. Grasp the leg gently behind the knee; your back should be flat against the floor. You should feel the stretch down the back of your thigh. Hold for 20–30 seconds. You can stretch your calf, too, by flexing your foot. Lower and repeat with the left leg.

Groin stretch

Sit on the floor and put the soles of your feet together with your heels at a comfortable distance from your groin. Holding your ankles, use your elbows to push down gently on your knees, producing a stretch that you should feel in the groin area. It is important to perform this stretch slowly and gently—don't force it. Hold for 10–15 seconds. With practice, the stretch will become easier.

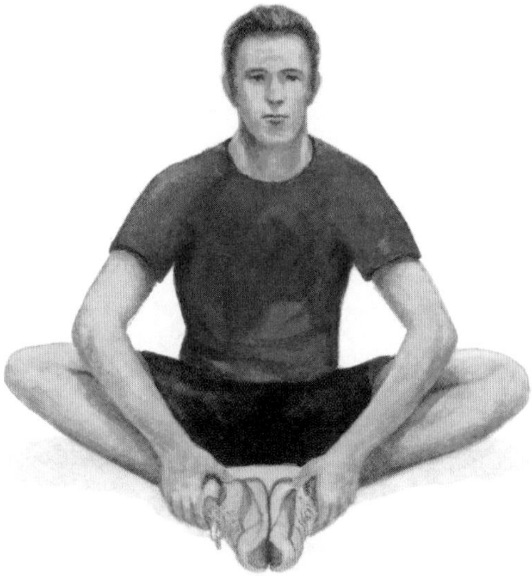

SUBLINGUAL IMMUNOTHERAPY

use for ✓ ***Allergies*** ✓ ***Insect bites and stings*** ✓ ***Sinusitis***

COMMON ANTIALLERGY MEDICATIONS suppress unpleasant symptoms such as itching or sneezing. Immunotherapy works by mitigating the body's response to the invading allergen. Unlike subcutaneous immunotherapy (SCIT), which is administered by injection, sublingual immunotherapy (SLIT) is largely a home treatment in which the medication is taken orally. Although SLIT was first explored as early as 1927, it became widely used only in the last decade, following clinical trials in the 1980s and 1990s. Early reviews suggest it could be as effective as SCIT, with a lower risk of serious reactions and the advantage, for those with a phobia, of being needle-free.

How it works

Allergies develop when the immune system reacts to usually harmless substances, such as grass pollen, producing so-called IgE antibodies that trigger allergy symptoms. Like SCIT, SLIT encourages the immune system to tolerate a specific allergen by introducing tiny amounts of it, in gradually increasing doses. The patient takes the allergen extract daily, holding it under the tongue before swallowing it.

To date, SLIT has proved effective for combating dust-mite and seasonal allergies, and allergic reactions to insect bites and stings. Research suggests it can reduce the risk of a severe reaction to a sting from 60 percent down to less than 10 percent. SLIT may also be useful for treating sinusitis patients, whose symptoms are often linked to seasonal allergies. Research into its use for food allergies is ongoing.

How to use

SLIT is expensive and generally prescribed only for severe cases when other medications are not effective. Once the allergen has been identified, the specialist can prescribe a customized preparation. Treatment usually begins in the doctor's office but can then be continued daily at home. Guidelines suggest taking the medication each morning on an empty stomach and holding it under the tongue for at least two minutes before swallowing. Missed doses should not be taken later in the day but simply continued the following morning. The therapy, which can be suitable for children as well as adults, usually continues for three to five years.

Safety first *While SLIT is considered very safe, it can produce mild side effects, including swelling, irritation or itching in the mouth as well as nausea. These normally subside within a few weeks. Severe side effects are rare.*

Where to find *For an accurate diagnosis and effective treatment, seek professional medical advice as some allergy tests and treatments have not been scientifically validated. Ask your doctor to refer you to a qualified practitioner.*

TAI CHI

use for ✓ ***Fall prevention*** ✓ ***Frequent illness*** ✓ ***Osteoarthritis*** ✓ ***Sleeping problems***

LEGENDARY TALES SURROUND THE ORIGINS of tai chi, a form of exercise combining deep breathing and relaxation with slow, gentle movements. Developed centuries ago as a Chinese martial art, it is said that a Taoist monk conceived it after dreaming of a crane and snake locked in a sinuous battle for supremacy. Tai chi is similar to **qigong** *(p. 266)* but has subtle differences, one of which is that it is normally practiced in a set sequence of moves. In keeping with traditional Chinese medicine, tai chi aims to balance body and mind to achieve well-being. Its popularity has spread from China around the world with an increasing body of clinical evidence to support its many benefits.

How it works

Tai chi movements exercise all the major muscle groups in a slow, controlled way, which is particularly effective for improving balance and mobility in older people, as a 2014 US review spanning 20 years of research concludes. Practicing tai chi can also help reduce the pain and stiffness of osteoarthritis, and has proved a safe and beneficial activity for people with cardiovascular disease.

The therapeutic combination of exercise, relaxation and deep breathing can also help people at risk of or suffering from type 2 diabetes as a recent Australian study has shown. With tai chi sessions three times a week, the 52 participants, aged between 41 and 70, reduced their blood glucose on average by 6 percent, blood pressure by 9 percent and waist circumference by 3 percent. In a 2007 US study, older people who practiced tai chi had significantly higher immunity to the varicella virus, which causes both chickenpox and shingles. This and other studies also suggest the mental benefits of tai chi, such as reducing depression and psychological stress, and aiding sleep.

How to use

To learn the best technique, join a regular class led by an experienced instructor. Once you are familiar with the movements, you can also practice daily at home. Though benefits may be experienced immediately, it can take many years to perfect the tai chi sequence. Discuss any health needs with your instructor as programs can often be modified to accommodate injuries or chronic pain.

Safety first *Tai chi is very safe and people of all ages and fitness levels can benefit. But it is worth checking first with your doctor if you are pregnant or have a serious medical condition.*

Where to find *Ask about classes at a local health club, library or health provider; or visit the Taoist Tai Chi Society of the USA website (www.taoist.org/usa) for information on classes in your area.*

MOVING MEDITATION

PERFECTING A SEQUENCE In tai chi, one movement flows into another, creating a set sequence or "form." There are several traditional forms, which can comprise 100 or more movements. The poses shown below are just a small part of a sequence that begins with "bird's beak" (1) and moves into "strumming the lute" (6). A full routine can take up to 40 minutes or so to perform and can take many years to learn. Some teachers maintain that a sequence is never truly mastered but with time and practice you will gradually become more fluent. You will need to memorize the moves as you would a choreographed dance. This is best done in a tai chi class where a teacher will take you through each move, often starting with a shortened form for beginners. Wear comfortable clothing that doesn't restrict your movements and keep your feet bare, or wear thin-soled soft shoes. Though tai chi takes a long time to learn, the benefits are often felt immediately. The breathing, movement and concentration help to calm the mind and cultivate a feeling of relaxed alertness.

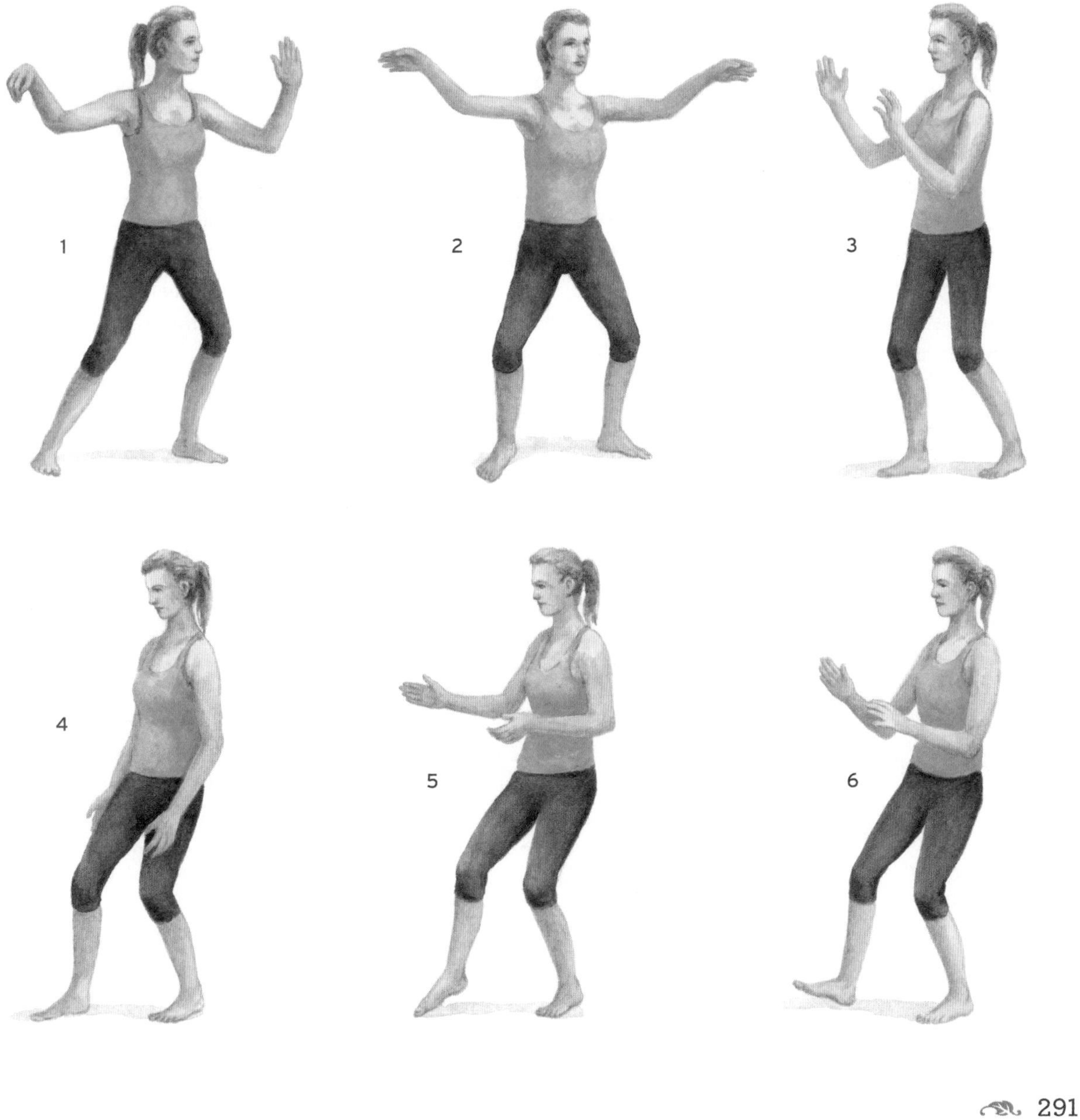

TEA *Camellia sinensis.* Also called: Black tea, Green tea

use for ✓ ***Bad breath and body odor*** ✓ ***Cancer support*** ✓ ***Dementia*** ✓ ***Fatigue*** ✓ ***Scalp and hair problems*** ✓ ***Stroke prevention*** ✓ ***Tooth and gum disorders***

LEGEND HAS IT THAT THE SECOND EMPEROR of China, Chen Nung, discovered tea when leaves from a bush accidentally drifted into his cup of boiling water. He wrote of his finding: "It quenches thirst. It lessens the desire to sleep. It gladdens and cheers the heart." Tea, whether green, black, Oolong or white, comes from the leaves of the tea bush. The difference is what happens after the leaves are picked: The longer they are left to dry and ferment, the darker or blacker the tea.

How it works

Although many studies have focused on green tea, all teas have similar health benefits–but with slightly different compositions of antioxidants and flavonoids. These substances protect the body from harmful free radicals that are thought to be responsible for many illnesses. Tea's reputation as being simultaneously soothing and invigorating is thanks to its high theanine content–which helps the body manage stress–coupled with a small amount of caffeine, which increases concentration, memory and mental acuity. Such attributes mean that tea may be of possible benefit in dementia. Meanwhile its abundance of polyphenols are thought to have cancer-fighting potential.

Safety first *Avoid excessive quantities of tea if you are sensitive to caffeine, or have premenstrual syndrome. If you are at risk of low iron levels, do not drink tea close to mealtimes as it may reduce iron absorption from food.*

Where to find *Tea is available in health food stores, supermarkets and specialty tea shops. Green tea supplements are available in health food stores and some pharmacies.*

With all these active ingredients, it is no wonder that the health benefits of tea are many, including reducing the risk of different cancers, dental decay, gum problems, fatigue and bad breath. It may help lessen the chances of heart disease and stroke in three ways: by lowering blood pressure, reducing triglycerides in the blood and preventing blood clots. One study showed that men and women who drank one or more cups of tea (black or green) per day had a 44 percent reduction in heart attack risk.

Tea may help fight obesity, too, by helping to boost the metabolism and therefore providing a mild fat-burning effect. Tea's astringent (tightening) tannins make it a useful topical remedy for irritated eyes, puffiness, swellings, insect bites and minor burns. Tea contains naturally high levels of fluoride, too, which hardens and protects teeth from decay.

How to use

Make the beverage from loose leaves or tea bags according to label instructions, and personal preference. Green tea is available as a freeze-dried extract in tablet or capsule form. When using green tea supplements, follow label instructions or take as professionally prescribed. Store tea in airtight containers away from heat and light to maintain potency and freshness.

TEA TREE *Melaleuca alternifolia.*

use for ✓ ***Acne*** ✓ ***Bad breath and body odor*** ✓ ***Bronchitis*** ✓ ***Colds and flu*** ✓ ***Cuts and scrapes*** ✓ ***Fungal infections*** ✓ ***Insect bites and stings*** ✓ ***Nail problems*** ✓ ***Scalp and hair problems***

CAPTAIN JAMES COOK IS SAID TO HAVE brewed up the aromatic leaves of *Melaleuca alternifolia*, calling it "tea tree" on one of his 18th-century antipodean voyages. Traditionally, the Budjalong Aborigines of New South Wales, Australia, crushed the leaves and used them on wounds and to treat coughs, colds, sore throats and skin ailments. "Healing lakes" into which the leaves had fallen and decayed were part of Aboriginal oral history.

Tea tree's therapeutic potential became more widely recognized in the 1920s when chemist Arthur de Ramon Penfold published research on the powerful antiseptic properties of the leaves' volatile oils, rating them 11 times more active than carbolic acid—the standard disinfectant of the day. A new industry was born and today the oil and a wide variety of tea tree formulations are available worldwide.

How it works

Tea tree oil distilled from the leaves and branches is an essential oil with proven antimicrobial and anti-inflammatory properties. Studies show that it can effectively combat a range of bacteria, viruses and fungal infections, suffocating and destroying the tiny organisms that cause disorders such as acne, bad breath and athlete's foot. Its insecticidal effects also make it useful for killing head lice and preventing further outbreaks.

In higher concentrations, tea tree oil has shown promise against antibiotic-resistant infections such as methicillin-resistant *Staphylococcus aureus*. While some people have suggested that regular use of the oil—like regular use of antibiotics—might make organisms more resistant to it, researchers say this is unlikely because the oil has so many active components that infectious microbes would have to develop multiple mutations.

Safety first **Tea tree essential oil should not be taken internally.** *Used topically, tea tree oil may trigger an allergic reaction in susceptible individuals. Tea tree oil has not been widely tested during pregnancy or breastfeeding and so it is best avoided or used only under medical supervision during these periods.*

Where to find *Tea tree products are available in pharmacies, health food stores, supermarkets and from a qualified herbalist.*

How to use

Tea tree essential oil is regulated by an international standard for "Oil of Melaleuca-terpinen-4-ol type" to ensure uniform biological activity. It should be stored in cool, dry, dark conditions to preserve its composition. Tea tree oil can be applied directly to insect bites and fungal nail infections, or diluted and used topically on rashes and sunburn. It can also be added to water to make an all-purpose cleaner.

For a simple mouthwash, add 20 drops of tea tree essential oil to 1 cup (250 ml) of water. Swill and spit out. To prepare an inhalation for treating colds, add 2–3 drops of oil to a bowl of boiling water. When using other tea tree products, such as soaps, deodorants and cleansers, follow the label instructions or use as professionally prescribed.

TENS AND ELECTROACUPUNCTURE

use for ✓ ***Chronic pain*** ✓ ***Neuralgia*** ✓ ***Shingles***

ELECTRICAL STIMULATION TO RELIEVE PAIN is a surprisingly ancient concept. Egyptian stone tomb carvings from 2500 BC show a patient being treated with a species of catfish that emitted an electrical charge. Modern therapies, such as TENS (transcutaneous electrical nerve stimulation), became more widely practiced following publication of the "gate control" theory of pain management in the 1960s, which suggested that selectively stimulating certain nerve fibers could suppress the sensation of pain.

How they work

The gate theory says that pain is the result of the interaction of signals from large and small nerve fibers travelling through a "gate" into the spinal cord (and to the brain where pain is perceived). The large fibers carry information about pressure and touch; the small fibers are connected to pain receptors and so carry pain signals. Since nerve impulses travel more quickly along the larger fibers, it is possible to flood the gate with signals from the larger fibers, preventing the pain signals from getting through.

In TENS, pads placed on the skin transmit electrical pulses. Set to a high frequency (90–130 Hz), and applied to larger nerve fibers, TENS reduces pain by closing the gate in the spinal cord to the pain signals coming from small nerve fibers. Set to a low frequency and applied to small fibers in muscles, it can prompt the release of neurotransmitters, such as gamma-aminobutyric acid (GABA) and serotonin, as well as opium-like endorphins, which dull the sense of pain. A burst mode stimulation is sometimes used to achieve both effects simultaneously.

In electroacupuncture, which also works by blocking pain signals and triggering the release of pain-relieving chemicals, electrical pulses are transmitted through needles or directly to electrodes placed at acupuncture points. Because several points are then stimulated simultaneously and continuously, the treatment may relieve pain more effectively than regular **acupuncture** *(p. 112)*.

While many patients report a beneficial effect for neuropathic (nerve), post-operative and chronic pain, as well as the pain of childbirth, scientific reviews of TENS and electroacupuncture treatments are mixed.

Safety first *Occasionally people suffer an allergic skin reaction to the electrode material, tape or conductive gel. Using newer pre-gelled electrodes may help. Never place electrodes over the eyes or over broken skin. Do not use if you have a Pacemaker or suffer from epilepsy. Do not use when pregnant, unless during labour.*

Where to find *Contact a pain clinic or physiotherapist for TENS advice or treatment, and a traditional Chinese medicine practitioner for electroacupuncture. Devices are available in pharmacies and clinics.*

How to use

There are many small, portable TENS devices that are designed for home use and use conductive pads. Electroacupuncture devices designed for use with needles are best kept for practitioner use. Consulting a practitioner and experiencing the treatments can help you decide what works for you. When using the machines at home, follow the manufacturer's instructions carefully.

TIGER BALM

use for ✓ ***Headaches*** ✓ ***Strains and sprains***

THE COLORFUL NAME, DISTINCTIVE LABEL and fiery action of this potent rub has attracted attention for more than a century. It was created by Aw Chu Kin, a Chinese herbalist at the Emperor's court, who moved to Rangoon and set up a medicine shop in the late 1870s, selling the ointment as a remedy to ease aches and pains. When his two sons took over the business, one of them christened the balm after his own name Boon Haw ("gentle tiger") and together they marketed the product across Asia. Today it is renowned worldwide, with some scientific backing and considerable personal testimony of its efficacy from users.

How it works

Tiger Balm contains five active ingredients—camphor, menthol, cajuput oil, mint oil and clove bud oil—in a unique aromatic blend, which can ease muscle strains and tension headaches. Camphor, a skin rubefacient ("making red"), dilates the blood capillaries and numbs the peripheral nerves. Both camphor and cajuput oil have a warming effect and are traditional ingredients in muscle liniments, while clove bud oil, mint oil and menthol have a local analgesic (pain-relieving) action. Rubbed on the chest, the balm's essential oils release a powerful vapor that helps clear nasal congestion.

Safety first **The ointment is for external use only and can be toxic if ingested.** *Avoid contact with the eyes and wash your hands immediately after use. In sensitive people, Tiger Balm may irritate the skin or trigger an allergic reaction. It has not been widely tested during pregnancy or breastfeeding so it is best avoided or used only under medical supervision during these periods. Keep out of reach of children and do not use on infants under two years of age.*

Where to find *Tiger Balm products can be found in health food stores, pharmacies and some supermarkets.*

How to use

The product is applied topically and comes in three different formulations of its main ingredients. Tiger Balm White is regular strength, suitable for headaches and muscle pain, and the only one that should be used as a chest rub. Tiger Balm Red, which also includes cassia oil, is an extra-strength ointment that induces greater skin warmth and is used mainly for muscle problems. Tiger Balm oil, with a similar composition to Tiger Balm White, is useful for covering larger areas of skin. Follow label instructions or use as professionally prescribed.

TINOSPORA CORDIFOLIA Also called: Guduchi

use for ✓ ***Hay fever***

THE CLIMBING, DECIDUOUS SHRUB, which often grows entwined around mango or neem trees, has a long history in Ayurvedic medicine. Tinospora, also known as guduchi, is a so-called adaptogen that balances and revitalizes the body. Its Hindi name "amrita" comes from ancient mythology: amrita was the gods' elixir of immortality. The herb is said to increase longevity, purify the blood, destroy toxins and boost strength and sexual potency. Ayurvedic practitioners prescribe it to speed convalescence and to treat a variety of disorders, including liver disease, diabetes and arthritis. Scientific studies indicate a range of therapeutic actions, including its potential for suppressing allergic symptoms.

How it works

Scientists have isolated a number of biologically active constituents from the root, stem and whole plant. Several of these have the potential to modulate the immune system, either boosting or suppressing the body's immune response. During allergic attacks, suppression is helpful because the immune system overproduces substances such as neutrophils and eosinophils, which trigger the unpleasant symptoms. In a 2005 study of 75 people with allergic rhinitis (sneezing, watery eyes and runny nose), those treated with *T. cordifolia* had a reduced neutrophil and eosinophil count, and experienced considerably fewer allergy symptoms.

Studies also support the herb's potential as an anti-inflammatory agent for relieving arthritic conditions, one of its traditional Ayurvedic uses. In a few recent Indian studies, Ayurvedic formulations containing tinospora were shown to be effective for treating rheumatoid arthritis and osteoarthritis. In Ayurveda, tinospora is also prescribed for diabetes, and animal research confirms that the herb can mildly reduce blood glucose levels, possibly by increasing glucose storage in the liver and limiting its release into the blood.

Safety first *No significant side effects have been reported. Tinospora has not been widely tested during pregnancy or breastfeeding so it is best avoided or used only under medical supervision during these periods. Because it can affect blood glucose levels, consult a doctor before taking if you have diabetes.*

Where to find *Formulations of the herb are available in health food stores or direct from a qualified Ayurvedic practitioner.*

How to use

Tinospora is usually available as capsules. Follow label instructions or take as professionally prescribed. Ayurvedic practitioners may prescribe the herb fresh or as a powdered or liquid extract.

TOMATO PASTE

use for ✓ ***Cancer support*** ✓ ***Prostate problems***

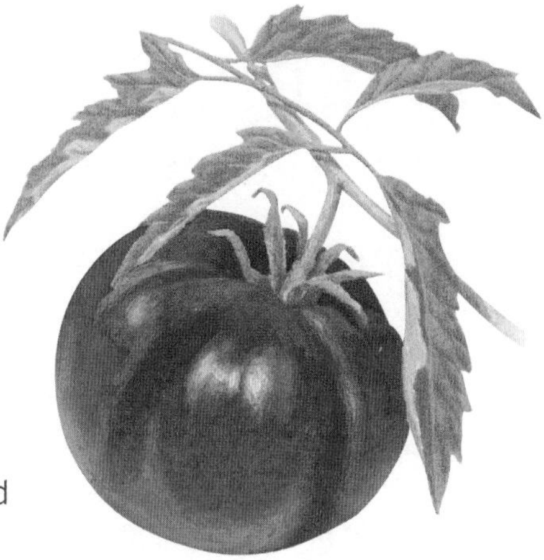

YOU MIGHT THINK THAT THE healthiest form of tomato was its fresh, rich-red, natural state. In fact scientists have discovered that one especially protective constituent—a pigment called lycopene—is present in much greater quantities in processed tomato products, particularly tomato paste. Back in the 1960s, scientists had largely dismissed lycopene as "physiologically inert." They considered it a bit of a substandard carotenoid—neither good nor bad but present in various organs because, unlike beta-carotene, the body could not convert it into vitamin A. That view changed when population studies began to indicate that people who ate a lot of tomatoes or tomato-based products had a generally lower risk of certain cancers—especially prostate cancer.

How it works

Besides the evidence from population studies, other research has linked low blood levels of lycopene to a higher risk of digestive tract, bladder and breast cancers, further supporting the belief that consuming lycopene-rich tomato products may have a protective effect. With 55 mg per 3½ ounces (100 g), tomato paste has more than six times the lycopene content of fresh tomatoes. The lycopene from processed tomatoes is also more readily absorbed because cooking breaks down the tomato's cell walls making the lycopene more available.

Like all carotenoids, lycopene is a powerful fat-soluble antioxidant with the potential for destroying free radicals, the unstable molecules that damage cells, triggering dangerous mutations. Studying its action on prostate cells, researchers have discovered that lycopene enhances the cells' own antioxidant response, destroys mutant cells and limits the capacity of cancerous cells to spread elsewhere in the body. Having more lycopene present in the skin may also provide enhanced protection against ultraviolet (UV) damage from sun exposure. Although effects have not yet been shown conclusively in human subjects, a 2013 US study did suggest that tomato products might help prevent breast cancer.

Safety first *Tomato and tomato products are safe when consumed in food.*

Where to find *Supermarkets carry a range of tomato pastes, sometimes described as tomato purée, passata or tomato concentrate.*

How to use

Add tomato paste to pasta sauces, spread it thickly on pizzas, blend it in Virgin Bloody Marys and include it in salad dressings and sandwiches. It's best to follow the Mediterranean diet and eat tomatoes with olive oil (as lycopene is fat-soluble, the addition of some oil increases its absorption). Some research also suggests that the combined effect of constituents in tomato concentrates is more potent than its lycopene content alone.

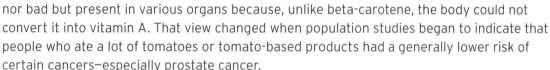

TURMERIC *Curcuma longa*

use for ✓ ***Cancer support*** ✓ ***Gall bladder problems*** ✓ ***Strains and sprains***

TURMERIC, THE SPICE THAT GIVES curry its rich, golden hue, has been a mainstay in India's ancient system of Ayurvedic medicine for thousands of years. It has traditionally been used to reduce inflammation, calm stomach disorders, heal laryngitis, control diabetes, stop diarrhea and was even thought to slow the aging process. The potent medicinal properties of turmeric led to US researchers being awarded a US patent for its use in wound healing. This was seen as an act of "biopiracy" by the Indian government who demonstrated that this application was not new and subsequently had the patent revoked.

How it works

The source of turmeric's rich, yellow-orange color is curcumin, a fat-soluble antioxidant that also has anti-inflammatory and antitumor properties. In one 2009 study of people with painful osteoarthritis of the knee, published in the *Journal of Alternative and Complementary Medicine*, turmeric extracts had pain-reducing powers on par with ibuprofen. Its pain-soothing, inflammation-squelching abilities may also be useful for treating strains and sprains. Curcumin's traditional use in digestive disorders has also been backed up by research. In one study of 440 people with digestive problems, those who took curcumin supplements daily reported a 67 percent improvement in abdominal pain, bloating, pressure and a feeling of fullness. This compound also helps keep cholesterol dissolved in bile acid, a digestive fluid, which may reduce the risk for gallstones.

A growing stack of research suggests that curcumin also may have cancer-fighting talents. In two studies from Germany, researchers found that by reducing inflammation, curcumin could have the potential to slow the spread of prostate and breast cancers. In another strand of research, scientists from the UK think that curcumin may make radiation and chemotherapy more effective against treatment-resistant cancers, according to results of a laboratory study. However, cancer experts advise against taking turmeric or curcumin supplements without medical supervision during cancer treatment, because it may make some drugs less effective as well.

Safety first *The use of turmeric in foods is generally considered safe. Since turmeric may interfere with blood clotting, do not take it as a supplement without discussing this with your doctor. Avoid in medical doses during pregnancy as it may stimulate early labor. Turmeric has not been widely tested during breastfeeding so it is best avoided in medical doses during that time.*

Where to find *Turmeric can be bought in supermarkets. Supplements are available in health food stores or from a qualified herbalist.*

How to use

Herbal healers say the best way to enjoy turmeric is to start by using this warm, slightly bitter spice in food. It's delicious in curries, soups, on meat, in salad dressings and in sautés. Turmeric is also available in capsules, tinctures and as a tea. Recently researchers have been able to make a highly absorbable water-soluble form of curcumin called Theracurmin, which may be up to 30 times more potent than regular curcumin. If you choose to take a supplement, follow label instructions or take as professionally prescribed.

UVA-URSI *Arctostaphylos uva-ursi.* Also called: Bearberry

use for ✓ ***Urinary tract infections***

BEARS LOVE TO MUNCH THE BRIGHT RED berries of this low-growing plant, as indicated by its Latin name—uva-ursi—which means "bear grapes." Uva-ursi grows wild in mountainous regions of North America and northern Europe. Native Americans and Europeans alike used its glossy green leaves as a remedy for urinary tract infections for hundreds of years. In fact, it remained a popular treatment for bladder infections until the discovery of antibiotics in the 20th century.

Today, uva-ursi is widely promoted as a bladder-infection remedy and even as a way to prevent recurrent infections. Respected herbalists agree that this herb can ease symptoms of mild infections—but they're unanimous in adding that uva-ursi must be used carefully. They discourage the long-term use of this herb.

How it works

Uva-ursi contains arbutin, which is converted by the body into an antimicrobial compound that's swiftly eliminated in urine; when it reaches the bladder, it seems to help fight infection in several ways. In laboratory studies, uva-ursi has demonstrated potential for killing several forms of bacteria; it also seems to interfere with the ability of bacteria to latch on to the inner wall of the bladder. Meanwhile, uva-ursi may also act as a mild diuretic, increasing urine production, which may help to flush bacteria out of the body. This herb also contains tannins that calm inflamed mucous membranes.

Safety first *Do not give uva-ursi to children. Pregnant women should not take uva-ursi because it may start early labor. It has not been widely tested during breastfeeding so it is best avoided or used only under medical supervision during this period. Skip this herb if you have high blood pressure, Crohn's disease, digestive problems, kidney or liver disease, ulcers or take the drug lithium.*

Where to find *Uva-ursi is available in health food stores or from a qualified herbalist.*

How to use

The herb comes as a tea, tincture or capsule. Follow label instructions or take as professionally prescribed. Do not use uva-ursi for more than a week at a time and don't use it more than five times in a year. The arbutin in this herb is converted into hydroquinone in the body. It battles infection, but in laboratory studies has caused liver damage.

Uva-ursi works best when urine is alkaline, herbalists say. So skip acidic foods such as citrus fruit, tomatoes, strawberries and pineapple while using it and eat plenty of vegetables, which can raise the pH of your urine.

VALERIAN *Valeriana officinalis*

use for ✓ ***Jet lag*** ✓ ***Sleeping problems***

VALERIAN ROOT STINKS. THE ANCIENT Greeks dubbed it *Phu* (pronounced Phew!), with good reason as it smells like a very stinky sock. But this herb can help if you're stressed or unable to sleep—a use that dates back thousands of years in Greece, Rome and China. Valerian's sedative powers gained popularity in Europe in the 1600s; as late as the 1940s, it had a place in the US National Formulary as a sleep aid and anxiety remedy.

How it works

Valerian's calming, sleep-inducing properties and distinctive aroma share a single source: isovaleric acid, found in the plant's roots. Herbalists and researchers alike note that it works well for some people, but not for all. And the only way to find out is to give it a try.

Nightly tablets of valerian root extract helped about one in 13 insomniacs enjoy a longer night's sleep, with fewer middle-of-the night wake ups, in one 2007 study conducted by the Norwegian Knowledge Centre for the Health Services. In a promising study from Iran of 100 women with insomnia related to menopause, 30 percent of those who took a valerian extract daily for four weeks reported improvements in sleep quality. Combined with **hops** *(p. 206)*, another sleep inducer, it may help counteract the effects of jet lag by helping you get some shut-eye—either on the plane during a long, overnight flight or once you've reached your destination.

In Switzerland, University of Zurich researchers found that valerian compounds boost the effects of gamma-aminobutyric acid (GABA), a soothing brain chemical that eases fear and anxiety. In laboratory studies, it has calmed stressed-out mice, rats and zebra fish. But it has proved less effective in human studies. Some have found no benefits, while a remedy that combined valerian with lemon balm, another anxiety soother, did ease stress in a small 2006 study of 24 people from the UK's University of Northumbria.

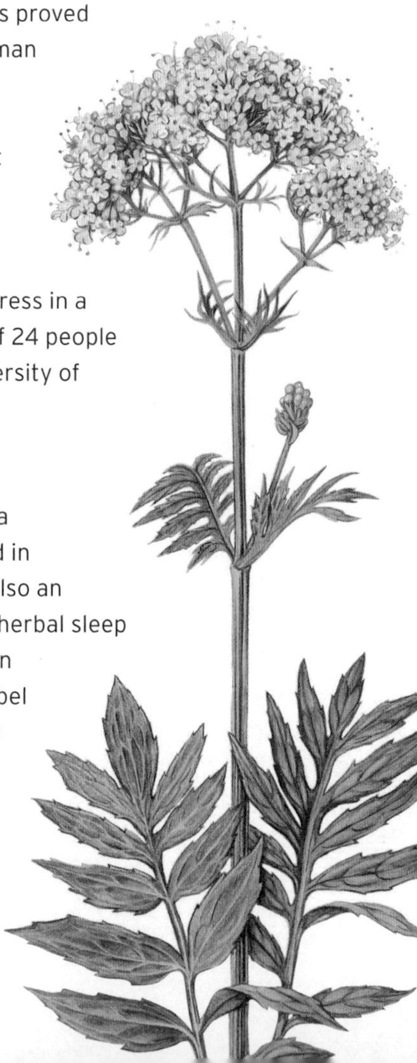

Safety first *Valerian has not been widely tested during pregnancy or breastfeeding so it is best avoided or used only under medical supervision during these periods. Do not take within two weeks of scheduled surgery; valerian slows down the central nervous system and should not be used with anesthesia or other medicines with the same effect. Do not take if driving or operating heavy machinery.*

Where to find *Valerian products are available in health food stores, pharmacies or from a qualified herbalist.*

How to use

Valerian is used as a tea, in tinctures and in capsule form. It is also an ingredient in some herbal sleep and stress-reduction remedies. Follow label instructions or take as professionally prescribed.

VITAMIN A

use for ✓ ***Acne***

AROUND A CENTURY AGO, AS SCIENTISTS began to isolate nutrients and assess their significance, vitamin A was among the first to be explored. The antioxidant vitamin which, among other essential functions, protects eyesight and keeps skin healthy, is available from meat, eggs, fish oils and dairy products, as well as fruit and vegetables. The body readily absorbs vitamin A from animal foods in the form of retinoids and produces its own vitamin A from beta-carotene, obtained from dark-green or deep orange-red vegetables and fruit. Deficiency is rare in developed countries but is the major cause of preventable blindness in children in the developing world.

How it works

The fat-soluble vitamin, which is stored in the liver and other fatty tissues, plays an important role in immune function, growth, reproduction, and bone and tooth formation. It helps the eyes adjust to light and is vital for keeping the eyes, skin and mucous membranes of the nose, mouth and lungs moist.

A diet rich in vitamin A may help prevent cataracts and help to protect premenopausal women against breast cancer. Vitamin A also aids skin repair. Research suggests that supplements may boost immune response and accelerate the healing of surgical wounds. Severe acne is sometimes treated with a cream or pills containing synthetic retinoids that reduce the amount of sebum produced and prevent dead skin cells from clogging hair follicles.

How to use

It's best to get your vitamin A from food, preferably in the form of beta-carotene from plant sources. For adults (19+), the US Recommended Dietary Allowance (RDA) is 900 mcg/day for men, and 700 mcg/day for women, with an upper limit of 3,000 mcg/day.

See your doctor before taking it as a supplement. To avoid excessive intake of vitamin A, look for a supplement or multivitamin that has it in the form of beta-carotene. Follow label instructions or take as professionally prescribed.

Safety first *Normal dietary levels are not dangerous but pregnant women should avoid retinoid creams and rich retinol sources, such as liver or cod liver oil; high intakes have been linked to birth defects. Like all fat-soluble vitamins, vitamin A is stored in the body and can be toxic if too much is absorbed. (Natural beta-carotene from plants, on the other hand, is nontoxic as the body converts it into vitamin A only as it needs.) Consult a doctor before taking vitamin A supplements.*

Where to find *Foods rich in beta-carotene and vitamin A are available in supermarkets. Supplements are found in health food stores and pharmacies; creams are available on prescription from your doctor.*

If you suffer from acne ask your doctor about topical medications containing synthetic retinoids. Weaker forms of retinol are widely used in cosmetic products, especially "anti-ageing" creams; a 2007 study showed that retinol could reduce the appearance of wrinkles in older skin.

VITAMIN B_6

use for ✓ ***Concentration, improved*** ✓ ***Menstrual problems*** ✓ ***Nausea and vomiting***

VITAMIN B_6, ALSO KNOWN AS PYRIDOXINE, is a water-soluble vitamin found in a wide variety of foods and added to others such as fortified breakfast cereals. It should be possible to get all you need from a well-balanced diet. However, the vitamin cannot be stored in the body so it must be consumed daily.

A deficiency in vitamin B_6 is rare; a lack is usually associated with low concentrations of other B-complex vitamins such as B_{12} and folic acid. Those most at risk of a deficiency are: individuals with impaired kidney function; people with autoimmune disorders; and people with malabsorptive conditions.

How it works

Vitamin B_6 performs many functions within the body. It is involved with more than 100 enzyme reactions, mainly connected with protein metabolism, during which protein is converted to glucose. It enables the body to use and store energy from carbohydrates as well as proteins, and for this reason can help reduce tiredness and fatigue.

It is essential for red blood cell formation and normal brain development and function as it helps the body make several neurotransmitters—the chemicals that carry signals from one nerve cell to the other. The vitamin's other functions include maintaining normal levels of the amino acid homocysteine, high levels of which are a risk factor for cardiovascular disease, and maintaining a healthy immune system.

Safety first *Larger doses of vitamin B_6 up to 200 mg/day have been used in some studies but only for short periods. Since high doses can result in nerve damage, skin rashes, sensitivity to sunlight and nausea, always consult your doctor first.*

It is also possible that vitamin B_6 could interact with some antibiotics and antiepilepsy medications, among others. Check with your doctor first if you are taking medication.

Where to find *Foods containing vitamin B_6 are available in supermarkets. Find supplements in health food stores, pharmacies and supermarkets.*

How to use

For adults (19+), the US Recommended Dietary Allowance (RDA) is 1.3 mg/day, rising to 1.7 mg/day in men and 1.5 mg/day in women over 50, with an upper limit of 100 mg/day. Good sources include fish, meat, whole cereals, bananas, chickpeas and yeast extract, as well as fortified foods.

A lack of vitamin B_6 has been shown to play a part in the cognitive decline in some older adults, with research demonstrating a link between the vitamin and brain function in the elderly, so taking a supplement could improve concentration.

There is some evidence that vitamin B_6 could reduce the symptoms associated with premenstrual syndrome, including forgetfulness, bloating and anxiety. In trials, taking 30–75 mg/day was also shown to reduce morning sickness in pregnant women. Some studies, however, suggest that while it improves nausea it does not reduce vomiting.

Vitamin B_6 is available in tablet, capsule and liquid form and is often found in multivitamin and B-complex formulations. Follow label instructions or take as professionally prescribed.

VITAMIN B_{12}

use for ✓ ***Anemia*** ✓ ***Celiac disease*** ✓ ***Dementia*** ✓ ***Depression*** ✓ ***Eczema and dermatitis*** ✓ ***Mouth ulcers***

ONE OF EIGHT B VITAMINS, B_{12} IS ESSENTIAL to create red blood cells, maintain healthy nerve cells and build DNA and RNA, the body's genetic material. Although animal-based foods are the only natural sources, other foods may be fortified with the vitamin. The body stores of B_{12} last a long time and deficiencies are rare in younger people.

Vegans are potentially at risk of deficiency and older people may become deficient because they cannot properly absorb the vitamin. Vitamin B_{12} deficiency is also a feature of pernicious anemia where the immune system attacks the parietal cells in the stomach responsible for producing intrinsic factor, which is necessary to absorb B_{12}. While low levels cause tiredness, weakness and moderate cognitive problems, more serious deficiencies can result in dementia and life-threatening anemia.

How it works

The replication of red blood cells requires an adequate supply of vitamin B_{12} and folate. Both also help the body utilize iron and produce DNA and RNA. Vitamin B_{12} is further involved in maintaining the protective myelin sheath around nerves and like other B vitamins assists in converting food to energy.

Absorbing the vitamin is a relatively complex process. Our digestive enzymes and stomach acids must first separate and release it from proteins in the ingested food. Then the vitamin has to combine with a protein in the stomach lining called "intrinsic factor" before traveling into the small intestine from where it is absorbed.

In older people, the condition atrophic gastritis, which thins the stomach lining and reduces the secretion of stomach acids, may hamper absorption as can low levels of intrinsic factor. People with celiac or Crohn's disease or those who have undergone gastrointestinal surgery are at risk as these conditions can affect the functioning of the small intestine. Some experts recommend that people over 50 should get most of their B_{12} from fortified foods or supplements because the vitamin is more easily absorbed from these sources.

Safety first *Vitamin B_{12} is generally considered safe and nontoxic.*

Where to find *Foods containing vitamin B_{12} are available in supermarkets. Supplements can be found in health food stores, pharmacies and supermarkets.*

How to use

For adults (14+), the US Recommended Dietary Allowance (RDA) is 2.4 mcg/day. Good natural sources include shellfish, fish, dairy foods, offal, beef, pork and eggs, as well as fortified foods.

People with pernicious anemia, celiac or other gastrointestinal disorders may be prescribed supplemental B_{12} to correct a deficiency. Supplements may also help those whose symptoms, such as depression or dementia, are linked to low B_{12} levels. Taking vitamin B_{12} may also help prevent common mouth ulcers. Topical B_{12} creams have been shown to relieve atopic dermatitis as the vitamin scavenges nitric oxide, which is involved in the inflammatory response.

Vitamin B_{12} is generally available as a tablet or capsule. Follow label instructions or take as professionally prescribed.

VITAMIN C

use for ✓ ***Allergies*** ✓ ***Colds and flu*** ✓ ***Cuts and scrapes*** ✓ ***Shingles*** ✓ ***Skin rashes*** ✓ ***Stroke prevention***

VITAMIN C, ALSO KNOWN AS ASCORBIC acid, is vital for growth and development. The body is not able to make vitamin C–and cannot store it–but a well-balanced diet should contain plenty of the nutrient. Fruit and vegetables are good sources of the vitamin. In addition, some cereals and drinks are fortified with vitamin C. Raw or uncooked foods are the best source of the vitamin, the levels of which decline if foods are cooked or stored for long periods.

Groups of people most at risk of a vitamin C deficiency include smokers–smoking affects the absorption of the nutrient–older people with a less varied diet, people with medical conditions that affect digestion and absorption and those on a poor diet.

How it works

Vitamin C is the body's primary water-soluble antioxidant, helping to protect cells from the effects of free radicals, the unstable molecules that damage cells, triggering dangerous mutations. The vitamin is needed to make collagen, the main structural protein in the body's various connective tissues. This gives it an important part to play in wound healing, repairing cuts and scrapes and preventing bruising.

How to use

It's best to get your vitamin C from food. The US Recommended Dietary Allowance (RDA) for adults (19+) is 90 mg/day, 75 mg/day for women who are pregnant, and 120 mg/day while breastfeeding. Good sources include all types of fresh fruits and vegetables.

Long considered a remedy for the common cold and flu, research suggests that while vitamin C won't prevent you from catching a bug, it can alleviate symptoms and shorten the duration of the illness. Its antiviral properties augment the body's immune system so it can help to treat viral syndromes such as shingles.

A 20-year research project undertaken in Japan and published in 2000 showed a clear relationship between higher levels of vitamin C in the body from a diet rich in fruit and vegetables and a decreased risk of stroke. Previous studies had demonstrated that foods rich in vitamin C and potassium were associated with lower rates of stroke.

Combined with grape seed extract and the flavonoid quercetin, vitamin C can also be used to relieve the symptoms associated with hay fever and asthma by counteracting the inflammation caused by such conditions due to its natural antihistamine properties. However, this involved taking a dose of 500 mg/day or more. These antihistamine properties also make it a useful ally against skin rashes or hives.

Vitamin C supplements are available in capsule, effervescent and chewable forms. Follow label instructions or take as professionally prescribed.

Safety first *Taking large amounts of vitamin C–more than 2000 mg/day–could cause stomach pain, diarrhea and flatulence. These symptoms normally disappear once a normal intake of the vitamin is resumed.*

Where to find *Buy vitamin C-packed fruit and vegetables in supermarkets. Supplements are available in health food stores, pharmacies and supermarkets.*

VITAMIN D

use for ✓ ***Chronic pain*** ✓ ***Celiac disease*** ✓ ***Diabetes and insulin resistance*** ✓ ***Fall prevention*** ✓ ***Frequent illness*** ✓ ***Incontinence*** ✓ ***Osteoporosis*** ✓ ***Psoriasis*** ✓ ***Raynaud's disease***

VITAMIN D IS SOMETIMES CALLED the "sunshine vitamin" because it is formed in the skin with the help of sunlight. It was once considered important only because of its role in skeletal health and development, where it helps maintain bone density and reduce the risk of fracture. However, scientists are discovering that it also affects at least 35 other types of human tissue, and has far-reaching effects on health.

In recent years it has also become clear that vitamin D deficiency is much more common than was previously believed. For example, a 2010 Nutrition Journal study found 42 percent of US adults deficient in Vitamin D, with highest rates among African Americans and Hispanics. The Archives of Pediatric and Adolescent Medicine reported that 52 percent of US children had insufficient Vitamin D levels.

Are you getting enough?

Vitamin D is present in different forms and scientists are still determining exactly how much vitamin D we need for optimal health. It is generally agreed that in order to maintain bone density and muscle function, vitamin D should be present in the blood at levels of at least 50 nmol/liter (20 ng/ml)—and that much higher levels may be preferable.

Relatively small quantities of vitamin D are consumed in the diet (from foods such as oily fish, liver, eggs and fortified dairy foods), and ideally the remainder of our requirements should come from the action of sunlight on the skin. However, getting enough vitamin D this way is not always easy, and the amount of sunlight your skin needs to produce adequate amounts of vitamin D is highly individual. It depends on many factors, including where you live and your skin tone. Ask your doctor about how much exposure is suitable for you.

Many people need to take supplements in order to address deficiency and/or maintain adequate levels of vitamin D. Those at particular risk of deficiency include pregnant and breastfeeding women, people whose skin is rarely exposed to sunlight (such as nursing home residents and people who wear covering clothing for religious reasons), people with certain health conditions (including celiac disease), and those taking certain medications. People who are obese require greater quantities of vitamin D.

How it works

Once converted into its active form by the body, vitamin D acts more like a hormone than a vitamin. Its core roles are enhancing the absorption and utilization of calcium, ensuring there are adequate amounts of calcium and phosphate in your bloodstream, and helping to build and maintain bone. In addition, vitamin D is required for the growth and development of the cells, and the normal functioning of the nerves, muscles and immune system.

As the body of scientific research into vitamin D has grown over the last decade, new information has emerged suggesting that vitamin D deficiency is associated with many serious health problems (including diabetes, Alzheimer's disease and some forms of cancer). However, in some cases it is not yet known whether vitamin D deficiency contributes to the development of the disease or occurs as a consequence of the disease process.

continued on page 306

VITAMIN D *continued*

How to use

When consumed in food and supplements, vitamin D is measured in micrograms (mcg) or international units (IU). The US Recommended Dietary Allowance (RDA) is 15 mcg (600 IU)/day for adults aged 19–70 years and 20 mcg (800 IU)/day for those older than 70 years.

In practice, many people need to consume vitamin D in quantities significantly greater than the RDA in order to address deficiency states, and can benefit from taking vitamin D capsules or drops, often in doses of 25 mcg (1,000 IU)/day.

In older people, vitamin D deficiency increases the risk of falls and the likelihood of developing osteoporosis. Taking vitamin D reduces those risks by improving bone density, balance, and muscle mass and strength, consequently reducing the likelihood of bone fracture. In most cases, calcium should be taken along with vitamin D.

Many people who suffer with chronic pain (e.g., fibromyalgia) are deficient in vitamin D. Supplementation significantly reduces pain levels in some chronic pain sufferers, and may lead to improvements in sleep and vitality.

Low vitamin D levels are common in type 2 diabetes, doubling the risk of heart disease. In people with insulin resistance who are vitamin D deficient, taking high-dose vitamin D supplements has been shown to improve the condition—particularly when doses are sufficient to increase vitamin D levels in the blood to more than 80 nmol/liter (32 ng/ml). Having adequate vitamin D during fetal development and early childhood may also help protect some children from developing type 1 diabetes.

Vitamin D deficiency may contribute to the development of many other conditions, too, including cardiovascular disease, Alzheimer's disease, inflammatory bowel disease, autoimmune conditions, some forms of cancer, and susceptibility to frequent respiratory infections. Low levels of vitamin D are also common in people with incontinence and Raynaud's phenomenon. Supplements may be beneficial in many instances, but in some cases large doses are necessary. In those circumstances medical supervision is required.

Topical treatment with creams containing natural or synthetic versions of vitamin D can be used to relieve psoriasis, but sometimes cause side effects. Vitamin D supplements come in capsule, tablet and liquid form. Choose supplements containing vitamin D_3, which is more readily absorbed than the synthetic form, D_2. When using supplements, follow label instructions or take as professionally prescribed.

Safety first *Unless advised to do so and supervised by your doctor, do not take vitamin D supplements if you suffer from hypercalcemia, parathyroid disease or sarcoidosis. Vitamin D may interfere with the actions of some prescription medicines, including digitalis and calcium-channel blockers (medications used to treat high blood pressure, Raynaud's disease and migraine). Talk to your doctor before use.*

Like all fat-soluble vitamins, vitamin D is stored in the body and can be toxic if too much is absorbed. Normal intake of vitamin D-containing foods is safe, but when using supplements, do not exceed the recommended dose.

Where to find *The action of sunlight on skin is the best source of vitamin D. When required, supplements are available in health food stores and pharmacies. Higher doses may need a prescription and should only be taken under medical supervision.*

Vitamin D-based creams are available in pharmacies, and may require a prescription.

VITAMIN E

use for ✓ ***Eye disorders***

THIS FAT-SOLUBLE VITAMIN IS A POWERFUL antioxidant that helps to protect the body from free radicals, the unstable molecules that damage cells. It also supports the immune system and helps prevent blood clots. As the body cannot make vitamin E, we must get it from dietary sources. Wheat germ, nuts (especially almonds), seeds and vegetable oils, including sunflower oil, are among the best sources. Green vegetables provide some vitamin E and a number of foods are fortified with the vitamin. Vitamin E comes in different forms (called tocopherols) with the natural form (alpha-tocopherol) being more potent than synthetic forms. Deficiencies are rare and tend to occur only in people with Crohn's disease or other disorders that impede absorption.

How it works

During digestion and other body processes, unstable electrons called free radicals are formed, which combine with oxygen to create molecules that damage cells, contributing to major diseases and disorders. Vitamin E, the most abundant fat-soluble antioxidant in the body, protects against this destructive process by scavenging free radicals before they cause damage. Its preemptive action may help prevent heart disease and cancer, as some population studies suggest. The vitamin is also involved in immune function, and helps dilate blood vessels and reduce blood clotting, which further indicates a potentially cardio-protective effect.

Safety first *Because of the vitamin's anticoagulant effect, supplements could potentially cause bleeding and may interact with blood-thinning medications. Consult your doctor if you take such medications. Like all fat-soluble vitamins, vitamin E is stored in the body and can be toxic if too much is absorbed. Normal intake of vitamin E-containing foods is safe, but when using supplements, do not exceed the recommended dose.*

Where to find *Vitamin E-rich foods are available in supermarkets. Supplements can be bought in pharmacies and health food stores.*

How to use

It's best to get your vitamin E from food. The Recommended Dietary Allowance (RDA) for vitamin E is around 4 mg/day for children and 15 mg/day for adults (14+), with an upper limit of 1,000 mg/day. Despite some evidence that a vitamin-E rich diet can protect against cardiovascular diseases and some cancers, research in high-risk groups indicates that supplementation is generally not beneficial.

Taking supplements may, however, help combat two major eye disorders, due to the vitamin's scavenging ability with free radicals. US research suggests that taking vitamin E together with vitamin C, beta-carotene and zinc can reduce the progression of age-related macular degeneration (AMD) and that vitamin E, together with lutein and zeaxanthin could significantly reduce the risk of cataracts. **(See Multivitamins,** ***p. 240.*****)**

Vitamin E supplements come in capsule, tablet, oil and liquid form. Vitamin E is also formulated into skin creams. Follow label instructions or take as professionally prescribed.

VITAMIN K

use for ✓ ***Celiac disease*** ✓ ***Fall prevention***

FIRST DISCOVERED IN 1935 BY A DANISH biochemist who was investigating blood-clotting problems in chickens, vitamin K regulates blood clotting in the body like a conductor directing a symphony. In fact, the "K" stands for *koagulation*, the Danish word for coagulation. More recent research has led to a new understanding of this important vitamin, revealing another big benefit, this time for your bones.

Vitamin K deficiency is rare as it is easily obtained through the diet. It is packed into green, leafy vegetables. One serving of cooked kale, spinach, broccoli or other leafy greens provides more than your basic daily requirement. Fish, liver, meat, eggs and fortified breakfast cereals also provide vitamin K and your body has a backup system: Friendly bacteria in your gut produce a form of vitamin K, bolstering your levels.

Vitamin K deficiency can happen to people with digestive disorders including celiac disease and Crohn's disease, both of which interfere with absorption of this important nutrient. A deficiency can cause extra bleeding (a warning sign is bleeding at the gum line or lots of unexplained nosebleeds).

How it works

Blood clotting is a complicated, multistep process. Without vitamin K, the cascade of chemical changes that leads to coagulation cannot happen. The vitamin also plays a role in protecting your bones. Your body needs sufficient vitamin K to activate a protein called osteocalcin, which helps add a rock-hard mineral layer to the inner framework that keeps bones sturdy and fracture-free.

Low levels of vitamin K have been linked to an increased risk of osteoporosis (thin, brittle bones), while Harvard University researchers found that women who get plenty of vitamin K are 30 percent less likely to suffer a hip fracture during a fall. This is important, because a hip fracture after the age of 50 can lead to a loss of independence.

Safety first *Be careful with vitamin K if you take anticoagulant medication. Talk with your doctor about the best strategy for you. Do not take high doses of vitamin K during pregnancy and breastfeeding. Like all fat-soluble vitamins, vitamin K is stored in the body and can be toxic if too much is absorbed. Normal intake of vitamin K-containing foods is safe, but when using supplements, do not exceed the recommended dose.*

Where to find *Find vitamin K-rich foods in supermarkets. Supplements can be found in health food stores and pharmacies.*

How to use

It's best to get your vitamin K from food. The US Adequate Intake (AI) for adults (19+) is 90 mcg/day for women and 120 mcg for men. Most people will not need a supplement to get their fill of vitamin K. Ask your doctor whether you would benefit from supplemental K. Supplements come in liquid or tablet form. Follow label instructions or take as professionally prescribed. The amount in a multivitamin may be enough, but in some cases your doctor may recommend a vitamin K shot to raise your levels. Don't take separate vitamin K supplements on your own.

WALKING

use for ✓ ***Anxiety*** ✓ ***Constipation*** ✓ ***Depression*** ✓ ***Diabetes and insulin resistance*** ✓ ***Fall prevention***

IN TODAY'S SEDENTARY WORLD, THE SKILL we learn in the first 18 months of life is greatly underused. Yet walking is arguably the easiest, most convenient and most pleasant form of **exercise** *(p. 175)* and one that confers many physical and mental benefits. Human bodies are designed to move, and function best when we are active. While most adults take 3,000–4,000 steps a day, health experts recommend a daily total of at least 10,000 steps including a few bouts of vigorous walking.

How it works

Like any exercise, walking can raise your heart rate, improve blood flow, strengthen muscles and bones, and help keep your weight in check. But to reap these benefits we have to walk enough. Back in the early 1960s, Japanese researchers calculated that taking 10,000 steps a day was a helpful target for better health and one that most people could attain. That goal is now promoted by the World Health Organization and health authorities across the globe.

Studies suggest that this level of activity reduces blood pressure, waist circumference, and diabetes and cardiovascular risk. If you weigh 154 pounds (70 kg), walking 10,000 steps at a brisk pace can burn about 430 calories and could help you lose weight, provided you burn more calories than you consume. Regular walking also benefits digestion and helps prevent constipation by stimulating intestinal muscles to move food more quickly through the body.

The more you walk, the more energetic you feel and the better your mood. During exercise the brain releases "happy" hormones called endorphins that help lift depression, banish anxiety and help us relax and sleep better. In older people, regular walking can help slow mental decline and prevent dementia.

Walking with poles, called Nordic walking, further enhances the health benefits and is suitable for people of all ages and abilities, according to a 2013 review of studies. Using poles as you walk exercises the upper body, takes the weight off the knees and lower body joints, and helps improve balance.

Safety first *If you have health concerns, consult your doctor before you begin a new exercise regime.*

Where to find *Everywhere. For added interest, join a walking club and explore the world with walking vacations.*

Step to it

Investing in a pedometer will help motivate you to increase the number of steps you take each day. Those with an accelerometer mechanism are considered to be the most accurate. Pedometers sense your body motion and convert this into distance; newer models can do this at any angle, and can be worn, carried on a lanyard or in a pocket. Record your daily step count over several days and work out the average to see how far it is from the 10,000-step-a-day good health target.

If you don't walk regularly, start gently. Wearing loose, comfortable clothes and flat, well-cushioned shoes will make the experience all the more pleasurable. Choose shoes that are designed to absorb shock, that support your feet and ankles well and have uppers made of a breathable material. Then, however busy your schedule, build a little more walking into each day.

continued on page 310

WALKING *continued*

It's easy to add more walking to your daily routine—opportunities are everywhere. All you need to do is create some healthier habits:

- Walk up and down stairs rather than taking an elevator or escalator.
- When shopping or commuting by car, park far enough away to allow a short walk. If traveling by public transport, get off a stop early.
- Walk a dog or take children to school on foot.

Build your step count whenever and wherever you can. If walking alone, make it more fun by listening to music or favorite podcasts on your MP3 player. Walk with friends or family in attractive surroundings; research suggests that forest environments are especially therapeutic, reducing stress hormones and lowering blood pressure.

Up the pace

As your daily step count increases you can start to work a little harder. To reap the full health benefits, your walk must be a moderate-intensity aerobic activity which means faster than a stroll—the sort of pace that increases your heartbeat and makes you gently perspire, but you should still be able to hold a conversation without gasping for breath. Keep this up for a few minutes at first, then include a sizeable period of fast walking in every trip. Start slowly, build up your pace, then slow down toward the end of your walk. Finish up with some gentle **stretching** ***(p. 286)*** while your muscles are still warm to avoid post-exercise aches and pains.

The 12-week walking program (opposite) is suitable for people of all ages who are generally healthy. If you have a heart condition or other form of serious illness, check with your doctor first. From a gentle start, step up the pace to include the periods at a higher heart rate as indicated. As a general gauge, your maximum heart rate is 220 beats per minute minus your age; this rule of thumb is widely used by medical experts.

To check how your heart rate varies—at rest and during exercise—take your pulse; this indicates heart rate because each heartbeat pumps blood around the body, which can be felt in the blood vessels close to the skin's surface. Place the tips of two fingers over the inside of your wrist, on the thumb side, then press down lightly until you feel the pulsing. Using the second hand on your wristwatch, count the number of beats in 15 seconds, then multiply by four to get your rate per minute. You can also buy wristwatch-style heart monitors—those that include a chest strap tend to be more accurate.

The Nordic style

Activate more muscles, build upper body strength and burn up to 40 percent more calories with Nordic walking. What originated as a summer training regime for cross-country skiers has grown rapidly in popularity and Nordic walking groups can now be found across the world. Light, fixed-length, shock-absorbent Nordic poles made of carbon composites are recommended and it makes sense to seek out an instructor to ensure you use the correct technique.

STEP IT UP: 12-WEEK WALKING PROGRAM

This program requires you to monitor your heart rate. If you are generally of good health, your safe maximum heart rate is roughly 220 minus your age. You can measure your heart rate with a monitor or use the second hand of your watch. Remember to build the intensity gradually and keep within your limits.

WEEK	FREQUENCY	WARM-UP	WALK	COOL-DOWN
1	5 times a week	5 minutes	10 minutes at 50–60% max heart rate	5 minutes
2	5 times a week	5 minutes	15 minutes at 50–60% max heart rate	5 minutes
3	5 times a week	5 minutes	20 minutes at 50–60% max heart rate	5 minutes
4	5 times a week	5 minutes	20 minutes at 50–60% max heart rate	5 minutes
5	5 times a week	5 minutes	20 minutes at 50–60% max heart rate	5 minutes
6	5 times a week	5 minutes	20 minutes at 50–60% max heart rate	5 minutes
7	5 times a week	5 minutes	25 minutes at 60–70% max heart rate	5 minutes
8	5 times a week	5 minutes	25 minutes at 60–70% max heart rate	5 minutes
9	5 times a week	5 minutes	30 minutes at 70% max heart rate	5 minutes
10	5 times a week	5 minutes	35 minutes at 70% max heart rate	5 minutes
11	3 times a week	5 minutes	35 minutes at 70% max heart rate	5 minutes
	2 times a week	5 minutes	30 minutes at 70% max heart rate, including 5 minutes of hills or stairs	5 minutes
12	3 times a week	5 minutes	35 minutes at 70% max heart rate	5 minutes
	2 times a week	5 minutes	30 minutes at 70% max heart rate, including 10 minutes of hills or stairs	5 minutes

WHITE WILLOW BARK *Salix alba*

use for ✓ ***Back and neck pain*** ✓ ***Bursitis and tendonitis*** ✓ ***Chronic pain*** ✓ ***Headaches*** ✓ ***Strains and sprains***

FOR THOUSANDS OF YEARS HEALERS in Europe, North America, Egypt and China turned to the willow tree's pain-relieving prowess–advising their patients to chew the bark to ease pain, soothe inflammation and help cool fevers. In the early 1800s, chemists in France and Italy identified and isolated this bark's soothing compound and called it salicin, in honor of willow's botanical name. Salicin and salicylic acid became wildly popular as remedies for rheumatism, gout and joint pain, but there was a catch: Willow compounds were also high in irritating tannins that caused vomiting and stomach upset. By the late 1800s, a low-tannin source of salicin was isolated from the herb meadowsweet, which became the basis for the world's first Bayer aspirin. Willow bark was once again a herbal "folk" remedy, as it is today.

How it works

The combination of pain-easing salicin and inflammation-cooling flavonoids in willow bark help explain its use for many painful conditions where swelling or inflammation may be a factor. In a recent study from Israel's Technion Institute of Technology of 210 people with chronic low back pain, 39 percent of those who took a willow bark supplement daily for four weeks were pain-free by the last week of the study compared to 6 percent of those who took a placebo.

Willow seems to work more slowly than aspirin, but may keep pain at bay longer. Herbal healers also recommend it for headaches, chronic pain, strains and sprains and bursitis.

How to use

Willow bark is available as a tea, tincture or in capsule form. Products are often formulated from a mix of several willow species, which have similar properties to white willow. Follow label instructions or take as professionally prescribed.

Safety first *Willow bark has not been widely tested during pregnancy or breastfeeding so it is best avoided or used only under medical supervision during these periods. Do not give willow bark to children younger than 16 due to the risk of developing Reye's syndrome, a serious illness linked to aspirin use. Skip it if you're allergic or sensitive to salicylates, have stomach ulcers or stomach inflammation (gastritis), if you're taking pain-relieving nonsteroidal anti-inflammatory medicines (aspirin, ibuprofen, naproxen or prescription types) or if you take a blood-thinning medication.*

Where to find *Buy willow bark in health food stores or from a qualified herbalist.*

WHOLE GRAINS

use for ✓ ***Cancer support*** ✓ ***Diabetes and insulin resistance*** ✓ ***Eye disorders*** ✓ ***Heart and circulatory health***

FROM WHOLE-WHEAT BREAD AND STEEL-CUT oats to lesser-known, minimally processed grains such as millet, sorghum and teff, whole grains have taken center stage in the arsenal of healthy lifestyle changes proven to protect against serious illnesses including cancer, diabetes, heart disease and more.

Until a few hundred years ago, the grains most people ate were always "whole." That is, the grain still contained its fiber-rich outer shell called the bran and inner "germ"—the seed and surrounding nutrients including vitamins, minerals and "good" fats. In contrast, those healthy elements are removed when a grain is refined, leaving behind the starchy endosperm middle layer that contains a grain's carbohydrates. This is what we eat when we have white bread, white rice or any other food made with refined grains.

How they work

Whole grains offer many health advantages. Fiber in the bran layer (and sometimes, as in the case of barley, distributed in other layers as well) helps you feel full and speeds bowel movements. One type, called soluble fiber, also helps mop up excess cholesterol. That, plus the smidge of "good" fats and vitamins B and E found in whole grains seem to team up to ensure better heart health.

Meanwhile, fiber slows the absorption of glucose into your bloodstream, helping you avoid blood glucose spikes and dips that can lead to cravings and can make glucose control difficult. According to researchers from the Harvard School of Public Health, swapping just some of the refined grains in your diet for brown rice could lower your risk for diabetes by 36 percent.

Munching whole grains can even reduce your risk for a common, vision-robbing condition called age-related macular degeneration (AMD). In a landmark study in the *American Journal of Clinical Nutrition*, researchers found that people who ate the most whole grains were 32 percent less likely to develop AMD than those who ate the least. They speculate that the protective effect may be associated with the way whole grains help to tame blood glucose. Keeping blood glucose low, whole grains help reduce inflammation associated with a buildup of fatty deposits called plaque under the retina in AMD.

How to use

Choose whole grains over refined types as often as you can. Look for whole grains as the first ingredient in bread, breakfast cereal, crackers and pasta. Try brown rice, barley, steel-cut oats and other grains, too. It's true that these grains can take longer to cook, but even quick-cooking varieties, available in the supermarket, offer benefits.

Safety first *Talk with your doctor if you think you may have a gluten intolerance (celiac disease), in which case you should avoid grains and opt for substitutes such as buckwheat.*

Where to find *Whole grains are available in supermarkets and health food stores.*

continued on page 314

WHOLE GRAINS *continued*

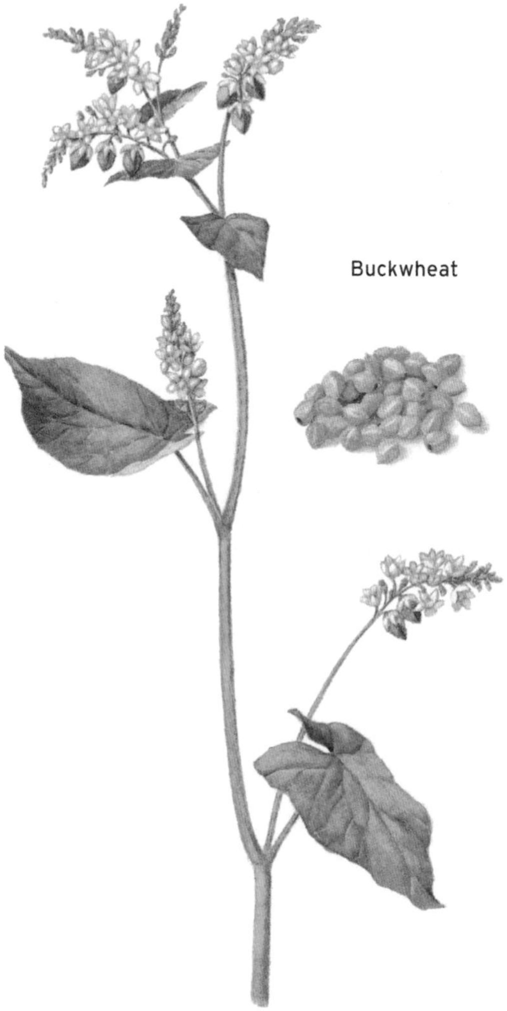

Buckwheat

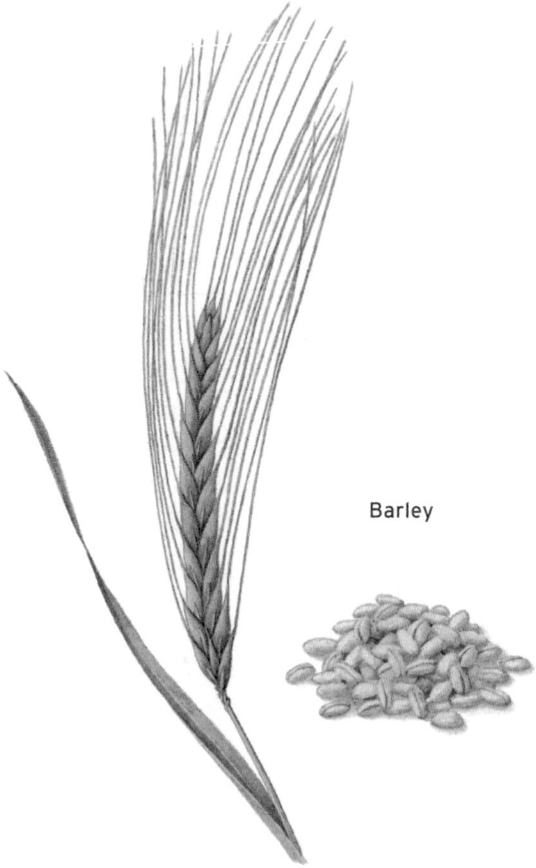

Barley

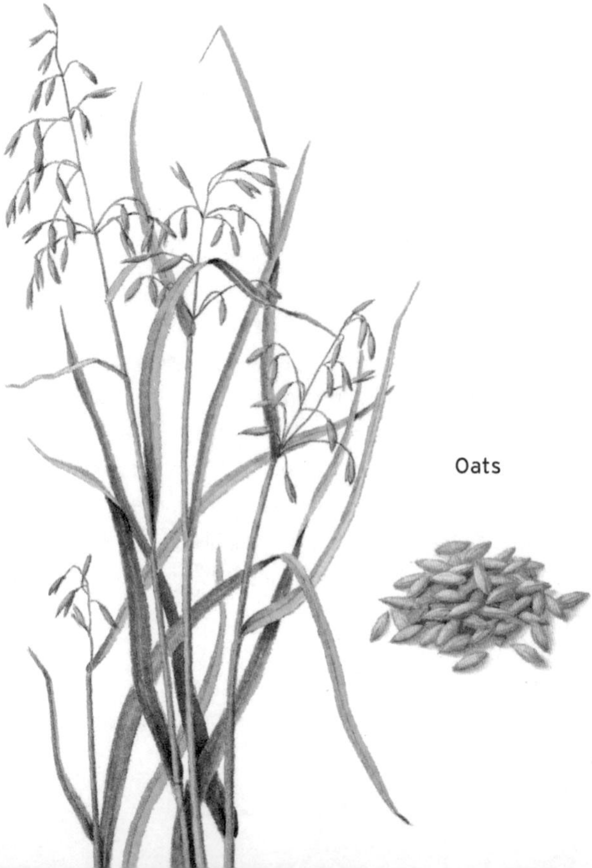

Oats

Wholesome grains

Most grains, including oats and barley, belong to the grass family and are cultivated as cereal crops all over the world. But some, such as buckwheat, belong to a different plant family. These seeds can be used in the same way as grains and are useful substitutes for people who have a sensitivity to gluten.

WITCH HAZEL *Hamamelis virginiana*

use for ✓ ***Bruises*** ✓ ***Cuts and scrapes*** ✓ ***Hemorrhoids*** ✓ ***Insect bites*** ✓ ***Varicose veins***

APPEARING ON LEAFLESS TWIGS, witch hazel's flowers look like an explosion of delicate yellow fireworks, brightening gardens in early spring. But preparations made from this plant's dried leaves, bark and twigs serve a far different purpose—easing the painful "fireworks" of hemorrhoids, healing minor cuts and scrapes and perhaps even helping to lessen the appearance of small varicose veins.

Native Americans used witch hazel for these purposes for hundreds of years. In fact, one of the first witch hazel patent medicines sold in North America—called Golden Treasure and later, Pond's Extract—was developed by a New York State businessman who heard about its powers from healers of the area's Oneida Nation in the 1840s.

How it works

Witch hazel is rich in two tannins: hamamelitannin and proanthocyanidin. These astringent compounds make skin and blood vessels tighten up. This can ease hemorrhoid pain, stop minor bleeding, ease itching and help minor skin problems heal. Recent research suggests proanthocyanidins in witch hazel may also have antiviral and anti-inflammatory effects.

Japanese researchers report that compounds in witch hazel also seem to neutralize cell-damaging free radicals in the skin—a discovery that could pave the way for this plant's use in antiageing skin products of the future.

How to use

Witch hazel ointment on a cotton pad can be applied to hemorrhoids, minor cuts and scrapes, bruises, insect bites and stings or even varicose veins. Witch hazel is an ingredient in products for hemorrhoids and in salves, creams and skin toners, too. Follow label instructions or use as professionally prescribed.

Safety first **Witch hazel is toxic if ingested.** *Don't use witch hazel on serious burns, cuts or wounds and keep away from the eyes—as witch hazel products usually contain a small amount of alcohol. Witch hazel has not been widely tested during pregnancy or breastfeeding so it is best avoided or used only under medical supervision during these periods.*

Where to find *Witch hazel is available in pharmacies and health food stores.*

YOGA

use for ✓ ***Anxiety*** ✓ ***Asthma*** ✓ ***Blood pressure, high*** ✓ ***Bursitis and tendonitis*** ✓ ***Cancer support*** ✓ ***Depression*** ✓ ***Heart and circulatory health*** ✓ ***Jaw pain*** ✓ ***Memory problems*** ✓ ***Phobias*** ✓ ***Sleeping problems***

THE WORD YOGA MEANS TO YOKE or joint together and, indeed, this ancient path to self-realization provides profound mind-body benefits. But just how old is this system of poses, breathing exercises, meditation, relaxation practices and chanting? The answer is: ancient. A set of soapstone carvings discovered in India depicts what appear to be yoga poses, dating to 3000 BC. And the first writings about yoga are in Sanskrit scriptures, also from India, called the Vedas, which are 4,500 years old. Today, tens of millions of people of all ages around the world practice yoga. Its growing popularity has inspired researchers to explore the science behind yoga's benefits. The verdict: You don't have to be fit, flexible or thin to get a health boost from the right yoga routine.

How it works

Even the shortest, simplest yoga routine can leave you feeling deeply calm. It's a wonderful feeling with far-reaching effects. In a 2009 US study, gentle poses and breathing exercises, performed just twice a week for 25 minutes each session, reduced blood pressure readings by 5 points. Yoga seemed to help by activating the body's parasympathetic nervous system, associated with relaxation, thereby decreasing heart rate and allowing arteries to dilate.

In another US study, from Boston University School of Medicine, one hour of yoga increased levels of the calming, mood-elevating brain chemical gamma-aminobutyric acid (GABA) by 27 percent. That's important news for people with depression, who often have low GABA levels. Other studies suggest yoga dials down activity in the sympathetic nervous system, associated with the body's high-stress, "fight-or-flight" response—significant if you're living with anxiety or have a phobia.

A regular yoga practice that included time for relaxation (called *yoga nidra*) helped people with insomnia fall asleep faster and get more nightly sleep in a Harvard Medical School study. Chronic stress also interferes with memory formation and recall, so easing tension with a regular yoga routine could help you sidestep memory lapses.

Yoga breathing exercises work their own particular magic. In people with asthma, these routines—called *pranayama*—have been shown to improve lung function and reduce wheezing and shortness of breath (when used alongside prescribed

Safety first *If you have a health condition such as asthma, back pain, brittle bones cancer, knee pain, neck pain or high blood pressure, talk with your doctor first about poses and types of yoga that are good for you and types to avoid. Seek out a yoga instructor with experience of working with people with your condition. If you take a yoga class, tell the instructor if you are pregnant and mention any medical condition you have. The instructor can modify poses so that they're safe and effective for you.*

Where to find *Look for classes in your community taught by a qualified yoga teacher; one organization that lists registered teachers is the Yoga Alliance (www.yogaalliance.org).*

medications). Meditative yoga routines, calming body and mind, have been shown to ease symptoms of obsessive-compulsive disorder.

In people with cancer, simple yoga routines can ease fatigue, reduce stress, improve sleep and reduce the need for sleeping pills during and after treatment. Gentle yoga stretches that increase flexibility and reduce muscle tension may also protect joints from a recurrence of bursitis, while relaxing moves can even help relieve jaw pain.

How to use

Don't fall for the myth that you have to be able to twist your limbs into a pretzel shape to experience yoga's benefits. In a US study of 400 cancer survivors, volunteers got results with just two short, weekly sessions of gentle Hatha or restorative yoga. A consistent routine that fits your schedule and ability level is best—don't push your body to the point where you may injure yourself. If you're new to yoga, look for a class for beginners.

WHICH TYPE OF YOGA?

There are many types of yoga and you may need to try several forms before you find a style—or a teacher—that suits you. Remember that yoga is essentially noncompetitive; you will be encouraged to progress at your own pace.

STYLE	LEVEL	DESCRIPTION
Iyengar	Beginner to advanced	Slow moves with a focus on good body alignment
Kripalu	Beginner to advanced	Slow, gentle movements; meditation
Viniyoga	Beginner to advanced	Postures are adapted for the individual
Hatha	Beginner to advanced	A gentle, slow-paced introduction to basic yoga postures
Restorative	Beginner to advanced	Passive, restful poses that are deeply rejuvenating
Vinyasa	Intermediate to advanced	Fast-paced, vigorous, flowing—with ever-changing routines
Kundalini	Intermediate to advanced	Uses postures, meditation, breathing exercises and chants to increase awareness
Ashtanga	Advanced	Physically demanding, set sequence of postures linked with breathwork
Bikram	Advanced	Takes place in a hot room, where you encouraged to sweat and this helps to remove toxins

continued on page 318

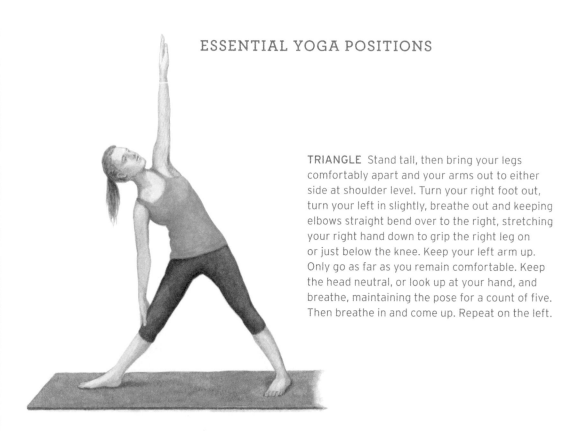

ESSENTIAL YOGA POSITIONS

TRIANGLE Stand tall, then bring your legs comfortably apart and your arms out to either side at shoulder level. Turn your right foot out, turn your left in slightly, breathe out and keeping elbows straight bend over to the right, stretching your right hand down to grip the right leg on or just below the knee. Keep your left arm up. Only go as far as you remain comfortable. Keep the head neutral, or look up at your hand, and breathe, maintaining the pose for a count of five. Then breathe in and come up. Repeat on the left.

DOWNWARD DOG Start on hands and knees. Tuck your toes under, breathe out and raise the hips to form an inverted "V." Keep your head in line with the torso and your arms and legs straight, with heels lifted off the ground. Push the chest up and back off your hands as you breathe out to flatten the curve in the upper back. Breathe, maintaining the pose for a count of five, then release and return to your starting pose to relax.

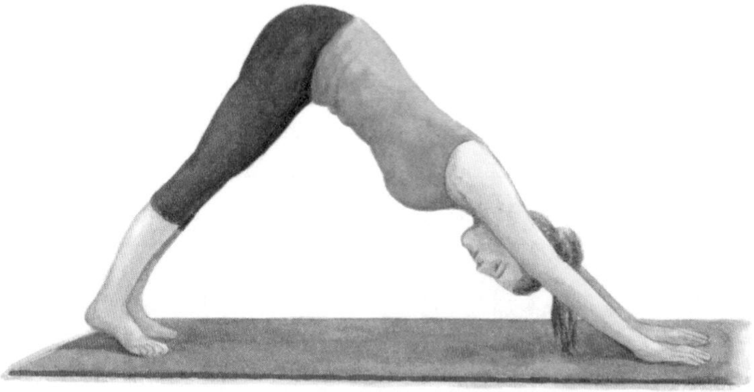

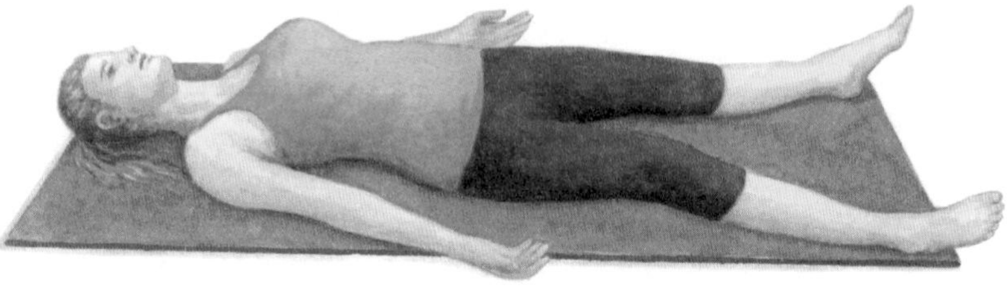

CORPSE POSE This relaxing posture is usually performed at the beginning and end of a yoga session. Lie down on your back, allowing legs and feet to fall naturally open. Let your arms rest limply at your sides, your palms facing upward. Relax the facial muscles and begin to take slow, deep breaths. Remain in position as long as you like, but take care to get up slowly.

ZINC

use for ✓ ***Celiac disease*** ✓ ***Colds and flu*** ✓ ***Cuts and scrapes*** ✓ ***Frequent illness*** ✓ ***Hair loss*** ✓ ***Natural fertility management*** ✓ ***Osteoporosis*** ✓ ***Wound healing***

TOPICAL APPLICATIONS OF ZINC HAVE BEEN used medicinally for thousands of years, but it wasn't recognized as a vital micronutrient until 1963. Meat, poultry and seafood (especially oysters and shellfish) are the best dietary sources of zinc.

Severe zinc deficiency is uncommon in the developed world, but many people have a mild deficiency, which may cause symptoms such as delayed growth, pregnancy complications and impaired immunity. People with malabsorption conditions (such as celiac disease) are at increased risk of low zinc levels. Others at risk of zinc deficiency include the elderly, vegetarians and pregnant and breastfeeding women.

How it works

Zinc is incorporated into many enzymes and body structures and plays numerous roles in the body. Among other functions, it is required for digestion, growth, immunity, reproduction, blood glucose regulation and helping to maintain the structure of the skeleton (thus helping prevent osteoporosis).

How to use

The US Recommended Dietary Allowance (RDA) of zinc for adult men (19+) is 11 mg/day. Women need 8 mg/day, increasing to 11 mg/day during pregnancy and 12 mg/day while breastfeeding. The upper limit of zinc intake is 40 mg/day. As well as meat, poultry and seafood, zinc is also present in plant foods such as whole grains, legumes, pumpkin seeds, sesame seeds and cocoa, but is poorly absorbed from them.

People who experience frequent colds and flu may benefit from daily zinc supplementation—especially if elderly. As well as helping to prevent respiratory infections, it can also be used to treat colds, and may reduce their duration by up to two days. Dissolve zinc gluconate lozenges in your mouth every two hours as soon as symptoms develop.

If you have a leg ulcer or are undergoing surgery, taking zinc supplements may help promote wound healing and reduce your risk of developing an infection. Topical zinc oxide can be applied to ulcers and burns for the same reasons.

Zinc is closely involved in reproductive health and may be beneficial for men and women who are planning conception. For men, taking zinc with folic acid may increase the production of healthy sperm, as was found in a Dutch study. Meanwhile, women who are pregnant or planning to conceive should guard against zinc deficiency, which may increase the risk of miscarriage, preeclampsia and other complications.

If you have alopecia, ask your doctor whether zinc might be beneficial for you. In clinical research, taking high doses of zinc over several months has triggered hair regrowth in a large percentage of sufferers. Zinc supplements come as capsules, tablets, liquids, lozenges and lotions. Follow label instructions or use as professionally prescribed.

Safety first *Zinc supplements interfere with some prescribed medicines and nutritional supplements. Ask your doctor for more information. Unless under the advice and supervision of a health professional, do not take high doses of zinc long term; doing so may induce copper deficiency.*

Where to find *Buy zinc-rich foods in supermarkets. Zinc supplements are sold in health food stores and pharmacies.*

GLOSSARY

Acid Having a pH value below 7, pH being a measure of the acidity or alkalinity of a substance or a solution.

Adaptogen A type of herb that helps the body adapt to mental or physical stress.

Adequate Intake (AI) This is an indication of how much of a nutrient people should obtain from their diets. It is given when there is insufficient scientific evidence available to calculate an average requirement known as the Recommended Dietary Allowance (RDA).

Alkaline Having a pH value above 7, pH being a measure of the acidity or alkalinity of a substance or a solution.

Allergen A substance that can trigger an allergic reaction in those sensitive to that substance.

Allicin A chemical that forms when garlic is crushed or cut and helps reduce low-density lipoprotein (LDL) cholesterol levels. Responsible for garlic's pungent smell, allicin produces numerous sulfur compounds, possibly with antibacterial properties.

Allyl sulfides Sulfur compounds, found in garlic, onions, leeks and other members of the onion family. They are thought to help lower the risk of heart disease, stimulate the immune system, and are under review for their potential to fight cancer.

Alpha-linolenic acid (ALA) An essential fatty acid linked to a range of health benefits. It cannot be made in the body and must therefore be obtained from foods. ALA is important for the maintenance of cell membranes and for creating substances in the body that protect against inflammation. ALA converts in the human body into two omega-3 fatty acids: eicosapentaenoic acid (EPA) and docosahexaenoic acid (DHA).

Amino acid The building block of proteins. Twenty amino acids are necessary for proper human growth and function. Nine amino acids are termed essential, because they must be obtained from the diet; the body produces the remaining 11 as they are needed.

Analgesic A substance that prevents or reduces the sensation or perception of pain in the body.

Anthocyanins The red and blue pigments found in certain fruits and vegetables. Anthocyanins are flavonoids with the potential to suppress tumor-cell growth, to lower LDL cholesterol levels and to prevent blood from forming clots. They are found in apples, berries, cherries, black currants, red and purple grapes, plums and pomegranates.

Antiallergenic A substance that calms down or inhibits the symptoms of an allergic reaction.

Antibacterial Bacteria-fighting or inhibiting.

Antibiotic A drug that kills or inhibits bacteria.

Antigen A foreign substance that stimulates the body to defend itself with an immune response.

Anti-inflammatory A substance that fights inflammation, the body's response to injury or irritation, marked by redness, heat, pain and swelling.

Antimicrobial Against or inhibiting microbes such as bacteria, viruses and fungi.

Antioxidant A compound that protects cells from the damaging effects of free radicals, which steal electrons from normal cells, damaging them in the process. Antioxidants replace the missing electrons.

Antiseptic A substance that fights infection.

Antispasmodic A substance that prevents spasms or cramps in the digestive tract or elsewhere.

Arteriosclerosis The stiffening and hardening of the arterial walls.

Astringent A substance that has a tightening effect on the skin or blood vessels. It contracts the tissues and stops bleeding.

Autoimmune disorder An ailment, such as rheumatoid arthritis, in which the immune system mistakenly attacks the body's own healthy tissues.

Bacteria Single-celled microorganisms that are found in air, food, water, soil and in other living creatures, including humans. "Friendly" bacteria prevent infections and synthesize certain vitamins; others cause disease.

Beta-carotene One of the most studied of the carotenoids, it is a potent antioxidant, plentiful in red, orange and yellow plant foods (as well as in dark green vegetables where the orange color is masked by chlorophyll). It is converted by the body into vitamin A. Food sources include: apricots, carrots, brussels sprouts, dark leafy greens, butternut squash, baby spinach and sweet potatoes.

Beta-sitosterol A plant sterol similar in structure to cholesterol. Beta-sitosterol may help to manage benign prostatic hyperplasia (BPH), as well as protect against high cholesterol and cancer. It is found in avocados, rice bran, seeds, soy foods and wheat germ.

Bromelain An enzyme derived from pineapples that is believed to have anti-inflammatory and pain-reducing properties.

Bronchodilator A substance that relaxes the muscles around the bronchi, resulting in expansion of the air passages into the lungs.

Bronchus Either of the two main branches of the trachea (windpipe) that leads into the lungs.

Capillary A tiny blood vessel that links veins and arteries.

Cardiovascular system The parts of the body relating to the flow of blood. This includes the heart, arteries, veins and capillaries.

Carminative A substance that helps to expel gas from the stomach or bowel, so relieving flatulence and stomach cramps.

Carotenoids Pigments that give certain fruits and vegetables their characteristic orange, yellow and red colors. Many are thought to possess potent antioxidant properties. To date, more than 600 carotenoids have been identified, including alpha-carotene, beta-carotene, beta-cryptoxanthin, lutein, lycopene and zeaxanthin.

Catechins A group of powerful antioxidants found in green tea and other foods. Catechins increase metabolism and the rate at which the liver burns fat.

Cellulose One of the main components of plant cell walls, this indigestible carbohydrate is an important source of insoluble fiber.

Chlorophyll The green pigment of leaves and plants, chlorophyll not only helps to freshen breath but it may also help to prevent DNA damage to cells. Sources include dark leafy greens, parsley, peas and bell peppers.

Cholesterol A fat-like substance that circulates in the blood and helps to maintain cell membranes. High levels are a major risk factor for heart disease.

Coenzyme A compound that works with enzymes to speed up chemical reactions in the body.

Collagen A fibrous protein that helps form bone, cartilage, skin, joints and connective tissue in the body.

Complementary protein A protein that lacks one or more of the essential amino acids but which when paired can supply a complete protein. For example, grains are high in the essential amino acid methionine, but they lack lysine. This essential amino acid is plentiful in legumes, which are deficient in methionine. So by combining a grain with a legume, a complete range of amino acids can be obtained.

Complete protein Contains all the essential amino acids. It is found in single animal foods; it can also be made by combining two or more complementary plant foods.

Complex carbohydrate Fiber and starch in legumes, vegetables and grains are complex carbohydrates. A diet that emphasizes complex carbohydrates can help protect against cardiovascular disease, stabilize blood glucose, relieve diarrhea and ease insomnia. Sources include fruit, grains, legumes and brown rice.

Decoction A water-based preparation, used to release active constituents from the tough parts of herbs, such as the bark, roots and seeds. The woody parts of the herb are cut into small pieces and simmered in water.

Digestive A herb or medication that promotes digestion.

Disaccharide A member of a group of carbohydrates that are formed from two monosaccharides.

Diuretic A substance that draws water from body tissues and increases the total output of urine.

Docosahexaenoic acid (DHA) An omega-3 fatty acid that is important for all phases of the human life cycle. A major building block of human brain tissue and the primary structural fatty acid in the brain and retina, DHA is vital for brain and eye health. Studies indicate that DHA may have cardiovascular benefits as well as neurological benefits. Although the body has enzymes that convert alpha-linolenic acid (ALA) to DHA, you obtain it more efficiently by eating oily fish such as herring, mackerel and salmon.

Dyspepsia Indigestion.

E. coli Short for *Escherichia coli*, *E. coli* is the name of several types of bacteria. Some types are harmless, but some strains can cause diarrhea and other symptoms. Harmful types of *E. coli* can be passed through food, water and contact with infected animals or people. Washing hands, cooking meat thoroughly and avoiding cross-contamination between raw meat and other foods can help prevent *E. coli*-related illness.

Eicosapentaenoic acid (EPA) An omega-3 fatty acid that is linked to cardiovascular and cancer-fighting benefits, and may help improve inflammatory conditions such as rheumatoid arthritis. Although the body has enzymes that convert alpha-linolenic acid (ALA) to EPA, you can obtain it much more efficiently by eating oily fish.

Electrolyte A substance that separates into ions that conduct electricity when fused or dissolved in fluids. In the human body, sodium, potassium, chloride and other minerals are electrolytes essential for nerve and muscle function and for maintaining the fluid balance as well as the acid-alkali balance of cells and tissues.

Ellagic acid A phenolic compound with potent antioxidant capabilities, ellagic acid is thought to fight cancer by causing cancer cells to die as well as by neutralizing carcinogens such as tobacco smoke or air pollution. Sources include apples, apricots, berries, grapes, pomegranates and walnuts.

Emollient An agent that softens tissue, notably the skin.

Endorphins Natural painkillers made by the brain, with effects similar to those of opium-based drugs.

Enteric coated An enteric-coated pill has been given a protective coating so that it can pass intact through the stomach and reach the small intestine before the coating dissolves and the contents are absorbed.

Enzyme A protein molecule that speeds up certain chemical reactions and processes in the body.

Epidermis Outermost layer of the skin.

Epinephrine Also called adrenaline, this is an adrenal hormone that prepares the body to react to stressful situations.

Essential fatty acid (EFA) The building block of fats. The various EFAs must be obtained from foods. They help form cell membranes, aid in immune function and produce important hormones.

Essential oil A volatile, highly aromatic oil contained in certain herbs or other plants. The concentrated oil is extracted by steam distillation.

Expectorant A substance that makes it easier to cough up phlegm and mucus.

Flavonoids A large group of chemicals found in plants. They have antioxidant, anti-inflammatory, antispasmodic or diuretic properties. Flavonoid compounds include anthocyanins, hesperidin, isoflavones, quercetin and resveratrol.

Free radical An unstable, highly reactive molecule that is the product of metabolism and also forms as a result of environmental pollution such as cigarette smoke. Free radicals can damage cells, potentially leading to premature ageing and the onset of many diseases.

Fructo-oligosaccharide (FOS) An indigestible carbohydrate compound. Fructo-oligosaccharides are thought to encourage the growth of friendly bacteria in the body and may reduce the amount of toxins produced by unfriendly flora in the colon. They are found in asparagus, bananas, garlic, Jerusalem artichokes and onions.

Fungi Infectious agents that have no green chlorophyll, stems, roots or leaves. They live in or off living or dead organic material, sometimes causing disease. Examples include molds, tinea and Candida.

Galactolipids A group of compounds found in plants, where they are an important part of cell membranes. Several galactolipids have been shown in laboratory experiments to possess potentially health-promoting benefits such as anti-inflammatory properties.

Glucose A simple sugar (monosaccharide) that is the body's prime energy source. Blood levels of glucose are regulated by several hormones, including insulin.

Gluten A protein in barley, buckwheat, rye and wheat. Certain people, particularly those with celiac disease, have an intolerance to it and experience an adverse gastrointestinal reaction necessitating the avoidance of foods made with these grains.

Glycemic index A measure of how easily a type of food is broken down by the body into glucose. The higher the number, the more easily it is converted.

Glycogen A form of glucose stored in the liver and muscles, which is converted back into glucose when needed in the body.

Hemoglobin The iron-containing pigment in our red blood cells that carries oxygen.

Hesperidin A flavonoid found in citrus fruit and juices, hesperidin is thought to improve the integrity of capillary linings.

High-density lipoprotein (HDL) The "heaviest" lipoprotein, HDL transports cholesterol from the tissues to the liver where it is removed from the body. It is often called "good cholesterol," because high levels of HDL in the blood have been associated with a lower risk of heart disease.

Histamine A compound released during allergic reactions, causing characteristic swelling and itching.

Hormone A chemical secreted by an endocrine gland that serves as a messenger triggering a specific bodily activity. Hormones have numerous functions in the body, including growth, development and reproduction.

Hyperglycemia Higher than normal level of glucose in the blood.

Hypertension High blood pressure.

Hypotension Low blood pressure.

Immune system The organs, tissues, cells and molecules that protect the body against invading pathogens or abnormal body cells.

Incomplete protein A protein, usually from plant sources, that lacks one or more essential amino acids.

Indoles Partially responsible for the strong taste of broccoli and brussels sprouts, indoles are a class of chemicals present in cruciferous vegetables.

Inflammation A protective reaction by the body in response to injury, infection, allergy or disease. The affected tissue becomes hot, red, swollen and painful.

Insulin A hormone produced by the pancreas that regulates carbohydrate metabolism. Insulin causes cells in the liver, muscle, and fat tissue to take up glucose from the blood. Insulin resistance, a precursor to type 2 diabetes, occurs when insulin is no longer effective at removing glucose from the blood.

In vitro Experiments carried out in an artificial environment, such as in a test tube or in a laboratory.

In vivo Experiments carried out within a living organism.

Isoflavones A major class of phytoestrogens, plant chemicals with mild estrogen-like activity.

Laxative A herb or substance that stimulates evacuation of the bowels.

Leukotrienes A group of chemicals produced by the body as part of the inflammatory response. Leukotrienes are believed to play a major role in causing the symptoms of hay fever and asthma.

Lignans Phytoestrogens with mild estrogen-like activity. They may have antimicrobial benefits, provide relief from premenstrual syndrome (PMS) and are thought to offer some protection against osteoporosis. Good food sources include flaxseed (linseed), soy foods and whole grains.

Limonene A phytochemical found in lemons, limes and oranges.

Linoleic acid One of the omega-6 essential fatty acids.

Linolenic acid One of the omega-3 essential fatty acids.

Lipid A fatty compound made of hydrogen, carbon and oxygen. Lipids are insoluble in water. The lipid family includes fats, fatty acids, cholesterol, oils and waxes.

Lipoprotein A combination of a lipid and a protein that can transport cholesterol in the bloodstream.

Low-density lipoprotein (LDL) These lipoproteins carry about three-quarters of the cholesterol in the blood; they are known as "bad" cholesterol because high levels in the blood are associated with arteriosclerosis and a higher risk of heart disease.

Lutein A pigment in the carotenoid family that is thought to help protect against macular degeneration and cataracts. Lutein is found in green leafy vegetables such as baby spinach and watercress, as well as corn and egg yolks.

Lycopene A powerful antioxidant that lends a red color to numerous foods, lycopene is particularly abundant in tomatoes and tomato products. Studies have shown lycopene to be protective against prostate cancer, lung cancer and heart disease.

Metabolism The collective term for the body's physical and chemical processes that are needed to maintain life, including derivation of energy from food.

Micronutrient Required in small amounts from the diet. Micronutrients include essential vitamins and minerals. They are critical for normal growth, development and good health. Micronutrients promote and regulate chemical reactions vital for life and participate in all body processes, such as deriving energy from food, transmitting nerve impulses and battling infections.

Monosaccharide A simple sugar such as glucose or fructose.

Monoterpenes A family of phytochemicals with medicinal properties. They are found in most essential oils.

Monounsaturated fat Found in olive oil, canola oil, peanut oil, some margarines, avocados, nuts and seeds, heart-healthy monounsaturated fat is not easily damaged by oxidation, so is less likely than saturated fat and trans fats to clog arteries. When consumed in place of saturated and trans fats, monounsaturated fats help lower LDL cholesterol levels. These fats are a key part of the Mediterranean diet, which has been associated with lower rates of heart disease and cancer.

Nervous system The body's control system. The central nervous system (brain and spinal cord) connects to the vast network of nerve cells that makes up the peripheral nervous system to relay sensory and motor impulses throughout the body.

Neurotransmitter A type of chemical found in the brain and throughout the nervous system that relays messages among nerve cells.

Estrogen Female sex hormone secreted by the ovaries. It plays a major role in regulating the menstrual cycle.

Oleic acid When consumed in place of saturated fat, this monounsaturated fat is linked to healthier cholesterol levels. Food sources include avocados and olive oil.

Oxalates Found in the greatest quantities in green vegetables, oxalates are compounds that bind calcium, iron and zinc, blocking their absorption in the body. People prone to kidney stones should avoid foods high in oxalates since the compounds may fuel the formation of certain types of kidney stones. Food sources include Swiss chard, cranberries, nuts, parsley, rhubarb, baby spinach, strawberries, tea and wheat bran.

Oxidation A chemical process in which food is burned with oxygen to release energy.

Pectin A soluble fiber that helps to lower artery-damaging LDL cholesterol. Pectin may also be useful for managing diarrhea and diabetes. Sources include apples, apricots, bananas, carrots and figs.

Peristalsis Wave-like muscle contractions that help food and fluids move along through the digestive tract.

Phenols A family of organic compounds in plants. For example, salicylic acid (found in willow bark).

Phenylketonuria (PKU) A condition caused by a genetic defect that prevents metabolism of the amino acid phenylalanine. People with PKU must follow a phenylalanine-free diet and avoid the artificial sweetener aspartame.

Phytochemical A naturally occurring plant chemical. Some phytochemicals offer protection against a variety of diseases.

Phytoestrogens Compounds found in plants that exhibit estrogen-like activity. The two major classes of phytoestrogens are isoflavones and lignans. Food sources include beans and soy.

Placebo A substance that contains no medicinal ingredients. A placebo may be administered during controlled drug trials to act as a comparison to the active drug being studied. When the recipients and the administrators don't know if the medicine is the real drug or a placebo, the trial is said to be "double blind."

Plasma The clear yellow fluid that makes up about 55 percent of the blood and carries cells, platelets and nutrients throughout the body.

Platelet A minute body that circulates in the blood and is needed for blood clotting and wound repair.

Polyphenols A class of compounds that contain phenol groups. They often have antioxidant and antibacterial properties.

Polysaccharide A class of complex carbohydrates, whose molecules are made up of several monosaccharide molecules. Cellulose is an example.

Polyunsaturated fat A fat containing a high percentage of fatty acids that lack hydrogen atoms and have extra carbon bonds. Such fats are liquid at room temperature (vegetable oils, for instance) unless hydrogen is added.

Prebiotics These act as a food supply to probiotics. Examples of prebiotics include onions, garlic, leeks, legumes and whole grains. Prebiotics are also available in dietary supplements, and food manufacturers have started adding prebiotics to some processed foods.

Probiotics "Friendly" bacteria that live in our digestive systems, combat harmful bacteria and help maintain the health of the cells that line the gastrointestinal tract. There are many different probiotics with *Lactobacillus acidophilus, L. rhamnosus GG* and bifidobacteria, among those more commonly studied.

Progesterone A female sex hormone, made by the ovaries, that helps to regulate menstruation.

Prolactin A hormone produced by the pituitary gland that is involved in the menstruation. Prolactin is also involved in promoting lactation.

Prostaglandins Hormone-like chemicals produced naturally in the body in response to a stimulus. Their wide range of effects include inducing inflammation, stimulating uterine contractions during labor and protecting the lining of the stomach.

Purines Compounds that form uric acid when metabolized, purines are found in a number of foods, particularly high-protein foods, such as offal. Caffeine (in coffee and tea), theobromine (in chocolate) and theophylline (in tea) are related compounds. People prone to gout or kidney stones should avoid purines.

Pyridoxine One of the B vitamins, more commonly called B_6, this vitamin is essential for protein metabolism and the production of red blood cells. It is important for a healthy nervous and immune system. Food sources include meat, fish, whole grains, avocados, bananas and potatoes.

Quercetin A potent flavonoid that has been linked to a reduced risk of cancer, cardiovascular disease and cataracts. Red onions, apples, grapes, red wine and berries are rich sources of quercetin.

Recommended Dietary Allowance (RDA) The US recommended daily amount of a nutrient for an average adult according to nutrition experts. RDAs do not take into account individual nutritional needs and vary by age, gender and whether a woman is pregnant or breastfeeding.

Resveratrol A phytochemical particularly abundant in the skin of red grapes, resveratrol is under review for its potential to improve cholesterol levels, prevent arteriosclerosis and reduce the risks for stroke and cancer. Sources include red and purple grape juice, and red wine.

Ribonucleic acid (RNA) A substance present in every cell that translates the information contained in DNA into instructions telling the cell which proteins to synthesize.

Rubefacient A substance that causes a localized reddening and warming of the skin.

Salicylates Compounds related to salicylic acid that are used for making aspirin and other painkillers and as a preservative. Naturally occurring salicylates in fruit or vegetables may produce allergic reactions in people who are sensitive to aspirin.

Salicylic acid A compound found naturally in willow bark. It acts in a similar way to aspirin.

Salmonella A bacterium that is a frequent cause of food poisoning.

Saponin A type of plant compound that produces a soapy foam in water.

Saturated fat Fat found in animal products such as meat and full-fat dairy products. Consumption of saturated fats has been linked to an increased risk of heart disease, certain cancers and other diseases.

Sedative A herb or substance that has a calming effect on the nerves, relieving anxiety and tension. It may cause drowsiness.

Serotonin A neurotransmitter that helps promote sleep and regulates many body processes, including pain perception and the secretion of pituitary hormones.

Standardized extract A concentrated form of an herb that contains a set level of active ingredients. Standardization helps to guarantee a consistent dosage strength from one batch of herbs to another.

Stanol Found naturally in vegetables, nuts and seeds, stanols are plant compounds that help lower cholesterol by reducing the amount you absorb from food. Stanols are sometimes added to margarines and other foods to boost their health benefits.

Statin A drug that lowers the level of cholesterol in the blood. Statins work by blocking the enzyme in the liver that makes cholesterol.

Stomachic A substance that stimulates the secretory activity of the stomach. It can be used as a tonic to improve the appetite.

Sucrose Better known as table sugar, sucrose is composed of glucose and fructose. It is obtained from sugarcane and sugar beets; it's also present in honey, fruit and vegetables.

Tannin A plant compound that has astringent properties that can contract blood vessels and body tissues.

Testosterone The principal male sex hormone, produced in the testes. Testosterone induces changes at puberty and helps to build strong muscles and bones. Women also make a small amount of testosterone in their ovaries.

Tincture A liquid usually made by soaking a whole herb or its parts in a mixture of water and ethyl alcohol (such as vodka). The alcohol helps to extract the herb's active compounds, concentrating and preserving them.

Tonic A herb or substance that is used to "tone" the body, organ or system, imparting strength and vitality.

Toxin Any substance that when introduced into the body is capable of causing an adverse effect.

Trans-fatty acid A fat that forms when vegetable oils are processed (hydrogenated) to improve their stability and to make them more solid.

Triglycerides The most common form of dietary and body fat; high levels of triglycerides in the blood have been linked to heart disease.

Tryptophan An essential amino acid, tryptophan is converted by the body into the B vitamin niacin. Tryptophan stimulates production of serotonin, a neurotransmitter that supports mental health. Complex carbohydrates enhance the absorption and use of tryptophan in the brain.

Uric acid A nitrogen-containing waste product of protein metabolism, uric acid causes gout when it builds up.

Xylitol A plant-derived sugar that bacteria are unable to metabolize, xylitol is the sweetener for sugar-free gums. Xylitol helps block the cavity-causing process when bacteria creates acid.

Zeaxanthin A pigment in the carotenoid family that is linked to a reduced risk for macular degeneration and cataracts. Zeaxanthin is found in leafy greens, red bell peppers and corn.

INDEX

Page numbers in **bold** refer to major discussions of ailments and remedies.

A

B

C

D

E

F

G

H

I

N

O

P

Q

R

S

T

U

Doctors' Favorite Natural Remedies

Consultant Professor Marc Cohen, MBBS (Hons), PhD, BMedSc (Hons), is one of Australia's pioneers of integrative and holistic medicine who has made significant impacts on education, research, clinical practice and policy. He is a medical doctor and Professor of Health Sciences at RMIT University. He sits on the board of a number of national and international associations including the Australasian Integrative Medicine Association. He has published more than 80 peer-reviewed journal articles along with more than 10 books on holistic approaches to health.

Authors Pamela Allardice, Mim Beim, Diane Cross, Sari Harrar, Jayne Tancred, Mariska van Aalst, Rachel Warren Chadd

Project Editor Celia Coyne

Concept and Project Designer Susanne Geppert

Proofreader Susan McCreery

Indexer Glenda Browne

New illustrations:
Susanne Geppert (pages 212, 217)
Edwina Keene (pages 4, 5, 16, 123, 128, 132, 155, 184, 185, 226, 235, 314)
Guy Troughton (pages 17, 113, 115, 116, 153, 177, 178, 179, 181, 197, 254, 259, 267, 287, 288, 291, 318)

Page borders, chapter opener backgrounds and decorative graphics © Shutterstock.

All other illustrations © Trusted Media Brands, previously published in *Grow Your Own Fruit and Vegetables the Natural Way*, *Magic and Medicine of Plants* and *Nature's Medicines*.

Doctors' Favorite Natural Remedies was first published in 2015 by Reader's Digest (Australia) Pty Limited, 80 Bay Street, Ultimo, NSW, 2007

National Library of Australia Cataloging-in-Publication entry
Title: Doctors' favorite natural remedies : the safest and most effective natural ways to treat 90 everyday ailments.
ISBN: 978-1-922085-66-5 (hardback)
Notes: Includes index.
Subjects: Naturopathy. Nature, Healing power of. Alternative medicine. Therapeutics, Physiological.
Dewey Number: 615.535

ISBN 978-1-62145-319-2

We are committed to both the quality of our products and the service we provide to our customers. We value your comments, so please feel free to contact us.

Reader's Digest Trade Publishing
44 South Broadway
White Plains, NY 10601

For more Reader's Digest products and information, visit our website:

www.rd.com (in the United States)
www.readersdigest.ca (in Canada)

Printed in China

10 9 8 7 6 5